Lecture Notes in Medical Informatics 47

Editors:
O. Rienhoff, Marburg
D. A. B. Lindberg, Washington

W0043680

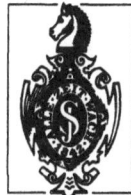

Jan L. Talmon   John Fox (Eds.)

Knowledge Based Systems in Medicine: Methods, Applications and Evaluation

Proceedings of the Workshop
"System Engineering in Medicine"
Maastricht, March 16-18, 1989

Springer-Verlag Berlin Heidelberg GmbH

Editors

Jan L. Talmon
Department of Medical Informatics, University of Limburg
PO Box 616, 6200 MD Maastricht, The Netherlands

John Fox
Advanced Computation Laboratory, Imperial Cancer Research Fund
Lincoln's Inn Fields
London WC2A 3PX, United Kingdom

Organized by:

The Department of Medical Informatics
University of Limburg
Maastricht
The Netherlands

Sponsored by:

Commission of the European Communities
under the
Medical and Health Research Programme

ISBN 978-3-540-55011-2   ISBN 978-3-662-08131-0 (eBook)
DOI 10.1007/978-3-662-08131-0

This work is subject to copyright. All rights are reserved, whether the whole or part of
the material is concerned, specifically the rights of translation, reprinting, re-use of
illustrations, recitation, broadcasting, reproduction on microfilms or in any other way,
and storage in data banks. Duplication of this publication or parts thereof is permitted
only under the provisions of the German Copyright Law of September 9, 1965, in its
current version, and permission for use must always be obtained from
Springer-Verlag Berlin Heidelberg GmbH.
Violations are liable for prosecution under the German Copyright Law.

© Springer-Verlag Berlin Heidelberg 1991
Originally published by Springer-Verlag Berlin Heidelberg New York in 1991

Typesetting: Camera ready by author

27/3140-543210 - Printed on acid-free paper

INTRODUCTION

This volume of the series Lecture Notes in Medical Informatics contains the proceedings of the Workshop on System Engineering in Medicine, which was held in Maastricht, The Netherlands, 16-18 March 1989.

This workshop was sponsored by the EC under the framework of the Medical and Health Research Programme.
The aim of the workshop was to assess whether there was sufficient support in the Medical Informatics community in the EC to establish a concerted action.

This proceedings contain papers of the presentations given at the workshop. These presentations were centred around three themes:
- Methods and Tools
- Applications in the domains of chronic care and critical care
- Evaluation of decision support systems

The papers were prepared after the workshop and therefore we were able to include the relevant parts of the discussions which were related to the presentations.

As a result of the discussions during the workshop, a proposal was prepared for the establishment of a concerted action, specifically addressing the development of guidelines for the evaluation of medical decision aids. This proposal was granted early 1990 under the same Medical and Health Research programme of the EC.
Over 40 institutes are participating in this concerted action.
It have been the outstanding presentations and the open discussions at the workshop that have been the starting point of this concerted action. The papers in this proceedings formed a starting point for the discussions in the meetings of the concerted action.

We believe that these proceedings contain valuable information for those active in the field of Medical Decision Aids. We, as editors, have carefully reviewed draft versions of these papers in order to achieve a consistent level of quality throughout the proceedings. In this we were assisted by Johan van der Lei, Erasmus University, Rotterdam, The Netherlands who reviewed the papers we were involved in. It is up to the reader to decide whether we succeeded in bringing together a series of papers which are relevant for the field.

Jan L. Talmon, John Fox
The editors

Medical and Health Research Programme of the EC

Biomedical Engineering in the European Community

The involvement of the European Community (EC) in the field of Medical and Health Research started in 1978 with the first programme which contained three projects. Since then, it has steadily expanded and it will include around 120 projects by the end of the fourth programme (1987-1991).

The general goal of the programme is clearly to contribute to a better quality of life by improving health, and its distinctive feature is to strengthen European collaboration in order to achieve this goal.

The main objectives of this collaboration are:
- increase the scientific efficiency of the relevant research and development efforts of the Member States through their gradual coordination at Community level following the mobilization of the available research potential of national programmes, and also their economic efficiency through sharing of tasks and strengthening the joint use of available health research resources,
- improve scientific and technical knowledge, in the research and development areas selected for their importance to all Member States, and promote its efficient transfer into practical applications, taking particular account of potential industrial and economic developments in the areas concerned,
- optimize the capacity and economic efficiency of health care efforts throughout the countries and regions of the Community.

The current programme consists of six research targets. Four are related to major health problems: *CANCER, AIDS, AGE-RELATED PROBLEMS*, and *PERSONAL ENVIRONMENT AND LIFE-STYLE RELATED PROBLEMS*; two are related to health resources: *MEDICAL TECHNOLOGY DEVELOPMENT* and *HEALTH SERVICES RESEARCH*.

Funds are provided by the Community for relevant "concerted action" activities which consist of research COLLABORATION and COORDINATION in the EC Member States and/or in other European participant countries. NETWORKS of research institutes can be set up and supported by means of meetings, workshops, short-term staff exchanges/visits to other countries, information dissemination and so on; centralized facilities such as data banks, computing, and preparation and distribution of reference materials can also be funded. The funds are not direct research grants; the institutes concerned must fund the research activities carried out within their own countries - it is the international coordination activities which are eligible for Community support. Each such research network is placed under the responsibility of a **PROJECT LEADER** chosen among the leading scientists in the network, with the assistance of a **PROJECT MANAGEMENT GROUP** representing the teams participating in the network.

The Commission of the European Communities is assisted in the execution of this Programme by a Management and Coordination Advisory Committee (CGC Medical and Health Research), and by Concerted Action Committees (COMACs) and Working Parties, composed of representatives and of scientific experts respectively, designated by the competent authorities of the Member States.

Other European countries, not belonging to the EC but participating in COST (Cooperation on Science and Technology) may take part in the Programme.

The present work was conducted according to the advice of **COMAC-BME** which supervises the coordination of research in biomedical engineering (BME) with the Medical Technology Development target.

More information may be obtained from:

Commission of the European Communities
Directorate General XII-F-6
200 Rue de la Loi
B-1049 Brussels
Tel: +32-2-2350034
Fax: +32-2-2350145 or +32-2-2362007
Telex: COMEU B 21877

CONTENTS

APPLICATIONS
Management of the critically ill

EVALUATION

AUTHORS INDEX

LIST OF PARTICIPANTS

METHODS

The Use of the KADS Methodology in Designing an Intelligent Teaching System for Diagnosis in Physiotherapy[1]

Joost Breuker and Radboud Winkels

Department of Computer Science & Law, University of Amsterdam, Amsterdam, The Netherlands

Abstract

In this article we present an overview of the KADS methodology for building knowledge based systems (KBS) and how it is applied in a paramedical domain: Diagnosis of physiotherapeutic disorders. We want to demonstrate that KADS's commitment to layered modelling of expertise provides a far more structured picture in domains which have traditionally a preponderant heuristic flavour, like medical domains. This has many advantages: not only does it provide a basis for systematic elicitation of knowledge from experts, it also enables a very modularised design of the KBS -which is particularly important for system maintenance. Moreover, the decomposition of knowledge and skills involved makes an articulate, semi-deep model a strong basis for an Intelligent Teaching System (ITS).This is illustrated by the description of the modelling and design of an ITS for physiotherapeutic diagnosis, the PhysioDisc system.
Several interesting conclusions can be drawn from this research on the acquisition and construction of knowledge bases for medical applications and on medical education.

Introduction

In this article we present an overview of the KADS methodology for building knowledge based systems (KBS) and how it is applied in a paramedical domain: diagnosis of physiotherapeutic disorders. One of the major principles in KADS is that the construction of a conceptual model of the expertise should precede the

---

1   The research reported here is partially funded by the Esprit Programme of the European Community (Contract P1098) and the Dutch INSP Programme (IIV-project). We like to acknowledge the contributions of colleagues in the P1098 project, in particular Bob Wielinga, and those in the IIV-Project, in particular Wilfred Achthoven and Armando van Gennip of Bolesian Systems, Helmond, NL.

design and implementation of a KBS. The construction of a conceptual model is supported by skeletal interpretation models for various types of expert tasks. For instance, in KADS several types of diagnostic tasks are distinguished. What we want to show here is that KADS's commitment to layered modelling of diagnostic expertise provides a far more structured picture in domains which have traditionally a preponderant heuristic flavour, like medical domains. This has many advantages: not only does it provide a basis for systematic elicitation of knowledge from experts, it also enables a far more modularised design of the KBS -which is particularly important for system maintenance. Moreover, the decomposition of knowledge and skills involved makes an articulate, semi-deep model a strong basis for an intelligent teaching system. As *Clancey, 1983* has shown, most 'flat' rule based systems do not lend themselves to teaching and coaching, because the rules contain mixtures of types of knowledge.

Space limitations prohibit to present more than a summary overview of both the KADS methodology and the IIV-project where the physiotherapeutic coach (PhysioDisc) was developed. We will often refer to articles and other documentation for more detailed descriptions. For recent publications on KADS see *Breuker & Wielinga (1989 and in preparation) and Hayward et al, 1989*.

Components of KADS[2]

KADS is a methodology for building KBS. The support tools are the Shelley workbench (*Anjewierden & Wielemaker, 1989*).
Any methodology should contain the following components:

- A task decomposition which provides guidance what to do when. This can vary from an enumeration of subtasks to a detailed sequence of instructions. For instance, in empirical research the specification of hypotheses should precede the plan for collecting and processing of data.
- A framework of concepts or Modelling languages which allow communication about the object(s) of the methodology. This is not the terminology of a specific domain, e.g. medical terms, but terms for conducting research (scientific methodologies) or constructing artifacts (engineering) in such domains. Formalisation (e.g. mathematics) and specification languages are typical examples.
- Methods, techniques and tools form the most practical part of a methodology. Application of a method or technique is associated with a particular (sub)task.

For supporting knowledge engineering these components can be summarised in KADS as follows:

- **Life Cycle Model.** Similar to software engineering, the task decomposition for knowledge engineering is called a life cycle model (LCM). The KADS LCM is to a large extent derived from software engineering models, which facilitates integration of software and knowledge engineering (*Edin et al, 1987*). In the next

---

2   KADS is an acronym that has lost its original meaning.

section we will discuss in particular where KADS differs from, or supplements, the software LCMs.

- **Modelling Languages**. In KADS there are three modelling languages. The first one -KADS Conceptual Modelling Language (KCML)- is used to construct a conceptual model of the expertise at hand (*Breuker et al, 1987; Breuker & Wielinga, 1989*). In the next sections we will present more details of KCML. For designing the artifact on the basis of the conceptual model, KADS has a Design Language in which the architecture of the KBS can be expressed (*Schreiber et al, 1987; 1988*). A third language is used for the specification of the task distribution and cooperation with the user and/or other systems a KBS is to be involved in. This Modality Framework results in a description of what, when and how communication with the user should occur and is the basis for the user interface design.
- Methods, techniques, tools of KADS consist in particular of the **Shelley workbench**[3], which contains editors for the various modelling languages and the knowledge base; tools which support the analysis of protocols of interviews; documentation facilities, and libraries.Much of what was part of the KADS Handbook (*Edin et al, 1987*) will be transferred to Shelley, as there are descriptions of elicitation techniques.

The development of KADS took about 6 years in time and 100 person years in effort, and there are still important gaps to be filled in. Moreover there are current efforts both in the direction of further founding and formalisation of the modelling languages, and in the direction of automatisation of knowledge acquisition processes. The KADS methodology has been tested in various field studies and is a standard in several software and knowledge engineering companies.

The Analysis Stage; KCML & Interpretation Models

KADS' LCM has the conventional stages like Design, Implementation, Operation, Maintenance. However the first stage, Analysis, differs from conventional LCM because it contains two parallel streams of activities. The 'external' stream is concerned with the specification of requirements similar to those in software engineering. The 'internal' stream consists of typical knowledge engineering activities: i.e. knowledge acquisition. Traditional systems can be designed from a set of functional specifications. For KBS this cannot be the case because it is not possible to derive models of how expertise works from its behaviour.

A predominant practice in knowledge engineering is to model the expertise directly from the verbal data elicited from an expert into some implementation formalism: in general a simple production system. This rapid prototyping approach suffers not only from the fact that there is in general not a simple mapping between these data and the code, but in particular that there is an insufficient level of abstraction that allows a coherent decomposition of the expertise involved. These abstraction and

---

3   A previous version of Shelley was called KADS Power Tools (see **Anjewierden, 1988**).

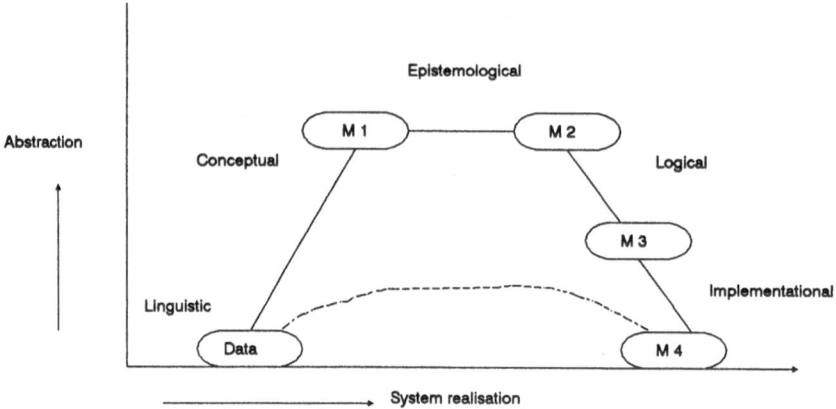

Figure 1:   The knowledge engineering space.

transformation dimensions form a 'knowledge engineering space' as is shown in Figure 1. The rapid prototyping trajectory in this space is presented as a dotted line. The solid line symbolises the KADS trajectory. It contains both higher levels of abstraction and a number of models (M1-M3) which function as stepping stones for bridging the gap between the data and the code.

The abstractions required for constructing a KBS are not arbitrary. They follow from views in AI on representing knowledge by layers of abstraction, as for instance argued by MINewell, 1982 in proposing the 'Knowledge Level' (cf. *Brachman's (1979)* epistemological level). For orientation we have marked in Figure 1 the positions of the levels of knowledge representation formalisms as identified by *Brachman, 1979*. These levels vary both in abstraction and distance from implementation formalisms.

This space can be vertically divided into an Analysis and a Design space. Analysis activities result in a Conceptual Model of the domain of expertise (M1). This model is expressed to a large extent graphically in KCML. KCML can be viewed as an interlingua between conceptual ('psychological') abstractions and the AI methods on which the system Architecture (M2) is based.

In the design stage of KADS' LCM the Conceptual Model is transformed in an architecture (M2), whose terms are more suited to comply with known implementation formalisms and -languages. M1 describes the competence in expert problem solving and has a cognitive flavour. By specifying M2, i.e. during KADS' design stage, the knowledge engineer takes decisions on modularisation and implementation formalisms for control, inference and knowledge representation, whereby external requirements such as speed, available target hard- and software, etc. are taken into account.

M3 is a detailed design model, which has the same structure as M2, but a more detailed specification of the knowledge base and the inference mechanisms.

M2 is not necessarily isomorphic to M1. One reason is that the problem solving methods used by real life experts may not be the optimal ones from the point of view of the machine. For instance, the information management capacities of the machine may enable it to handle hypotheses spaces which pose problems to even very skilled human experts. There are moreover reasons to believe that also the Conceptual Model cannot reflect the way human expertise operates, but rather provides a rational reconstruction of expertise in a domain (for details see: *Breuker & Wielinga, 1989*).

In the next section we will focus on KCML, because it lends itself easily for expressing the competences and types of knowledge involved in expert tasks.

KCML and Interpretation Models

Developing a KBS involves modelling of expertise, i.e. the structuring of the required knowledge, inference competence and (flexible) use of knowledge. These elements of expertise can be expressed in KCML because it is based on distinguishing these types of knowledge in (four) functionally different layers. The role of a Conceptual Model is similar to a functional specification.

KCML is based on a "four layer" theory on flexible expert problem solving. Flexibility is one of the hallmarks of expertise. In human expertise some forms of flexibility are based upon networks of knowledge with a very fine mesh. This detail is hard if not impossible to elicit and to model. Other forms of flexibility are obtained by variations in strategies to exploit domain knowledge. This kind of flexibility can be modelled in the **rational reconstructions** by the use of metalevels which allow strategic reasoning.

The four layers of KCML form the framework in which metalevel reasoning can be specified. A summary of these four layers is presented in table 1.

Layer	Elements	Relation with lower layer
Strategy	Plans; Metarules	controls
Task	Goals, controls statments	applies
Inference	Metaclasses; Knowledge sources	describes
Domain	Concepts; Relations	

Table 1: Layers of expertise (see Wielinga & Breuker, 1986).

- The first layer contains the static knowledge of the domain. This layer stands for what is generally viewed as 'the knowledge base' of a KBS. In KADS this layer does not necessarily consist of one uniform network or rule base, but there can be various heterogeneous structures (types of domain knowledge) which may be used for different functions. This layer may contain domain concepts, relations and complex structures such as models of processes or devices.

- The second layer is the inference layer. It describes the inference making competence in a particular domain. It provides the generic view on knowledge, i.e. exactly that aspect that makes a KBS different from a conventional software system, and lends power to the facts that constitute the knowledge at the domain level. The inference layer specifies what (types of) inferences can be made; not when or how they are made. The 'how' is dependent on the nature of the domain layer structures and the inference method(s) that can be applied. The 'when' is specified at the next, task layer. The inference layer specifications are pivotal in KADS: in fact most of the effort in constructing a Conceptual Model is in defining the structure of the inference layer. In the next section we will discuss the elements of the inference layer into more detail.

- The third layer is the task layer. At this level the basic objects are (sub)tasks, represented as goal statements, and control statements. The task layer describes the default control in the problem solving process and is more or less fixed.

- The fourth, strategy, layer is used for the specification of the variations that are to be foreseen in the problem solving process, and also in the communication processes with the user (*De Greef & Breuker, 1989*). Here specifications can be made as to what to do when data are lacking, what to do when an impasse occurs, how new task structures can be generated if an approach fails, how to match competence against the complexity of a problem (graceful degradation), etc. In practice, it is impossible, neither necessary to specify all these capabilities, which psychologists call intelligence. This is not only far beyond the state of the art of AI, but this full intelligence is not required in domains of specialised knowledge with a narrow range of types of problems.

These four layers are not to be conceived as successive metalevel structures; they are specification layers for the modelling of expertise. In terms of (human) problem solving only two levels of processing are involved: the object, or domain level reasoning, and the metalevel, strategic reasoning. The other two layers can be viewed as 'data'- or knowledge structures. The inference layer represents the abstraction of the domain knowledge that is used to plan a problem solving strategy given the identification of a what the current problem is about. This explains that people know how to solve a problem before actually solving it. They are for instance able to say in advance whether the problem is in their domain of competence or not, without trying actually to solve it. The task structure can be viewed as the result of this strategic reasoning. It is the plan of action in solving the problem. This view on the four layers is presented in Figure 2.

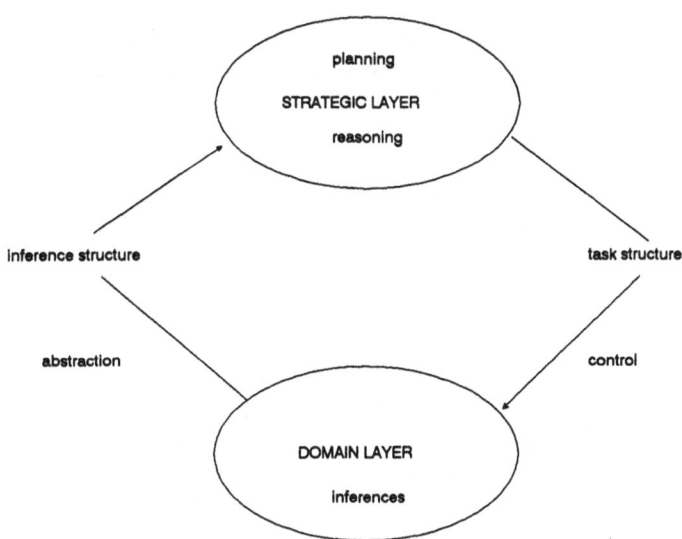

Figure 2: Processing and data layers in problem solving.

Elements of Inference structures

The vocabulary for the inference layer consists of three elements: Knowledge sources (KS), metaclasses, and the dependencies between these. A structure of these elements is called an inference structure (see also *Clancey, 1985*).

A *knowledge source* (KS) is a primitive inference making function, for which the metaclasses are the roles, or input/output parameters of this function. A *metaclass* stands for a set or structure of domain concepts and indicate what role these concepts can play in the problem solving process. Examples of such roles are: hypothesis, evidence, factor, diagnosis, plan, etc. This distinction between the meaning of a concept, i.e. its definition at the domain level and the role(s) it can play is important. Concepts can play various roles as is obvious by the fact that the same concept -say a particular disease- can play the role of a hypothesis, a diagnosis, and even evidence (e.g. in complications). These *dependencies* between terms such as hypothesis, evidence and diagnosis (solution) are not accidental: they form a pattern of states in the reasoning process. A KS identifies the type of inference that is required to go from one state in the problem solving process to another, e.g. to turn a set of hypotheses into a conclusion, to abstract evidence from data, etc. KCML specifies a typology of KS, which is summarised in table 2. For a justification of this typology see *Breuker & Wielinga, 1989*.

An example of an inference structure is presented in Figure 4. It represents the types of inferences and metaclasses in a typical **systematic** diagnosis task. Systematic means that there is some predefined way to generate hypotheses by decomposing the hypotheses space ('system model').

Group	Operation	Argument types
General concept	INSTANTIATE	description → instance
	CLASSIFY	instance → description
	GENERALISE	set → description
	ABSTRACT	description → description
	SPECIFY	description → description
Differentiate concepts	COMPARE	values
	MATCH	structures
Structure manipulation	ASSEMBLE	set → structure
	DECOMPOSE	structure → set
	SORT	set → set
	TRANSFORM	structure → structure
Change concepts	ASSIGN_VALUE	values

Table 2:   Typology of Knowledge Sources.

Interpretation Models

The inference structure in Figure 4 is not a very detailed one: in a particular domain, the inference structure is far more detailed. This structure is only a top-level abstraction which characterises typical diagnostic tasks. It is a generic model for these tasks, which means that this structure can be viewed as an initial structure for constructing a Conceptual Model in a particular domain, when it is obvious that this domain is a typical diagnostic domain. In this way, this structure can function as an initial model -an interpretation model- for analysing and modelling the expertise in a particular diagnostic domain.

Expertise comes in many varieties. This concerns not only the domain of knowledge, but also the type of task. An expert can design, monitor, repair, diagnose, configure, etc. an artifact, say audio-equipment. Although the knowledge required to perform these tasks may overlap to a very large extent, the skills involved in performing these tasks may be completely different. So different that they are often performed by different experts.
The types of generic tasks which are distinguished in KADS and for which interpretation have been constructed (*Breuker et al, 1987; Breuker & Wielinga, 1989*), are presented in Figure 3.

This taxonomy has some resemblance with the ones proposed by *Hayes-Roth et al, 1983* and *Clancey, 1985*, but it is far more worked out (see for a discussion on these taxonomies: *Wilson, 1989*). The major distinction is between analytic tasks and synthetic tasks. In synthetic tasks the solution consists of a new assembly of elements, while in analytic tasks the solution is a particular element, e.g. a disease, which has to be identified instead of constructed.

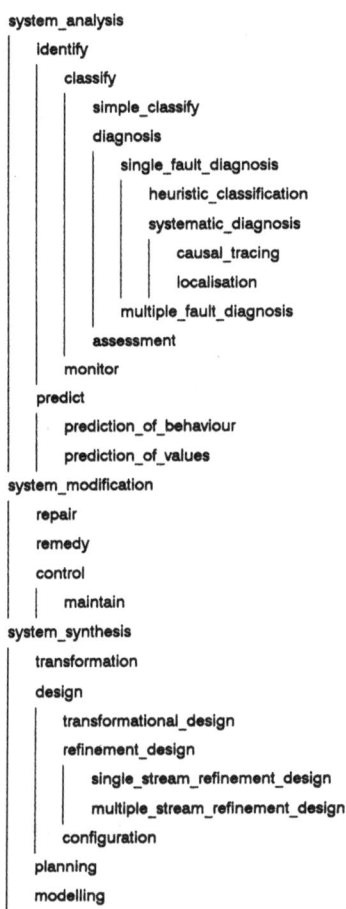

```
system_analysis
  identify
    classify
      simple_classify
      diagnosis
        single_fault_diagnosis
          heuristic_classification
          systematic_diagnosis
            causal_tracing
            localisation
        multiple_fault_diagnosis
      assessment
    monitor
  predict
    prediction_of_behaviour
    prediction_of_values
system_modification
  repair
  remedy
  control
    maintain
system_synthesis
  transformation
  design
    transformational_design
    refinement_design
      single_stream_refinement_design
      multiple_stream_refinement_design
    configuration
  planning
  modelling
```

Figure 3:   Taxonomy of Generic Tasks.

In *Breuker et al, 1987; forthcoming* for each of these generic tasks and interpretation model is presented. Here we will focus on diagnostic tasks because these play a very important practical role, also in medical applications.

Models For Diagnostic Tasks.

Systematic and heuristic diagnosis.

In the library of Interpretation models of KADS (Breuker et al, forthcoming) one will find two different interpretation models for diagnosis: systematic and heuristic. In figure 4 the inference structures of both models are presented. The heuristic model is *Clancey's (1985)* which appears to be particularly applicable in medical domains (e.g. *Chandrasekaran & Mittal, 1983*). The systematic model is developed particularly for domains which consist of the diagnosis of artifacts (devices) for which defective components can be localised. At first sight the two structures look very different, but we will argue that many of these differences are not inherent to

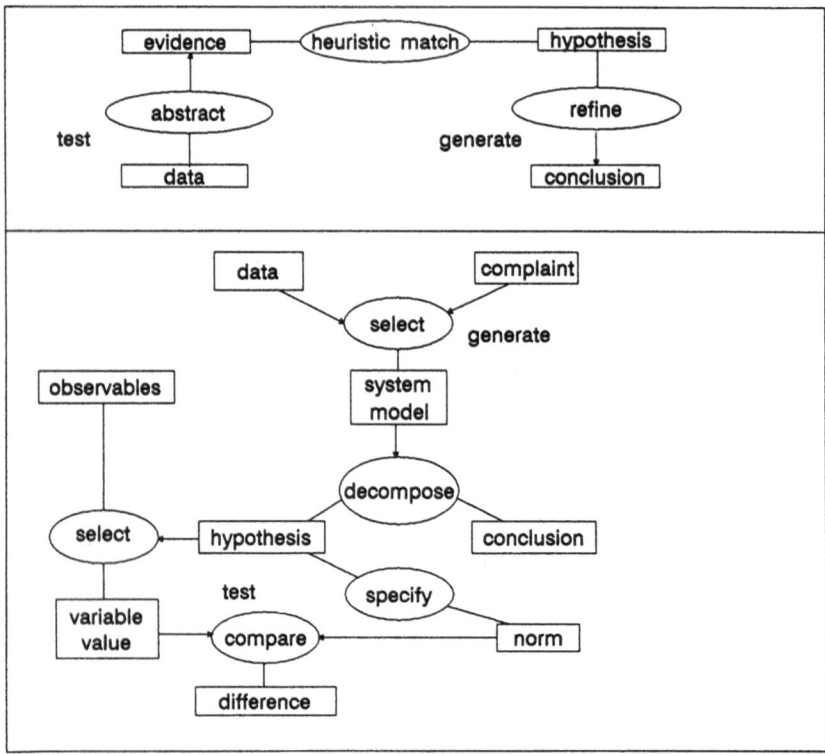

Figure 4: Inference structures for Heuristic (above) and Systematic (below) Diagnosis. Ellipses are knowledge sources. Boxes are metaclasses and arrows indicate dependencies.

the models, but can be attributed to the way experts and knowledge engineers view these types of domains.

Diagnosis consists of two subtasks: the *generation of hypotheses* on a malfunction or a defect and the *testing* of these hypotheses. In both models the generation of hypotheses consists of a successive refinement, i.e. focussing on more specific hypotheses. However, the inference structures differ strongly among the models.

Systematic Diagnosis.

In the systematic diagnosis model these generate and test subtasks can be easily distinguished. The major knowledge source (KS) for hypothesis generation is 'decompose'; for testing it is 'compare'. Both subtasks are interfaced via the metaclasses 'set of hypotheses' and 'expected value'.

The decompose KS assumes there is a hierarchical structure of parts or components at the domain level. A part stands for some function or process. In artifacts this relation between function and component is a very explicit one, but many (simple) natural systems can be decomposed in a such a way that there is a good correspondence between structure and function (*De Kleer & Brown, 1984*). This is called a component, structural, or 'system' model (*Clancey, 1988; Bredeweg & Wielinga, 1988*)[4].

In principle the diagnostic process is very simple. Partition the system according to its compostion and eliminate the correctly functioning parts in a top down (refinement) manner. The process of eliminating hypotheses can in fact be very complicated. As suggested by the systematic model, it may simply be a comparisson between an observed and an expected value. However, the model becomes far more complex -i.e. more detailed- if these data are not given, but have to be derived. For instance, observables may be obtained by experimental procedures, which may involve (re)configuration of a system. We have identified at least 5 different major types of hypothesis testing procedures (Breuker & Wielinga, forthcoming). Also, the derivation of expected values may follow complex paths of 'qualitative reasoning'.

Heuristic Diagnosis.

In the heuristic diagnosis model of Clancey hypothesis generation and testing overlap. The reason that they can overlap is that the same inference mechanism is used to link hypotheses and evidence: associations (see figure 4.). Instead of deriving values and designing 'experiments', data are directly coupled to hypotheses or conclusions. These associations can be the result of empirical correlations or of compiled out inference paths; hence the label 'heuristic'[5]. The use of associations indicates that there is little understanding of how things work in a domain. Lack of insight of how things work makes also the hypothesis generation process far more difficult. In principle there are several solutions, dependent on the amount of abstraction that can be accomplished.

- The simplest case is where data and hypotheses are associated in such a way that they form a decision tree. This will only work in very simple domains. The refinement is achieved by sequencing the choices in a strategic way (e.g. 'binary chopping'). The decision tree can be implicit in the rules of a production system -as in MYCIN-, but then there is not necessarily a basis for refinement.

- A second type of organising hypotheses is the use of associative paths, which may represent semi-causal links between intermediary (pathological) states. The associations are viewed as transitions between states. These states may be observable or assumed ones, and function in the process of diagnosis to partition the hypothesis space in a meaningful way.

- A third way of organising hypotheses to enable refinement is by the use of taxonomies. Taxonomies are abstraction hierarchies with intermediary concepts. Distinguishing 'viral' from 'bacterial' infections, or 'acute' from 'chronic' leukemia are simple examples. A taxonomy combines the advantages of a decision tree

---

4   Structural or qualitative models are certainly not the only type of models. Mathematical models are another type, but in understanding processes in the world we prefer structural models. This is one of the reasons that for instance quantum mechanics looks less elegant and appealing than relativity theory.

---

5   It is very deplorable that the terms 'heuristic' and '(empirical) association' have been confused in Clancey's paper. Heuristics refer to algorithms or methods that do not ensure that a (right) solution is obtained. Empirical association means that knowledge is linked on the basis of co-occurrence of events. Heuristic is to algorithm as association is to relation.

(distinctive attributes) and of state transitions (intermediary concepts). A state transition view is appropriate where the malfunctions are distinctive processes (e.g. syndroms); a taxonomy where a malfunction is relatively static.

Combinations of models.

In summary, systematic and heuristic models of diagnosis differ in two ways. First there is a difference between the way data and expected values are obtained or interpreted. Second, the structures of the hypotheses-spaces differ. In the systematic model it is a component hierarchy (part-of), while in the heuristic model it is at best a (is-a like) subsumption hierarchy. These differences are correlated in the sense that in a largely empirical domain associations, and abstractions of associative links perform the role of mechanisms or processes.

From the point of view of validity, systematic diagnosis is to be preferred to heuristic diagnosis. This is no surprise, but it requires the availability or constructability of a structural model. Note that a structural model will embody both the processing and the abstraction view. i.e. can have both a state transition and an abstraction hierarchy view.

Medecine is to a very large extent an empirical domain, which easily fits the heuristic framework. Both solutions for structuring the hypothesis space -state transition (e.g. *De Haan, 1989*) and taxonomies (e.g. *Sticklen et al, 1985; Fox et al, 1987*)- are used in medical KBS. Structural models are present in medicine (e.g. *Kuipers & Kassirer, 1987*), but we do not know of examples where both types of diagnosis are integrated.

Diagnosis in Medicine: combinatorial explosions, likelihoods and decompositions.

Although medicine is based to a large extent on theory about processes, its practice has a strong empirical flavour: both in the scientific as in the skill acquisition sense, i.e. becoming a doctor. The theories and models are very complex and local ones, based upon general principles of physics, chemistry, physiology, etc., but these models are used rather to explain or justify why a particular combination of processes is possible, than for generating and testing hypotheses. Contrary to many other domains of expertise where knowledge about first principles gets compiled out and becomes less accessible, in medical expertise this compilation and empirical association does not lead to forgetting of underlying models (*Boshuizen, 1989*).

This may seem paradoxical in a very empirically oriented task, but the major reason is probably that the construction of a model justifies hypotheses, which are selected on the basis of empirical associations. A model can be constructed which explains the data. This testing-by-justification instead of testing-by-collecting-new-evidence is a methodologically not well founded step, but (only) in the face of lack of data probably the better alternative.

This empirical basis for diagnosis may not have been intended in medicine-as-a-science, but it is the only alternative, when the general 'system model' consists of many and permanently dynamic, interacting processes[6] of which the manifestations (behaviour) can only be observed in an indirect and accumulated way. As a consequence there are not only time dependencies in the manifestations of malfunctions, but also the 'observables' or symptoms are to a large extent mediated by generally applicable (e.g. immunological) processes, so that their specificity is highly attenuated. This means that complaints and symptoms are unspecific for the underlying cause, and that there is a high degree of variation in manifestations of the same cause (disease) among individuals cases. In this respect medicine is hardly better off than social sciences where justifications (models) are far less established. As a consequence, the associative links are probabilistic ones, representing likelihoods between manifestations and malfunctions. Likelihoods mean that the frequency of co-occurrence of events is not always or never, but in between. In making decisions these likelihoods are very important: however in reasoning they are not. As long as a likelihood is greater than zero, and for a good reason, it is a reasonable possibility, and should be part of the reasoning process. Therefore the notion of 'uncertain knowledge' etc. is a misconception or even a contradiction in terms. The knowledge is not uncertain, but whether it is applicable in the current event, and if there are no distinctive features to exclude possibilities, likelihoods can be used to gamble on the outcome, or to calculate the risk of not further pursuing a line of inference. Likelihoods -of which probabilities are an expression- are based on subjective or objective frequencies of occurrences of events. Descriptions of the world (i.e. representations of knowledge) are rather statements which allow making inferences into possible worlds. Therefore, there is no reason to have probabilities associated with (the representation of) knowledge. It not only leads to statistically ill defined problems and dubious solutions, but it is also epistemologically wrong. The only function of probabilities is to control the selection of profitable routes of inference, but is has nothing to do with the inference processes themselves. In terms of KADS, the likelihoods can be conceived of as probabilistic conditions at the task and strategic level: not at the domain level.

Why is this important? In the first place to see that likelihoods are used for no other purpose than to keep the explosion of inference routes constrained. In medicine it means that if unspecific symptoms are combined with other unspecific symptoms the result can be that the hypothesis space is not refined, but gets expanded. In other words, in a pattern matcher combinatorial explosions are tamed by the use of probabilities. However, from a statistical point of view this is a very unsound practice, because likelihoods of events are confused with their descriptions. For instance, in statistical theory the sequencing of events affects the likelihood of some final state, but it is ridiculous to have the outcome of a reasoning process being dependent on the sequence of steps in the chain of inferences. The chain either leads

---

6   The human body differs from a device which can be inactive, or has far sharper system boundaries, or far less interfaces with other component which prevents the propagation of malfunctions in an interacting way.

to the conclusion or not, and that is what we think valid reasoning is about. Otherwise we would have the ridiculous situation that the likelihood of a result is dependent on the particular order of the reasoning steps: it can only be dependent on the order and likelihoods of events in the world.

If there are too many potential conclusions, the state of affairs in the real world can be taken into account and cost-effective reasoning may lead to exploring only those routes which look promising from the start. The fact that there is something epistemologically wrong with probabilities associated with descriptions has a number of practical consequences.

In second generation expert systems where strategic reasoning is separated from domain reasoning (e.g. *Steels, 1988*), the use of statistical theory for computing combined likelihoods of events can at least be separated from the reasoning itself. This is not the case in flat rule based systems. The standard practice here is to propagate the probabilities with the inference chains, which is statistically not well founded and object of discussions about 'uncertain' or 'fuzzy' knowledge'.

The second practical, but important issue -as far as the validity of KBS is concerned- is where the likelihoods come from. In most expert system the likelihoods or weights are based upon estimates of experts. Experts are humans and humans are very bad statistical processors (*Tversky & Kahneman, 1974*) and it seems that this observation is hardly ever taken seriously. Even statisticians are prone to gambler fallacies. This means that experts in combining and modelling likelihoods do not give the right estimates in real life situations which can be modelled by the simplest of all models. How can one expect that domain experts will give valid and reliable weights to associations for which there is no transparent model at all. Therefore, if likelihoods are used, and are only used to select cost effective routes of inference, i.e. at the control level, than the only empirically valid way to put these numbers in the system is not by what an expert says, but by how real statistics 'lie'.

This means that we want to keep the role of probabilities as marginal as possible in medical KBS. Reliable, stable and valid statistics are scarce, and their use should be in accordance with the assumptions of statistical models. In order to minimise this role of probabilistic and pseudo-statistical inferences, other descriptive reasoning principles based upon abstraction and decomposition should first be fully explored: in particular partial structural models of a domain which lend themselves to the application of 'systematic diagnosis'.

With this purpose in mind we have analysed the domain of physiotherapeutical diagnosis; not only because a medical KBS may be far more tractable in its reasoning, but in particular because we had also to teach students how to cope with large hypothesis spaces.

An Analysis in Physiotherapeutic Diagnosis

In the Intelligent Interactive Video (IIV) project[7] the aim was to construct an Intelligent Tutoring System (ITS) to train students in physiotherapeutic diagnosis: the PhysioDisc system. The students interact with PhysioDisc to solve cases in physiotherapy. They can request tests (e.g. have the patient walk) that are recorded on video disc, propose hypotheses and eventually come up with a conclusion (a physiotherapeuticdiagnosis). The focus is on orthopedic complaints in arms and legs, and peripheral neural complaints (*Winkels et al, 1989*).

Any ITS is also an Expert System, at least for the domain it tries to teach, and possibly also for the teaching task itself. In modelling the subject matter expertise for the physiotherapeutic domain, we applied the KADS methodology described in the previous sections.

The problem solving behaviour of experienced physiotherapists in diagnosis is based on many empirical associations and heuristics which have been acquired by experience and are often very specific. It seems plausible to start modelling this behaviour, using the interpretation model for heuristic diagnosis and end up with a descriptive conceptual model of the diagnostic expertise in physiotherapy. However, it is very doubtful whether heuristic classification can or should be the method to be used in teaching (see next section). For teaching purposes we want to pursue a more systematic approach in which hypotheses are generated in a systematic way and tests are structured to their applicability to categories of hypotheses. Systematic methods have not only the advantage that they can be taught explicitly as in methodologies -, but also that their execution can be controlled: an important precondition for intelligent coaching systems. Therefore, it appears that systematic diagnosis provides a better 'prescriptive' model than heuristic diagnosis. Besides these advantages for tutoring systems, a systematic model also is easier to maintain, it provides means for justifying and explaining conclusions, and it will perform better for some difficult or even unsolvable cases ('graceful degradation'). In other words, it is provides the characteristics of second generation Expert Systems (*Steels, 1988*).

Interpretation models describe expertise by four layers of different types of knowledge (cf. section 3.3 and table 1). In the case of the PhysioDisc system these layers can be thought of as:

- **Domain Layer**: Static facts and relations. I.c. the anatomic knowledge, types of malfunctions and the knowledge about tests.
- **Inference Layer**: The abstract competence of making inferences at the domain level. 'Selecting a test', or 'generating hypotheses' belong at this level.

---

7   The IIV project ran in 1988 and the beginning of 1989 with several participants: The School of Physiotherapy 'Hogeschool van Amsterdam' provided the physiotherapeutic expertise; Media Design produced the video disc; knowledge engineering, design and implementation of the system was done by Bolesian Systems (Helmond) and the University of Amsterdam. The entire project took about 3.5 person years, including the effort of the experts. The project was partially funded by the ministries of Economic Affairs and Education & Science of the Netherlands as part of the INSP program.

- **Task Layer**: Specifies which inferences should or could be made at what time. For systematic diagnosis in the physiotherapeutic domain one or more task decompositions can be made and they are specified at this level (see figure 5 for part of the task structure of PhysioDisc).
- **Strategic Layer**: At this level decisions concerning task decomposition are made, the problem solving process is being monitored, etc. In the PhysioDisc system, this level is not present (yet). The task structure is fixed.

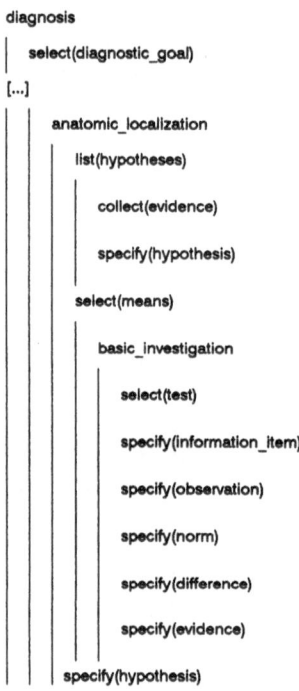

Figure 5: Part of the task structure of the IIV system. Except for the select' tasks, the system may decide to let the student skip (sub)tasks.

To find a systematic model of the problem solving behaviour of experts, one has to perform a 'rational reconstruction' of the heuristic behaviour. In the case of the physiotherapeutic diagnostic expertise, after a (partial) description of the domain layer, knowledge engineers together with experts tried to fit the interpretation model of systematic diagnosis (see fig. 4) on the domain. What constructs can perform the role of hypotheses, which decomposition principles for hypothesis generation can be identified, etc. At first we constructed 1 conceptual model for the entire diagnostic process, but that did not fit. It appeared that different ways of constraining the search or hypothesis space could be distinguished, and that a clever way of combining these 'methods' lead to a more or less systematic and controllable process of hypothesis generation and testing. These different decomposition methods are based on structures given in the domain, i.c. the hierarchical structure of the human anatomy and small and fixed numbers of types of tissues and pathologies. We ended up with 5 different models[8] that complement one another. The 'conclusions' of applying a partial domain model constraints the hypothesis space for another (next) model application.

Applying the five domain models correspond to different phases of the physiotherapeutic diagnostic process, which can be indicated by their outcome:

1. A description of the patient's complaint (e.g. trouble when walking)
2. An anatomical localization of the complaint (e.g. the left knee)
3. A specification of the tissue involved (e.g. muscle)
4. An instantiation of the specific tissue (e.g. musculus soleus)
5. A specification of the pathology (e.g. a rupture)

These outcomes are associated with different kinds of investigation. A description of the complaint is typically achieved in the anamnesis, the anatomical localization in what is called the 'basic investigation', specification and instantiation of tissue usually in the 'local anatomic investigation', and the pathology in the final phase by 'supplementary investigation'. The assembly of these heterogeneous elements constitutes a full diagnosis, e.g. 'The trouble with walking is caused by a rupture of the musculus soleus (a muscle) in the left knee'.

The order in which these models are used is very important. When one starts with instantiation of tissue for example, the hypothesis space is immense, while starting with tissue specification does not provide any constraints. Decisions about the order are taken at the strategic level, where the task structure is produced and the entire process is monitored. In some special cases the order does not matter, e.g. when both provide equal constraints.

Testing hypotheses is done in one or more test cycles within every phase of the diagnostic process. Given a hypothesis set, one or more investigations can be applicable, and, apart from pragmatic aspects, the physiotherapist picks any one of these. Besides that, certain tests are always performed, and some in a fixed order. In most cases there are many tests to choose from, so a physiotherapist does not have to fall back on testing hypotheses by justification (see section 4.2). If they cannot perform the test themselves, they can refer a patient to a specialist, e.g. for x-rays. Nevertheless, they are inclined to find models that explain their observations and inferred evidence.

---

8   Actually, the first phase in the diagnostic process, the anamnesis, has not been truly modelled, since none of the experts in the domain seem to agree on the right method to go about this part of the investigation. In the PhysioDisc system this phase has been implemented as traditional Computer Assisted Instruction, i.e. the system has no knowledge about how to perform an anamnesis, does not know what questions mean, etc. Everything is hardwired in the code.

Teaching Physiotherapeutic Diagnosis

As mentioned earlier, the aim of the IIV project was to build a Tutoring System to teach physiotherapeutic diagnosis. It was the experience of expert teachers at the School of Physiotherapy 'Hogeschool van Amsterdam' that students particularly had problems in applying the *theories* in specific cases, i.e. making the step from *support knowledge* to *operational knowledge (Clancey, 1983).*[9]

They learn about the human anatomy, about pathologies and about tests (or know were to find the information), but they do not know how to apply this knowledge to proceed from a patient's complaint to a physiotherapeutic diagnosis. In terms of the types of knowledge distinguished in KADS (see previous section), they seem to lack the strategic knowledge to come to a task decomposition, and sometimes they are unable to make inferences at the domain level. The primary goal of the PhysioDisc system is to teach the students exactly that knowledge. As the PhysioDisc system does not have an explicit strategic layer (yet), but a fixed task structure, that structure is the primary didactic goal. It specifies i.a. the order in which to apply different decomposition principles, it explicitly introduces hypotheses formulation phases, test cycles, etc. (see figure 5). Experiments with students and human tutors showed that students have a tendency to jump to conclusions (*Winkels & Breuker, 1988*). As soon as they have some information about the complaint, they focus on one or two possible causes, and it is very difficult to broaden their horizon. It seems they work according to a heuristic diagnostic model, like the experts do, but they obviously lack the experience and knowledge to handle this strategy. Since the Domain Expert of the PhysioDisc system works according to a more systematic model, we can keep the students from jumping to conclusions, and provide them with an alternative way of controlling the search space. The five steps in going from a complaint to a physiotherapeutic diagnosis keep the 'local hypothesis space' relatively small.

Moreover, we can support this systematic approach by providing continuous feedback on the state of the hypothesis space, the tests they have performed and the evidence they have gathered. The PhysioDisc System described runs on a PC-AT with 640 Kb and is written in Prolog. It has been positively evaluated by a physiotherapeutic, an educational and a programming expert by order of the funding ministries. After further evaluation with students in the autumn of 1989, the system will be used to support regular courses at all (10) Dutch schools of physiotherapy.

See figure 6 for a fragment of a session with the system (unfortunately one cannot see the rest of the screen).

---

9   Within our model of coaching, this linking of support and operational knowledge is achieved by providing students with explicit didactic relations between these different kinds of knowledge, i.c. an 'abstraction' link when acquired 'skill' (operational knowledge) is linked to support knowledge (e.g. a causal model), and a 'concretion' link when the opposite is done (Breuker et al, 1986).

OK.
WHAT HYPOTHESES DO YOU HAVE NOW?
> rupture of muscle in elbow
YOU SPECIFY 'RUPTURE OF MUSCLE IN ELBOW'. YOU SEEM
TO THINK THE CURRENT GOAL IS 'PATHOLOGY SPECIFICA-
TION'. IT IS HOWEVER 'ANATOMICAL LOCALIZATION'.
[skip]
> elbow shoulder
ELBOW AND SHOULDER ARE POSSIBLE, BUT THERE ARE
MORE JOINTS THAT MAY BE EFFECTED.
> wrist
VERY GOOD.
WHAT DO YOU WANT TO DO NOW?
- DESCRIPTION OF COMPLAINT
- ANATOMICAL LOCALIZATION
- TISSUE SPECIFICATION
- TISSUE INSTANTIATION
- PATHOLOGY SPECIFICATION
[student clicks 'tissue specification']
YOU CHOSE TISSUE SPECIFICATION. THAT IS NOT CORRECT.
DO YOU REMEMBER THAT 'ANATOMICAL LOCALIZATION' IS
DONE BEFORE 'TISSUE SPECIFICATION'?
[skip]
WHAT TEST DO YOU WANT TO DO NOW?
> wind watch
OK. HERE COMES 'WIND WATCH'. PLEASE WATCH THE MONI-
TOR.
[skip]
OK. WHAT HYPOTHESES ARE LEFT FROM YOUR ORIGINAL
SET?
[student now edits his hypothesis set and keeps all]
SHOULDER AND ELBOW ARE STILL POSSIBLE, BUT NONE OF
THE INVESTIGATIONS SHOWED ANY EVIDENCE FOR YOUR
HYPOTHESIS 'WRIST'.
[or the system may pose a diagnostic question to find a possible miscon-
ception of the student:]
WHAT INVESTIGATION PROVIDED EVIDENCE FOR YOUR
HYPOTHESIS 'WRIST'?

Figure 6: Example of a session with PhysioDisc. The system's remarks are in capitals.
Comments are between square brackets.

Conclusions

Two categories of conclusions can be drawn from the experiences with KADS in a medical domain. The first category applies to the acquisition and construction of knowledge bases for medical applications; the second to medical education.

However, it appears that the conclusions on these two issues are difficult to separate.Indeed, building an ITS is viewed as putting the highest demands on the explicitness of the knowledge in terms of qualitative models rather than straightforward sets of operational rules (*Clancey, 1983; 1988*). In principle, medical diagnosis does not lend itself easily for a modelling approach. There are relatively few ITS in this area. Medical diagnosis is characterised by very large hypothesis spaces, and unspecific evidence, based on indirect and sometimes expensive data. Physiotherapy may not be typical in the latter respect because many and simple tests are available, but the way diagnostic problems are solved has the same structure. Thinking aloud protocols show typical heuristic strategies based on local pattern matching in generating hypotheses. This means that at the start of the project there was the somewhat depressing prospective of collecting all these specific associations, very local models, and no apparent task structure. The only part that could provide a more global structure was the anatomy involved.

Anatomy lead itself perfectly for decomposition, so a systematic diagnosis model was indicated. Later it was found out that this model had to be combined with a more heuristic, classification based model for other types of knowledge that were involved. Combining models is standard practice in KADS, because in real life tasks hardly ever have a simple 'generic' form. However, combining these models as to partition the hypotheses space in this domain was new and appeared very effective. Combining these models made also clear that the models were sufficiently close that they could be integrated instead of cooperate with one another via interfaces (say: metaclasses in KADS).

It had a number of consequences. The first one is that we did not have to use probabilities. As we have stated in section 4, we would be inclined only to use these if there was no alternative -and then in a very careful way, i.e. as part of the control rather than the reasoning itself.[10]

Another consequence was that we had to make a **rational reconstruction** of the domain. This rational reconstruction has been driven by the need to make some standard strategy (task structure) explicit, so that students could at least acquire some way to hook operational associations to subgoals. This was achieved by separating the testing from the hypothesis generation task in the first place.As this was insufficient, we had to partition the hypothesis generation task further and discovered that 'any principle' could be applied as long as it would constrain next steps. Whether we can generalise this finding to other (medical) diagnostic domains is hard to say, but it is certainly a heuristic that has been insufficiently applied.

Rational reconstructions have an obvious disadvantage: the way experts say (or show) how they solve problems is no longer 'valid'. A new framework, consisting of an explicit task- or inference structure has to be created by the knowledge engineer.

---

10   Besides the theoretical and practical reasons why likelihoods were not very welcome, it is almost impossible to use these in an educational setting, where one rather wants to induce careful and systematic considerations rather than associated likelihoods.

This framework -or **interpretation model**- may enforce an organisation of the domain knowledge that has the risk of being inadequate. However, it is our experience that the validity of the framework is established very soon. The experts who used a completely different strategy in their problem solving behaviour than PhysioDisc became very valuable 'debuggers' of the models for the various types of knowledge.Moreover, as teachers, they were prepared to change their instruction before the system was even built. In this way the role of a knowledge engineer is similar to a librarian who finds heaps of books where the owners have no problem in finding their way. He can propose some subject matter dependent schema that may index these books in accordance with what the owner-experts consider to be relevant. More important: this indexing schema makes these books and their implied knowledge accessible by the lender-novices.

Although the role of trying to apply organisation principles and interpretation models in domains where knowledge engineers are laymen at best has certainly the risk of grossly erring by commission, it appears that there is little alternative in trying to model expertise.

References.

Anjewierden, A. (1988) Knowledge Acquisition Tools, AI-Communications, 0, pp. 29-38.

Anjewierden, A., & Wielemaker, J. (1989) Extensible objects. Paper for OOPSLA'89 (Esprit 1098; Tech. Report UvA-C1-TR-006a, University of Amsterdam.

Boshuizen, H.P.A. (1989) De ontwikkeling van medische expertise. Ph D Thesis, Rijks Universiteit Limburg.

Brachman, R.J. (1979) On the epistemological status of semantic networks. In: R. Findler (ed). Associative Networks, Academic Press, New York.

Bredeweg, B. & Wielinga, B. (1988) Integrating qualitative reasoning approaches. Proceedings of the European AI Conference, Pitman, London.

Breuker, J.A. (ed) (1987) Model driven knowledge acquisition: Interpretation models. Deliverable D1, Esprit 1098, University of Amsterdam.

Breuker, J.A., Winkels, R.G.F. & Sandberg, J.A.C. (1986) Didactic Goal Generator. Deliverable 2.2.3 of the ESPRIT Project P280, 'EUROHELP'. University of Amsterdam.

Breuker, J.A. & Wielinga, B.J. (1989) Models of expertise in Knowledge Acquisition. In: G. Guida & C. Tasso (eds). Topics in Expert System Design: methodologies and tools. North Holland, Amsterdam.

Breuker, J.A., Wielinga, B.J. (eds) (In preparation) The KADS Methodology for building knowledge based systems. Academic Press.

Chandrasekaran, B. & Mittal, S. (1983) Conceptual representation of medical knowledge for diagnosis by computer. MDX and related systems. In: Advances in Computers, Academic Press, New York, pp. 217-293.

Clancey, W.J. (1983) The epistemology of a rule based system: a framework for explanation. Artificial Intelligence, 20, pp. 215-251.

Clancey, W.J. (1985) Heuristic Classification. Artificial Intelligence, 27, pp. 289-350.

Clancey, W.J. (1988) The role of qualitative models in instruction. In: J. Self (ed). Artificial Intelligence and Human Learning, Chapman & Hall, London.

De Kleer, J.H. & Brown, J.S. (1984) Qualitative reasoning about physical systems. Artificial Intelligence, 24, p7.

Edin, G, Rooke, P., Breuker, J., Rangecroft, T. & Hayes, F. (1987). The KADS Handbook. Esprit 1098, J1, Scicon Ltd, London.

Fox, J., Myers, C.D., Greaves, M.F. & Pegram, S. (1987) A systematic study of knowledge base refinement in the diagnosis of leukemia. In: A. Kidd (ed). Knowledge Acquisition for expert systems: a practical handbook.

Greef, P. de & Breuker, J.A. (1989) A methodology for analysing modalities of system/user cooperation for KBS. Proceedings of EKAW '89, Paris, pp. 462-473.

Haan, N. den, (1989) DERMAX, een expertsysteem voor dermatologisch onderzoek. Master thesis, University of Amsterdam, Department of Computer Science.

Hayes-Roth et al (1983) Building Expert Systems.

Kuipers, B. & Kassirer, J.P. (1987) Knowledge acquisition by analysis of verbatim protocols. In: A. Kidd (ed). Knowledge Acquisition for expert systems: a practical handbook.

Newell, A. (1982) The Knowledge Level. Artificial Intelligence, pp. 87-127.

Schreiber, G., Bredeweg, B., Davoodi, M. & Wielinga, B. (1987) Towards a Design Methodology for KBS. Deliverable D8, Esprit 1098, University of Amsterdam.

Schreiber, G., Breuker, J., Bredeweg, B. & Wielinga, B. (1988) Modelling in KBS Development. Third European Workshop on Knowledge Acquisition. Steels, L. (1987). The deepening of expert systems. AI Communications, 0, pp. 9-16.

Sticklen, J., Chandrasekaran, B. and Josephson, J.R. (1985) Control issues in Classificatory diagnosis. Proceedings of the IJCAI-85, Los Angeles 1985, Morgan Kaufman, Los Altos, pp 300-306.

Tversky, A. & Kahneman, D. (1974) Judgement under uncertainty: heuristics and biases. Science, 184, pp. 1124-1131.

Wielinga, B.J. & Breuker, J.A. (1986) Models of Expertise. Proceedings of ECAI 1986.

Wilson, M. (1989) Task Models for knowledge elicitation. In: D. Diaper (ed). Knowledge elicitation: principles, techniques and applications, pp. 197-220.

Winkels, R.G.F., Achthoven, W.A. & Gennip, A. van (1989) Methodology and Modularity in ITS Design. Proceedings of the 4th International Conference on AI & Education, Amsterdam, May 1989.

Winkels, R.G.F. & Breuker, J.A. (1988) Een Computer Coach voor het IIV Project. Deliverable of the Intelligent Interactive Video System project.

Questions from the discussion.

Groth: I agree that knowledge acquisition is important, but equally important is the analysis of the needs of the user adn the impact of a decision support system on the user's working conditions. How does that fit into the KADS methodology?

Breuker: Your question suggests that there may be a conflict between the knowledge that is acquired and the needs of the (prospective) user. In principle there shouldn't be one of course, because it is assumed that the user needs this experience-support and what I presented were methods in KADS to transfer -or rather 'reconstruct'-

this knowledge in as much valid ways as possible. You meant probably with your question how in KADS we can specify the needs of the user. The Modality framework (De Greef & Breuker, 1989) is specifically developed for this purpose. I didn't have time to present this, but essentially this framework is concerned with the specification of how the system and user can cooperate within some task distribution; what and when should be communicated; how these issues can be empirically investigated, and what constraints this analysis provides for the design of the user interface.

Talmon: In KADS, several interpretation models have been defined, for example for several diagnostic and classification tasks. To what extent are these models general and is your library of models complete?

Breuker: The whole enterprise of trying to come up with a full, high level description of the various types of problem solving tasks borders to megalomania. Therefore, you should take the validity of these models with a grain of salt. In the article I have presented an example of the issues that are at stake in further testing and refining these models. In fact, I wanted to present all variations which concern ways of hypothesis generation and testing in diagnosis. We have identified at least 10 different ways of hypothesis testing which may range from simple observation to reconfiguration and repair of a device. I have even pointed to the practice in medicine of hypothesis testing by constructing a qualitative, 'deep' model, i.e. hypothesis testing by explanation -whether this is a valid way or not!.
However, the current state of the interpretation models is highly dependent on experience, within the KADS-project, but in particular in (commercial) practice outside the project. In general, our experience is that the models provide a strong initial guidance, even if the model selected is incorrect. Incorrect can both mean that the wrong model has been selected or that the model in the library is incorrect. We have found some errors in the models, these will be corrected in new versions, but we have found particular incompleteness, i.e. insufficient detail. Another problem is the fact that in practice a 'real life' task may be composed of various generic tasks, and that moreover these combinations of generic tasks may vary according to the type of task, which complicates the picture. Therefore, to put it simple: the models are not complete; in particular for a number of synthesis and modification tasks, they are often too general, and only partially validated and this process of validation is very complicated.

Talmon: Aren't the ideas behind the methodology, i.e. the description at different levels and the use of knowledge sources and metaclasses not more important than the collection of models that are available?

Breuker: Indeed it may turn out that KCML or the 'Four Layer Theory' is theoretically more important, and moreover, KCML is the tool that can also be used in a bottom up way. In practice, the model are highly valued, even for the wrong reasons, because they provide some initial structure. This may be partially a psychological phenomenon: the knowledge engineer may fear empty structures as much as writers abhor white paper. However, for a novice knowledge engineer the interpretation models are a real guidance. We shouldn't forget that there is still a lot of confusion of even the types of tasks that should be distinguished. The taxonomy of tasks we have developed is not self evident and by itself already very important to avoid confusion between the performance of a task and the way cooperation between the system and the user is arranged.

For instance, a large team of AI researchers (Hayes-Roth et al, 1983) of reputation has proposed a typology in which 'coaching' and 'diagnosis' are typical expertise tasks, while for the audience it didn't give rise to any confusion to talk about: the coaching of diagnosis in physiotherapy (instead of, for example: the coaching and diagnosis in physiotherapy, as comparable to: the planning and diagnosis in phsyiotherapy).

References:

De Greef, P. & Breuker, J.A. (1989). A methodology for analysing modalities of system/user cooperation for KBS. In: J. Boose, B. Gaines and J.G. Ganascia (eds), Proc. of the 3rd European Workshop on Knowledge Acquisition for Knowledge-Based Systems, EKAW-89, Paris, 1989, pp 452-474.

Hayes-Roth, F., Waterman, D.A. & Lenat, D.B. (eds) (1983), Building expert systems, Addison-Wesley, New York.

Machine Learning as a Tool for Knowledge Acquisition

R.A.J. Schijven and J.L. Talmon,

Dept. of Medical Informatics and Statistics, University of Limburg, Maastricht, The Netherlands.

Abstract

*K*nowledge acquisition is the bottleneck in building knowledge based systems. Experts have often difficulty in expressing the expertise they use for making their decisions. This paper describes the use of machine learning techniques for knowledge acquisition. With these methods one avoids the verbalization of the knowledge. The knowledge is derived from example cases that are solved by the expert. We will give a brief introduction in the different approaches to machine learning and describe in more detail a program developed by us. An example is given of the successful application of this program.

Introduction

Machine learning techniques are becoming increasingly accepted as tools for the knowledge acquisition process. Machine learning algorithms that address the problem of learning from examples are the most relevant ones for the development of knowledge based systems. Specifically for those systems that have to perform a classification or diagnosis task. The algorithms that learn from examples assume that at least the relevant features in the application domain are available for a set of cases together with the classification or diagnosis given by the expert. The task of the machine learning techniques is to derive a meaningful classification/diagnosis scheme. That scheme needs to mimic, as good as possible, the input-output relation of the classification task as performed by the human expert.

Within the domain of learning from examples, there are globally two different approaches. The first one is called conceptual clustering. It can be considered as a generalization process. The most well-known procedure of this type is AQ15 developed by the group of Michalski (see *Michalski et al, 1986* for 3 applications in the medical domain). In this approach, one example of a specific class is taken as the description of that class. The values for the different features act as constraints in the description of the class. These constraints are to be relaxed such that no examples of other classes fall within the description of the reference class. The best description is the one that covers most of the examples of the class. Those examples that are not covered form the new set of learning cases for the next description of the class. The sequence of induced descriptions goes from the most general to the most specific when ordered according to the number of cases covered. This method turns out to be search intensive and shows signs of combinatorial explosion when the number of examples and/or the number of features increases (*Rendell et al, 1987*).

The other approach uses specialization. Most of the work in this domain is based on or related to the approach described in *Quinlan, 1986*. In this approach one tries to divide the feature space recursively in smaller regions such that in the end each region contains (in principle) only examples of one a priori class. This approach results in a classification tree. As one descends the tree during the design phase, one defines more and more restrictions to describe the class of interest. Hence, one can speak of a specialization process. When the tree is used for the classification of new cases, one has to test one (or a combination) of the parameters against one or more thresholds at a node of the tree. One descends the tree according to the outcome of such a test. This process is repeated until one reaches a leaf node of the tree. This node has a class label that will be assigned to the case that is analyzed. This approach was not only developed in the domain of Artificial Intelligence. More or less independent of Quinlan's work, similar research was done in the domain of statistics (*Breiman et al. 1984*) and in the domain of pattern recognition (*Talmon 1986*). In the next paragraph we will describe the latter approach. We will demonstrate its successful application in the design of a system for the interpretation of data recorded during non-invasive testing of the arteries of the limbs.

Non-Parametric Partitioning Algorithm

Our Non-Parametric Partitioning Algorithm -abbreviated as NPPA- was developed when we were facing a classification problem that could be characterized as data rich. We had over 17,000 examples described by some 15 features (*Talmon 1983*). These features were real-valued but had highly non-normal distributions. Also the variance-covariance matrices of the classes that were considered were different and hence standard statistical classification techniques did not perform at a sufficiently high level of accuracy.
A limited review of the literature in the domain of pattern recognition and applications of decision algorithms for medical problems revealed several approaches. Each of these appoaches had some shortcomings that would be unacceptable for our application. The algorithms described in *Friedman 1977, Gleser and Collen 1972* and *Henrichon and Fu 1969* formed the basis for our approach.
In table 1, we have listed our design goals together with an indication in which of the above-mentioned algorithms these properties were explicitly mentioned.

The fact that a multi-class algorithm is needed is obvious. In many applications several possible outcomes have to be considered.
In many medical applications, several types of data may occur. Some of the features will be of the yes/no type, others will allow for a continuous range of numerical values, others will take a value out of an unordered set of possible values. The

	Friedman	Gleser	Henrichon	Quinlan
Multi-class		X		X
Multi-data type		X	X	X
Optimization of thresholds	X		X	X
Stopping rule		X		
Limited Branching	X			

Table 1: Properties of different approaches in non-parametric machine learning algorithms.

algorithm should be flexible enough to handle these different types of data in a consistent way.

During each step of the algorithm not only an optimal feature should be selected but also one or more optimal thresholds (given some criteria for optimality) are to be determined. In some of the above-mentioned algorithms the continuously valued features have to be categorized beforehand. Hence performance of the resulting classification tree will depend upon this categorization (See *Gleser and Collen 1972* for an example). Although *Henrichon and Fu 1969* propose some optimization of thresholds, an initial partitioning of each feature axis has to be determined for each step.

In many applications, it is impossible to separate all examples with the available features such that the resulting classification tree still has predictive value.

Therefore, a stopping rule is needed to decide when a proposed split of a region will have no predictive value.

Finally, we posed a restriction on the branching at each node of the tree. When a high branching factor is allowed, the set of example cases in a certain region becomes very small soon. Again the predictive value of such a split is not necessarily guaranteed. We decided to allow only a binary tree to be created by the algorithm.

In principle, the algorithm works as follows.

NPPA starts with all example cases that are submitted to the learning phase. It will recursively split the feature space in two regions based on a feature and a threshold that optimizes some performance criterion. Next it checks whether this performance is still significant. If not, no further splitting is done, otherwise the split is performed. Of course, when a region only contains examples of one class, no further splitting is done.

We use as a performance criterion the reduction in uncertainty in classification as measured by a reduction in the Shannon entropy. Let's assume that the probability of belonging to a certain class is p_i, $i = 1..C$. The Shannon entropy is given by

$$E = -\sum_{i=1}^{C} ln(p_i)$$

Assuming that we have a continuous valued feature with some threshold T, the
entropy in each region after splitting is given by

$$E_j = - \sum_{i=1}^{C} ln(p_{ij}), \text{ with } \begin{array}{l} j=1 \text{ for } \textit{feature value} < T \text{ and} \\ j=2 \text{ for } \textit{feature value} > T \end{array}$$

The reduction in entropy is given by

$$I(T) = E - \sum_{j=1}^{2} p_{.j} E_j$$

$p_{.j}$ being the probability of being in region j.
By systematically moving the threshold, I(T) can be optimized for each feature and
the feature with the largest value of I(T) is selected as the best one.
For features that have a value from a limited (un)ordered set of possible values, a
split of the learning cases is obtained by selecting the cases with a specific value and
compare then against the rest. The value that provides the largest I(T) is used to
compare the performance of such a feature with that of the other features. The
reduction of entropy is also used in the algorithms of Gleser and Collen and of
Quilan.

Although only for large numbers N of example cases, $2*N*I$ has a χ^2 distribution with
C-1 degrees of freedom, this measure is used to determine whether the obtained
reduction in entropy is significant (p 0.05).
When $2*N*I$ becomes too small for a certain region, the recursive partitioning of
that region stops.
When the partitioning is finished, the user has to provide a label for each region that
is created. Of course, regions that contain only cases of one a priori class are labelled
automatically.
NPPA presents the derived knowledge in the form of a classification tree. This
representation is easily converted into a set of rules by following a branch in the
tree and using the criteria for descending that branch in the condition part of the
rule. The label of the terminal node of the branch of the tree is used as the conclusion
of the rule.
The NPPA algorithm has been applied in several domains:

- ●ECG analysis (*Talmon 1983*)
- ●Analysis of questionnaires taken before endoscopy.
- ●Analysis of data from non-invasive testing in patients with peripheral vascular
  disease.

Some of the results of this last study will be presented in the next paragraphs.

Non-Invasive Vascular Testing

During the non-invasive testing in patients with peripheral vascular disease, three
tests are available to localize obstructions of the arteries of the legs and assess
their functional severity:

ZIEKENHUIS ST. ANNADAL MAASTRICHT VAATLABORATORIUM HEELKUNDE 043-862272	HAEMODYNAMISCH ONDERZOEK Patient identification

Datum onderzoek: 4-10-'82 ☐ Kliniek: ☒ Polikliniek: surgery

Aanvragend specialist: Dopplernr.: 6451082

Vaatoperatie(s): —

VERSLAG: Both pressure-response curves are pathological. Ankle/arm-index R = 75% at rest. After exercise: 27%. Ankle/arm-index L = 75% at rest. After exercise: 39%. Patient is able to walk 3 minutes on treadmill, then experiences pain in both calfs.
The right CFA-waveform shows deminished backflow, but a normal forwardflow. The waveform in the left CFA is highpitched (stenosis). There is a fall in pulsatility between the CFA and the PA on both sides, right more than left. After the treadmilltest the waveforms in the CFA's are registered again, confirming the existence of pathology in the aorto-iliac segments.
Conclusion: pathology at the aorto-iliac level on both sides. Occluded superficial femoral artery R. Stenosis in the left common femoral artery and in the left superficial femoral artery.

DOPPLERDRUKINDICES Loopafstand: 4 km/uur: 3 min, met/~~zonder~~ pijn calfs

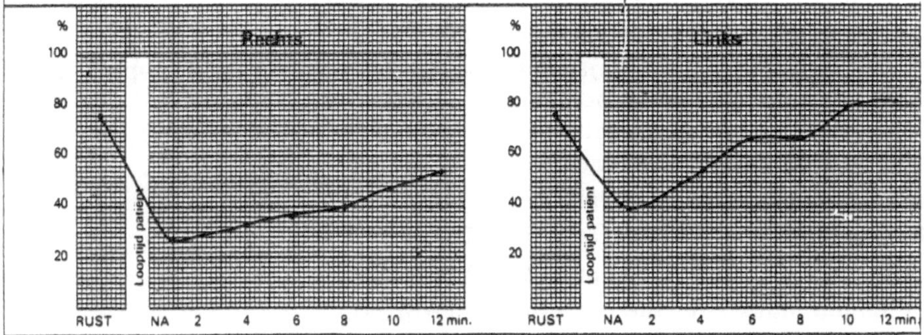

	Rechts							Links							
Brach.	145	205	165	150	150	150	140	Brach.	145	205	165	150	150	150	140
Tib.Post. Dors.Ped.	110	55	55	55	60	70	75	Tib.Post. Dors.Ped.	110	80	90	100	100	120	115

DOPPLERREGISTRATIES	Rechts	Links	Dopplerdrukken mm Hg R	L
A. Brachialis	(Norm) / Path. + ++ +++	Norm. / Path. + ++ +++	145	
A. Femoralis Communis	(Norm) / (Path.) (+) ++ +++	Norm. / Path. (+) ++ +++ stenosis	130	155
A. Femoralis Superficialis	Norm. / Path. + (++) +++	Norm. / Path. (+) ++ +++		
A. Poplitea	Norm. / Path. + (++) +++	Norm. / Path. (+) (++) +++	110	110
A. Tibialis Posterior	Norm. / Path. + (++) +++	Norm. / Path. + (++) +++	110	110
A. Dorsalis Pedis	Norm. / Path. + (++) +++	Norm. / Path. + (++) +++		

+ = Geringe afplatting, Geringe backflow, Minder pulsatiel
++ = Sterke afplatting, Geen backflow, Collaterale vulling
+++ = Als ++ doch veel meer uitgesproken

Figure 1: Example of a report of a non-invasive vascular test. The technicians report is on the top. The measurements are given in the lower part of the figure.

- The systolic blood-pressure readings taken from the upper arm, the thigh, the upper calf and the ankle, while the patient is at rest.
- The Doppler waveforms of the groin, the knee and ankle arteries, visually graded on a 7-point scale ranging from normal to very severely abnormal.
- A stress test. The patient has to walk on a treadmill for at most 5 minutes at a speed of 4 km/hour. Before and at regular intervals after the exercise, systolic blood pressures are measured at the upper arm and the ankles. The ratio of these blood pressures provide diagnostic information and result in a trend plot, which is used to determine the functional importance of obstructions.

These tests result in a report, made by the technician, describing the results of the three tests. At the end the technician adds the overall conclusions on the state of the arteries of the lower extremities (see figure 1).

The aim of the system is to support the interpretation of the test data and to automate the report generation process. This will result in a consistent, computer generated interpretation of the test results which may be used for subsequent higher level diagnostics and therapy planning. A more detailed description of this system is given in *Talmon et al 1988*[*] .

Machine Learning With Non-Invasive Vascular Test Data

From the hospital's archive we randomly selected 200 previously performed tests (providing test data of 400 legs)such that a representative patient population for the vascular laboratory was obtained.

In this paper we will restrict ourselves to the judgments of the pressure curves. For each curve, we determined five features:

- the ankle/arm ratio at rest (RIND),
- the first post exercise ankle/arm ratio (MIND),
- the difference between RIND and MIND (DIND),
- the minimum index after the exercise test (AMIN),
- the time needed for the pressure curve to recover (TIME).

These features were judged by the technicians to be of relevance for describing the degree of abnormality by the technicians of the vascular laboratory.

Two technicians independently judged all 400 curves on a five point scale, ranging from normal to very severely abnormal. In 340 cases, the classification of the two technicians was in agreement. In the other cases there was a difference of only one degree of severity among the classifications of the technicians.

The 340 cases on which the technicians agreed were used for the first analysis. A learning and test set of both 170 cases were made. With the learning set a classification tree with 5 terminal nodes was derived with NPPA, labelling 162 cases correctly. Testing the classification tree with the other 170 cases resulted in the misclassifica-

---

*   This project is carried out together with the Department of Surgery and the Vascular Laboratory of the Academic Hospital in Maastricht.

tion of 11 cases. However, the labelling of the wrongly classified cases differed only one class from the judgment of the technicians.

After this first phase, 60 cases were left in which the technicians disagreed as well as the 19 cases in which there was a difference between the classification of the technicians and that of NPPA. We gave the technicians the opportunity for a second opinion by providing them again the 79 cases but now accompanied by the different classifications that were given by them and the classification tree. This analysis resulted in an additional 44 cases in which the technicians agreed, yielding a total of 384 out of the 400 cases. Using this set of cases, a second analysis with NPPA resulted in a classification tree again with 5 terminal nodes. Agreement was achieved in 185 and 179 cases for the learning set and test set respectively.

In the last phase of the knowledge acquisition process, we discussed the 16 cases that where classified differently by both technicians to come to a consensus. Finally, the total set of 400 cases was used as a learning set. This resulted in a classification tree (see figure 2) with 10 terminal nodes and agreement in 386 cases (96%).

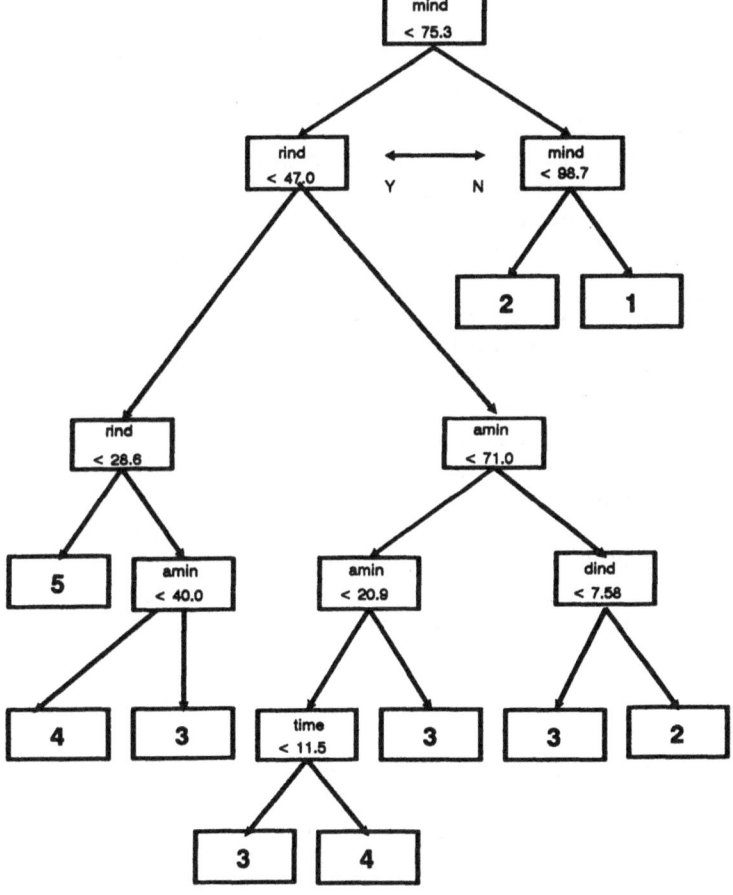

Figure 2: The classification tree derived from the total set of 400 example cases.

We felt it justified to use all cases as training examples since the analyses during the first and second phase showed good reproducibility. Currently this classification tree is under evaluation in a clinical setting.

The same machine learning technique has also been used for the analysis of the data that were obtained from the other noninvasive vascular tests.

The resulting classification trees were verified by the technicians. It turned out that the sequence in which the parameters were used differed from what they expected. They assumed that the arm-ankle ratio at rest would be the most important one. A low index indicates an abnormal curve. Since this parameter is the first one that becomes available during the test, it's relevance is easily overestimated.

Despite this discrepancy between the derived knowledge and the informally expressed knowledge of the technicians, the classification tree was accepted by the technicians. They judged it as describing a reasonable and accurate classification scheme which could be implemented in the system.

Conclusions

We may conclude that machine learning techniques can be very useful tools in the knowledge acquisition process. High agreement was achieved between the program and the consensus opinion of the technicians in our domain of application. Also previous studies in the domain of ECG analysis give similar results (see *Talmon 1983*). However, when large overlap between classes exists, also machine learning techniques will fail to find classification trees that will have sufficient predictive value for new cases. The power of the algorithm is it's independence of the underlying distributions of the feature values. Also the handling of different types of features is useful.

A disadvantage of using machine learning techniques as a knowledge acquisition tool is the difficulty to represent and use the knowledge of the expert. So far these techniques are mechanistic and hardly allow for the incorporation of the expert's knowledge in the learning phase. Integration of machine learning techniques in other methods for knowledge acquisition would certainly improve the quality of the derived knowledge, not only articulated by the expert, but also the knowledge derived from the examples.

Before a classification tree is used on new cases, experts need to verify the structure of the tree. In our opinion, such an analysis is mandatory to have the derived knowledge as well as the future predictions made by the tree accepted by both the expert and the potential user of the system.

References

Breiman, L., Friedman, J.H., Olshen, R.A, Stone, C.J.: Classification and regression trees. Wadsworth, Belmont, CA, USA, 1984.

Friedman, J.H.: A recursive partitioning decision rule for nonparametric classification. IEEE Trans. on Comp, C-26, 404-408, 1977.

Gleser, M.A. and Collen, M.F.: Towards automated medical decisions. Comp. and Biomed. Res., 5, 180-189, 1972.

Henrichon jr, E.G., Fu, K-S.: A nonparametric partitioning procedure for pattern classification, IEEE Trans. on Comp., C-18, 614-624, 1969.

Michalski, R.S., Mozetic, Hong and Lavrac: The multi-purpose incremental learning system AQ15 and its testing application to three medical domains. Proc. 5th AAAI-86, 1041-1045, 1986.

Quinlan, J.R.: Induction of Decision Trees, Machine Learning, Vol. 1, Nr 1, Kluwer Academic Publishers, pp 81-106, Boston, 1986.

Rendell, L., Benedict, P., Cho, H., Seshu, R.: Improving the design of rule-learning systems. Report no. UIUCDCS-R-87-1395, Dept. of Comp. Science, University of Illinois at Urbana-Champaign, Urbana, Ill, USA, 1987.

Talmon, J.L.: Pattern recognition of the ECG: A structured analysis. Thesis, Free University, Amsterdam, 1983.

Talmon, J.L.: A multiclass non-parametric partitioning algorithm, Pattern Recognition Letters, 4, pp 31-38, 1986.

Talmon, J.L., Schijven, R.A.J., Kitslaar, P.J.E.H.M., Penders, R.: An expert system for diagnosis and therapy planning in patients with peripheral vascular disease. In: Systemes Experts en Medicine, Dr. H. Joly (ed), EC2, 1988, pp 199-209.

Tools for Modeling Time-oriented Concepts

Applications for Retrieval of Liver Transplantation Data

Günter Tusch

Clinic for Abdominal and Transplantation Surgery and Institute for Medical Informatics Medical School Hannover, D-3000 Hannover, FRG

Abstract

Physicians and surgeons are able to interpret intensive care patients' data on a very sophisticated level. Patient data only reflect pathophysiological states, so that there is a gap between recorded data and clinical concepts evolved from this data. To support knowledge acquisition based on these time oriented data tools are described to be used for clinical research in the setting of liver transplantation. One tool incorporates a time model derived from Allen, 1984. Interactive definition and refinements of concepts can immediately be tested on the data. The first evaluation results are very encouraging. Some aspects of problem specific evaluation are discussed in this article using an example of a rejection concept.

Introduction

During the postoperative course of liver transplanted patients many different disorders of the transplanted organ can be observed. The most important ones are rejection, infections, toxic disorders of the liver caused by immunosuppression, obstruction of the bile ducts, or problems with the arterial supply. Also a coincidence of several disorders can occur in rare cases. Therefore the doctor has to cope for a multitude of clinical parameters and the high variability of the clinical course.
Furthermore, in the relatively young field of liver transplantation only a part of the phenomena can be explained by pathophysiological models.
The clinician often makes his decisions on the basis of constellations of symptoms and signs showing him similarities to previous courses as far as he memorizes them.

A computer support is indicated, because the variety and the many combinations of significant parameters make it error prone for the individual physician to remember important features of past cases. The most important aspect of decision support by computer in the transplantation setting is modeling time, especially time courses (see also *Tusch et al, 1989b*). I will describe in the sequel some common approaches for modeling time fitting into this environment, and after that will explain two tools being developed at the Medical School in Hannover for tackling with the problem. I will put a special emphasis on the aspect of evaluation from a problem oriented point of view. The general aspects will be provided by other articles in this volume. Although these methods are developed for problems in liver transplantation evaluation, they also may apply to other intensive care settings.

The LTX Documentation System

Since 1986 all courses of liver transplanted patients from the transplantation clinic of the Medical School in Hannover are documented in a prospective registry (*Tusch et al, 1988*). Daily acquired diagnostically important time dependent parameters, organ function scores, histological findings, and other aspects of liver transplantation are filed in this registry.
The data are stored in a data base that is part of an "departmental information system" (*Tusch et al, 1988*).

This documentation system serves two main aims: In the first place, it is a basis for clinical research and statistical investigations and also for retrospective judgment of patients' courses and classification of disorders by experienced clinicians (In lack of a sufficient gold standard the clinical judgments are used instead). In the second place, the system is planned to provide a computerized archive of patient courses to be used for comparison with actual cases. This may serve for clinical decision support in cases of doubt by comparing outcomes of "similar" historical cases *Tusch et al, 1988*. *Tusch et al, 1987*, mention that this way of decision making exhibits aspects similar to the procedure of the exploratory data analysis.

To approach the two aims I will discuss tools being developed to support both the generation as well as the application of clinical concepts on actual data. The process of concept generation may be used as part of the knowledge acquisition process for expert systems. Finally, this may result in a knowledge-based systems that "know" concepts of "similarity" in patient courses, and can be used for patient matching (*Tusch et al, 1987*) or case retrieval (*Bernauer et al, 1988*).

A Model for the Acquisition of Clinical Knowledge

To give a deeper insight into the problem and show what kind of tool may be needed, I will discuss in detail a modification of the model of the knowledge acquisition process given in *Tusch et al, 1987*. This model also will partly serve as a basis for the considerations of tool evaluation in a subsequent chapter. The model assumes a four step process:

- Selection of the problem domain (e.g. rejection episodes).

- Identification of episodes reflecting the problem. The underlying concept is that there exists a similarity between cases exhibiting the same problem and that they can be discriminated from all other cases. This similarity is intuitive, based on clinical experience, clinical concepts, and statistical perception. The concept's definition will become more concrete in a sequence of refinement steps. In doing so, the raw data, as a measurable reflection or subjective scaling of not directly observable pathophysiological processes, are interpreted in the clinical context. In a mathematical sense this might best be conceived as transformations.
- Exploratory data analysis on the basis of suitable mathematical transformations modeling the medical correlations, and afterwards searching for statistical correlations against a suitable gold standard.
- Development of a score or a stochastic model for the chosen cohort, and evaluation of this score or model in a prospective clinical trial for later use in clinical decision making.

Obviously a clinical decision making procedure is very similar to what is described in step 1 to step 3 (see also *Tusch et al, 1987*), however step 3 not completed. Decision making usually relies on models, judgments, and transformations appearing to be plausible by clinical experience and research. Obviously noise and measurement errors of the output signal do not cause serious trouble to the experienced surgeon. He is only interested in the shape or form of a curve and quantities and dimensions of the parameter values. The doctor will ignore measurement errors producing implausible results.

The tools I will describe are suited to support the clinician with this process, especially step 2. Reformulating the purpose of the tools in the light of this chapter I will conclude: The task is to find abstractions from the raw data that allow a description of shapes and forms of the curves as they are used typically by the physicians for conceptualization, and furthermore to develop a calculus that allows modeling of time relations on top. This approach aims at step 2 of the above model, while systems hitherto developed as RX (*Blum ,1982*) or the successor RADIX (*Walker and Blum, 1986*) support step 3 (exploratory data analysis).

Artificial Intelligence Approaches

Disorders in the peri-operative phase of liver transplantation develop within a few days and are to be treated immediately. The treatment modifies the clinical pattern of sign and symptoms. Therefore time series analysis and most of the usually applied filtering methods are not suitable. Only initial non-function of the donor organ could be successfully dealt with by discriminant analysis (see *Tusch et al, 1989a*). The problem is to appropriately localize the start of the disorder in the clinical course to find a reference point.

Despite of these problems a doctor finds meaningful interpretations in his cognitive process. This fact suggests the application of methods of artificial intelligence, because they are supposed to allow for a direct "translation" of cognitive processes into a computer representation. There are two developments for time oriented concepts, I will call them in the sequel "event oriented" and "interval based" approaches. Regarding the event oriented approach, calculations are performed for each possible time point separately, whereas using the interval based approach that can be traced back to work of *Allen, 1984* calculations are performed for a complete interval. *Berzuini, 1989* gives an overview of the interval based approach, therefore I will assume acquaintance with this topic.

Advantages of the event oriented approach are twofold: they are not so complex and expensive from a programmers point of view, and they can be embedded very easily in rule-based systems as realizations in VM (*Fagan et al, 1984*), RX (*Blum, 1982*) or ONCOCIN (*Kahn et al 1986*) have shown. An extension of ONCOCIN (only of prototypical character) recognizes distortions of oncological protocol schemata by an augmented transition network (ATN). In RX intervals are constructed from the single parameters of the patients' visits including missing values to gain interpretable units. Temporal functions and predicates are developed to retrieve a set of time points corresponding to intervals being processed in the knowledge base in an iterative manner. (Because of this point wise processing I will classify RX as event oriented).

An Event Oriented Prototype

In the above mentioned knowledge-based temporal classification applications a result is achieved by forward-chaining or by techniques starting from temporal facts. The tools investigated here are used to locate all intervals that match to a given pattern in terms of a "data base query" (patient matching, *Tusch et al, 1987*). A "query" of this kind represents relations of clinical concepts derived from raw data. Definitions of clinical concepts exhibit a quite formal structure as in the formulation: "Rejection of clinical type I is characterized by 'a predominant increase in transaminases' (*Gubernatis et al, 1988*) and absence of fever". Therefore also techniques for natural language data base query (as developed e.g. from *Allen, 1984*) might be suited.

Because of the advantages listed in the previous chapter, an event oriented approach was implemented (*Tusch et al, 1987*). The prototype was based on a two layer model: one layer of basic elements and one of clinical concepts.

Basic elements of a description language were represented by mathematical transformation procedures. On top of this basic layer the physician could formulate his clinical concepts. The different transformation procedures of the basic layer covered for the settlement of the raw data and a preprocessing according to the clinical context. For example, body temperatur is meaningless, when the blood of the patient is ultrafiltrated to withdraw water and at the same time cool fluid is substituted. Categorizations of variables as "bilirubin" ("normal", "increased", ...) could depend on the clinical status of the patient (e.g. "ventilated"), as it was implemented in VM (*Fagan et al, 1984*). From parameter values of previous or following days a trend could be calculated what was also categorized. The trend calculation was individually adjustable according to the clinical meaning of the parameter. This applied also to groups of parameters with a similar clinical meaning (e.g. transaminases).

Clinical concepts (the second layer) were formulated in frames. A slot in a frame could be linked to a transformation procedure or directly to the data base. The frame represented the structure of the clinical concept, whereas the value lists in the slots represented the typical instances of a concept. Each instantiation of a concept frame represented one day of a patient's stay for that the concept applied.

This prototype exhibited a series of disadvantages: Because only local temporal coherence was considered, therefore the procedure was susceptible to missing values in the data. For every time point the concepts were evaluated separately, for that reason it was difficult or even impossible to formulate complex temporal relations understandable to a clinician (e.g. "increase of bilirubin before increase of transaminases"). It also proved to be hard to reconstruct coherent phases from the resulting time points, when missing data caused gaps.

An Interval Based Tool

Interval based time logics have been developed by McDermott, 1982, and in main part by *Allen, 1984*. The basics of this approach are described by *Berzuini, 1989*. An overview in concern of our context also is provided by *Tusch at al, 1989a, 1989b*. Allen's approach is meant for applications in natural language processing, especially natural language data base queries, similar to the problem considered here.

Because most of the parameters in our application domain are acquired only once a day, the unit for measuring intervals is one day. It is reasonable to assume an equally distant basic scale for the time model, as one day for example (*Rading, 1988*) and not, as Allen uses, a continuous scale as a basis for measuring the intervals. Then closed intervals can be used avoiding the problem of representing point intervals (*Allen, 1984*), since the smallest interval has the length of the basic unit (in our case but not necessarily 1 day). Allen proposes thirteen possible *relationships of two intervals. Most of them can be considered as a refinement of the relationship "during". This differentiation may be useful in technical applications, however, in the medical field with its imprecision of models and data and as well the fixed basic scale in the first place the relationships "before", "after", "during", "overlaps", and their inverses should be considered. "During" and "overlaps" cover for "equal", "meets", "starts" or "finishes" (see *Allen, 1984*). Allen uses these relationships to define restrictions on intervals entered in the knowledge base propagated to the net of already established relationships. Now the "inconsistent labeling problem" may arise (*Allen, 1984*). In the transplant application area concepts are defined modular in a strict hierarchical manner. By allowing only convex time relations and hierarchical ordering using causal abstraction hierarchies the problem can be avoided (*Kohane, 1986*).

Each clinical concept is represented by a set of "occurrence intervals" in the data base, but two identical sets of occurrence intervals not necessarily represent the same clinical concept (*Rading, 1988, Tusch et al, 1989b*).

The user of the tool who wants to model his cognitive concepts and have them represented by intervals in the data base has two basic aims:

- To describe patterns as convex unions of occurrence intervals of basic clinical concepts (I will term this according to Allen's terminology "events")
- To specify clinical concepts dependent on a specific context (I will term these "concepts" in there strict sense).

Events adequately will be represented by the interval stemming from the unions of the constituent intervals. The event "Increase of transaminases" defined by "Increase of GOT" (see figure 1) or "Increase of GPT" is sufficiently represented by the union

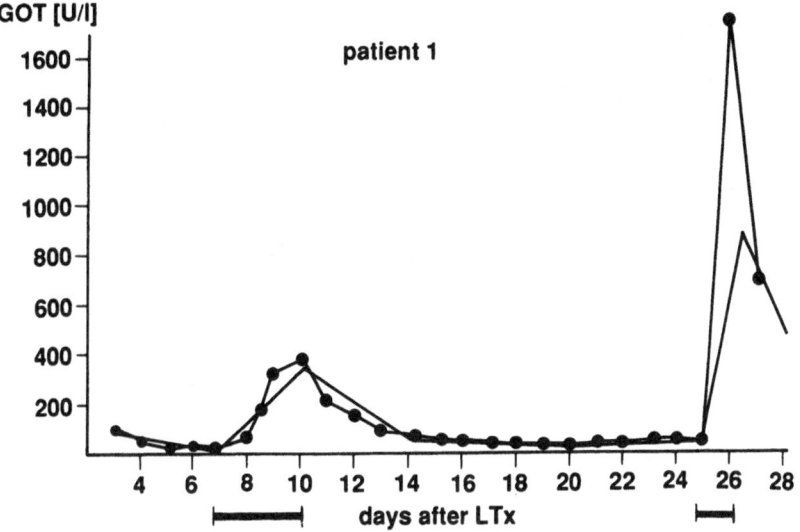

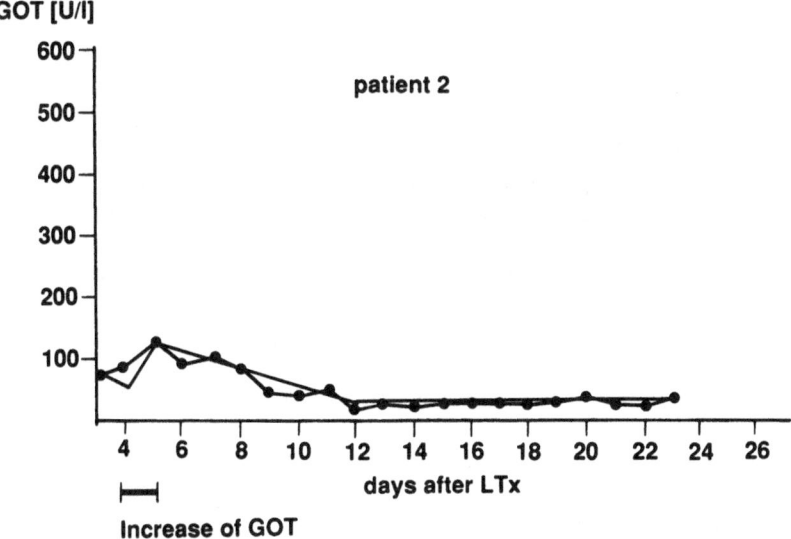

Figure 1: Example of a clinical concept and occurrences

of occurrence intervals of both events. A concepts like "Type-II rejection" characterized by a clinician as "a predominant increase in bilirubin and temperature" (*Gubernatis et al, 1988*) may adequately be modeled by the phase of bilirubin increase predominant over transaminases. This is represented by using a context-free language (*Rading, 1988*) on the basis of transformations as described in the last chapter.

There are two occurrences of "Increase of GOT" with patient 1 and only one with patient 2.

However, instead of point wise descriptions transformations and basic events are now based on intervals. "Events" are constructed from transformations and relationships of transformations, as an example see the event "Bili_Increase" in figure 2. A "concept" using this event may be the concept "High_Bili_Increase" in figure 3 (COMB and EXCL denote that events or concepts occur at the same time or exclude each other).

EVENT: Bili_Increase
        INCREASE(BILIRUBIN)"CONSTANT"

Transcript:
All occurrences of patient episodes with the occurrence interval representing increase of bilirubin.

Figure 2: Event "Bilirubin_Increase".

The Current State of Implementation

Syntactic issues of the language

For a better understanding of the current capacity of the tool here a brief look at the most important syntactic features of the language at its present state of implementation. Basic elements of the language are names of transformations as INTERPOL for a special type of interpolation of parameter curves, or interval mappings like INCREASE, DECREASE or LEVEL resulting in intervals limiting the phase of increase, decrease or a specific level of a clinical parameter.

In general, events have the following form (Backus-Naur-notation):

< event > :: [< transformation >] < clin. parameter > < relation >
          [< transformation >] (< Clin. parameter > ! < constant >)
< event > :: < interv. mapping > [< transformation >]
          < clin. parameter > < realtion > < value >

'Relations' are the usual ones $< =$, $<$, $=$, $>$, $> =$, 'values' may be "CONSTANT", "HIGH", etc. dependent on the mapping's definition. An example for the first event type can be found in figure 2 (the transformation INTERPOL is implicitly stated as standard transformation), an example for the second type in the concept 'Type-II_rejection' in figure 3. Combinations of both types of events by "AND" and "OR" are also events.

```
CONCEPT: Type-II_rejection
COMB Bili_Fever
    OVERLAPS
    (INCREASE(GOT)"CONSTANT" OR
    INCREASE(GPT)"CONSTANT")
COMB (4 , 21)
OCC_INTERVAL:
    BEGIN(Bili_Fever), END(Bili_Fever)

CONCEPT: Bili_Fever
    MAXTEMP37.5
    DURING
    High_Bili_Increase
OCC_INTERVAL:
    BEGIN(High_Bili_Increase), END(Bili_Increase)

CONCEPT: High_Bili_Increase
    (BILIRUBIN100 AND Bili_Increase)
    DURING
    Bili_Increase
OCC_INTERVAL:
    BEGIN(Bili_Increase), END(Bili_Increase)


Transcript:
Retrieve all occurrences of patient episodes, where the
interval representing increase of bilirubin with at least part-
ly fever episodes overlaps an interval representing an in-
crease of transaminases (GOT or GPT) within day 4 and 21
after liver transplantation.
This concept is characterized by the interval including the
whole course of increase of bilirubin.
The concept Bili_Increase represents the occurrences with
at least a small part greater than 100 umol/l.
```

Figure 3:   Concept "Clinical type-II rejection"

For concepts it is possible additionally to specify a minimum and maximum duration in days every component event. Allen's relationships as listed in the previous chapter only apply to concepts. COMB refers to concurrent, and EXCL to mutually excluding concepts. The result interval unique to concepts is usually described by the beginning and the end of events being components of the concept. For further details see *Bernauer et al, 1988, Rading, 1988.*

The user interface

The user interface consists of one part for graphical and one for text display. The most important features of the textual part include interactive modification of the parameters in the transformation and interval mapping functions to adjust, e.g. for half-life time of parameters or categorization of levels. Furthermore, interactive definition of events and concepts, as well of the display of parameter values is implemented.

The graphical part of the interface basically consists of a display of the clinical parameters from the database on the user's demand (y-axis = units of the parameter, x-axis = days of patient's course). Scale and datum line are interactively modified. Data of one or several patients (e.g. exhibiting one concept) will be displayed on the user's convenience. "Continuous" parameters, like enzymes, are figured by line graphs, discrete events, like medications, by arrows. Furthermore, occurrence and result intervals of all events and concepts may be shown immediately after modification, patient specific and as well for a group of patients.

Finally functions for database or knowledge base management are available. Figure 4 gives an overview over the complete system.

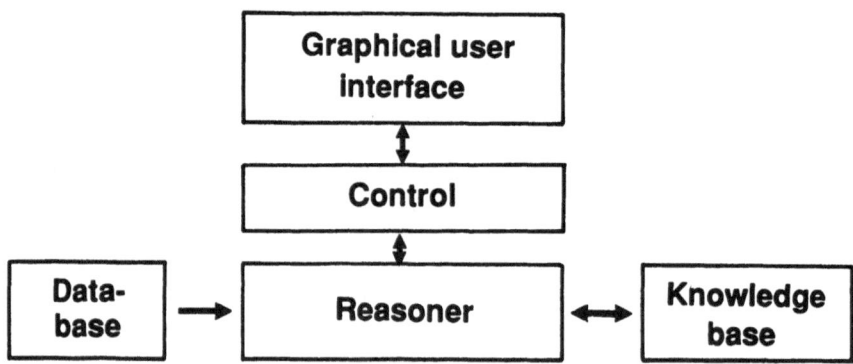

Figure 4:   Overview over the system (from **Tusch et al, 1989**)

Some Aspects of Evaluation

In principle, the use of every tool based on statistical or AI methods assumes the data contain the most important aspects of the problem to be solved. If for some cases this is not true, the additional information has to be specified or the cases are to be excluded from the analysis in the worst case. Furthermore, the information usable for modeling depends on the purpose: for decision support only the information can be used what is supposed to be available at the time of decision, for classification of historic cases the complete information (e.g. also on treatment or treatment effects) can be put to use.

Evaluation of knowledge-based systems is the topic of several papers in this volume. For that reason I will add only very specific aspects dealing especially with the problem of tool evaluation in this setting.
I will discuss three items here:

- Is the language sufficient for a formulation of the clinical concept?
- Does the translated formulation exhibit reasonable classification results?
- Is the (final) formulation (after some refinement steps) understandable to the expert and may be used by an explanation facility?

For a complete evaluation of the first question on sufficiency of the language all possible concepts in this environment should be investigated. This is impossible, so I will propose the 'tracer method', developed by *Kessner and Kalk, 1973*, and used for quality assurance problems. In this context it means using concepts that are "typical" for the field, occurring in a sufficient frequency, and known as a standard disorder. The language then hopefully copes for other clinical concepts related to liver transplantation.
A suitable tracer for liver transplantation fulfilling these requirements is early acute rejection. According to *Gubernatis et al, 1988*, two types of rejection can be distinguished, and type-II rejection is more frequent. Therefore type-II rejection may serve as a good tracer.

Proceeding according to the model in chapter 3 and especially to step 2 ("formulate-and-refine"), a concept of type-II rejection as shown in figure 3 (*Tusch at al, 1989a*) was formulated. Of course, the process is circular and the refinement could proceed. However, I think as a preliminary result it shows the power of the language and the adequacy of the formulation.
Answering the second question on classification, it is not only sufficient to apply the conventional measures as sensitivity and specificity as shown for the example in table 1. Furthermore a comparison to conventional statistical techniques must be included (see *Tusch et al, 1989a*) and an investigation of the stability of the procedure according to variations in input.

Considering both tools including the first prototype in chapter 5 the last question involves a trade-off. While the event oriented approach is not so expensive from a programmers point of view it allows only for complex clinical concepts to be modeled in a programming language style or even not to be model at all.Therefore the interval

Group	Type-II correct	Type-I as not Type-II	No rejection as not Type-II	Overall accuracy
Learning	14/14	6/7	14/16	34/37
%	100	86	88	92
Test	5/5	2/2	5/8	12/15
%	100	100	63	80

Table 1: Results of the evaluation (from **Tusch et al, 1989a**)

based method is more transparent to the expert and to the end-user as well.The structure of the interval concepts supports a generation of explanations.

Discussion

Patient matching and partly exploratory data analysis are techniques forcing a modification of classical AI methods and time oriented data. For reasons of transparency of the procedure and easy formulation of concepts an interval based procedure exhibits more advantages than an event oriented one.Because the refinement of concepts is an essential part of this process, the implementation described here uses a context-free grammar to provide a language for the formulation. ATN's as in *Kahn et al, 1986*, may be used for recognizing fixed concepts. Another feature to be used in complex time relationships is the explicit denotation of the intervals representing the whole concept.This often is not implicitly defined by the union or intersection of the constituent intervals.

The model also can be utilized for supporting decision analysis (see *Berzuini, 1989*) as shown in *Tusch et al, 1989b*.

Acknowledgements

This work was supported by the Deutsche Forschungsgemeinschaft.
I am indebted to my collegues in the LTX project Dr. Jochen Bernauer, Dr. Gundolf Gubernatis and Michael Rading for many valuable discussions.I also would like to thank the late Prof.Dr. P.L.Reichertz, Prof.Dr. R.Pichlmayr, and Prof.Dr. B.Schneider (Medical School) and Prof.Dr. D.Müller (University) in Hannover.

References

Allen, J.F.: Towards a General Theory of Action and Time Artificial Intelligence 23 (1984) 123-154.

Bernauer, J., Rading, M., Tusch, G., Reichertz, P.L., Gubernatis, G., Pichlmayr, R.: Case Description and Case Retrieval on Time Oriented Patient Data.In: Rienhoff, O., Piccolo, U., Schneider, B. (Eds.): Expert Systems and Decision Support in Medicine.Proceedings. Lecture Notes in Medical Informatics 36.(Springer, Berlin, Heidelberg, New York: 1988) 308-313.

Berzuini, C., Quaglini, S., Bellazzi, R.: Belief Network Representations of Temporal Knowledge for Medical Expert Systems. This volume, 49-67, 1990.

Blum, R.L.: Discovery and Representation of Causal Relationships from a Large Time-Oriented Clinical Database: The RX-Project. Lecture Notes in Medical Informatics 19.(Springer, Berlin, Heidelberg, New York: 1982)

Fagan, L.M., Kunz, J.C., Feigenbaum, E.A., Osborn, J.J.: Extensions to the Rule-Based Formalism for a Monitoring Task. In: Buchanan, B.G., Shortliffe, E.H. (Eds.): Rule-Based Expert Systems: The MYCIN Experiments of the Stanford Heuristic Programming Project. (Addison-Wesley, Reading: 1984) 397-423.

Gubernatis, G., Kemnitz, J., Tusch, G., Pichlmayr, R.: HLA Compatility and Different Features of Liver Allograft Rejection. Transplant Int. 1 (1988) 155-160.

Kahn, M.G., Fagan, L.M., Shortliffe, E.H.: Context-Specific Interpretation of Patients Records for a Therapy Advice System. In: Salamon, R., Blum, B., Jorgensen, M. (Eds): Medinfo 86. Proceedings of the Fifth Conference on Medical Informatics, Washington, October 26-30, 1986. (North-Holland Publ. Co., Amsterdam) 175-179.

Kessner, D.M., Kalk, C.: A Strategy for Evaluating Heath Services. Vol. 2, Washington, National Academy of Science, Institute of Medicine, 1973.

Kohane, I.S.: Temporal Reasoning in Medical Expert Systems. In: Salamon, R., Blum, B., Jorgensen, M. (Eds): Medinfo 86. Proceedings of the Fifth Conference on Medical Informatics, Washington, October 26-30, 1986. (North-Holland Publ. Co., Amsterdam) 170-174.

McDermott, D.: A Temporal Logic for Reasoning about Processes and Plans. Cognitive Science 6 (1982) 101-155.

Rading, M.: Ein operationales Modell zum Beschreiben und Erkennen von komplexen Ereignissen in zeitabhängigen Beobachtungen - entwickelt am Beispiel einer klinischen Verlaufsdokumentation. Diplomarbeit. (Fachbereich Mathematik der Universität Hannover: 1988).

Tusch, G., Bernauer, J., Reichertz, P.L.: Matching Patients: An Approach to Decision Support in Liver Transplantation. In: Fox, J., Fieschi, M., Engelbrecht, R. (Eds.): AIME 87 European Conference on Artificial Intelligence in Medicine. Proceedings. Lecture Notes in Medical Informatics 33. (Springer, Berlin, Heidelberg, New York: 1987) 25-33.

Tusch, G., Bernauer, J., Gubernatis, G., Lautz, H.-U., Farle, M., Reichertz, P.L., Pichlmayr, R.: Ein Departementelles Informationssystem zur Unterstützung der Lebertransplantation. In: Rienhoff, O., Piccolo, U., Schneider, B. (Eds.): Expert Systems and Decision Support in Medicine. Proceedings. Lecture Notes in Medical Informatics 36. (Springer, Berlin, Heidelberg, New York: 1988) 509-515.

Tusch, G., Bernauer, J., Gubernatis, G., Rading, M.: Knowledge Acquisition Using Syntactic Time Patterns. To appear: AIME 89 European Conference on Artificial Intelligence in Medicine. Proceedings. Lecture Notes in Medical Informatics. (Springer, Berlin-Heidelberg-New York: 1989a).

Tusch, G., Bernauer, J., Gubernatis, G., Rading, M.: A Knowledge-Based Decision Support Tool for Liver Transplanted Patients. To appear: In: Barber, B., Dexian, C., Wagner, G. (Eds): Medinfo 89. Proceedings of the Sixth World Conference on Medical Informatics, Beijing, October 16-20, 1989b. (North-Holland Publ. Co., Amsterdam).

Walker, M.G., Blum, R.L.: Towards Automated Discovery from Clinical Databases: The RADIX Project. In: Salamon, R., Blum, B., Jorgensen, M. (Eds): Medinfo 86. Proceedings of the Fifth Conference on Medical Informatics, Washington, October 26-30, 1986. (North-Holland Publ. Co., Amsterdam: 1986) 32-36.

Questions from the discussion:

Grant: How often did you need to refine the hypotheses of the experts during the definition of the events and concepts?

Tusch: Refinement steps were necessary for the discrimination of similar constellations, or in other terms, to increase specificity. In the rejection case there were two disorders with a similar pattern, so that two refinement steps were needed.

Wyatt: Can you accomodate situations where you have processes that run on different time scales like, for example processes that change quickly, say in seconds or minutes, and processes that change slowly, say in hours or days?

Tusch: The time scale is defined by the parameters of the transformation function or the interval mapping dependent on the underlying clinical parameter. Therefore, clinical parameters with different half-life time show different parameters of the same transformation function, e.g. interpolation. Of course, there is a limit in our application domain of one day as the smallest unit.

McNair: In your evaluation, about 15% of the cases were wrongly classified. Do you have a means to express how close a case is to a certain concept or event?

Tusch: No, we have not yet implemented a distance measure of that kind. We are still developing a distance model for that problem.

Belief Network Representations of Temporal Knowledge for Medical Expert Systems[1]

Carlo Berzuini, Silvana Quaglini, Riccardo Bellazzi

Dipartimento di Informatica e Sistemistica. Universita' di Pavia, Pavia, Italy.

Abstract

Bayesian belief networks can be effectively used to represent stochastic models of temporal processes for inclusion within expert system knowledge bases. Semi-markov models of progression provide a reasonably general framework in which many pieces of temporal knowledge, particularly in medicine, can be cast. A belief net can graphically depict basic conditional independence assumptions underlying a stochastic model, which facilitates confronting the model with available domain knowledge. Probabilistic distributional information characterizing the model is stored distributedly in the various frames of data associated with each node of the net. In this way the belief network becomes a powerful reasoning machine, capable of performing temporal reasoning both forwards and backwards in time, coherently with a probabilistic model of progression. Inferencing is accomplished by propagating probabilities on the network. A propagation algorithm using a sampling scheme is proposed, which overcomes some of the shortcomings of previously known algorithms. Simple examples from the clinical application field are used throughout. The style of exposition is informal.

Introduction

Most medical decisions involve concepts of *temporal evolution*. For example, a causal diagnostic explanation must account for the temporal latency of observed manifestations given the hypothesized aethiological factor. The choice of a medical treatment strongly hinges on notions such as the patient's past clinical course, current medical status and predicted future course. Patient's monitoring involves analyzing the timing of changes in the patient's manifestations.

---

1   This work was facilitated by support from MPI-40% and MPI-60% grants, and from C.N.R. grant no. 87.01829

Yet most current medical expert systems either neglect temporal considerations, or avoid dealing with them systematically. MYCIN-like systems 'squash' the temporal dimension into statements of the type 'symptom X evokes disease A', neglecting the *timing* of the symptom with respect to crucial events in the patient's history. Yet a clinician might judge the disease hypothesis irrelevant at a glance just because the observed timing is inconsistent with it.

Early practical solutions to this problem involved associating temporal qualifiers, such as PAST, RECENT-PAST, NOW, etc. to individual items of the symptoms' chronology. Such qualifiers can be straightforwardly embedded in a standard rule-based formalism, and enable the system to significantly reduce the search space by taking into account observed temporal patterns. This *ad hoc* solution, however, has limitations. *Quantitative* temporal information cannot be reasoned about. Moreover, the number of conceivable data patterns may increase dramatically, making it un-manageable with a standard rule formalism.

This motivated interest into new proposed approaches, such as interval-based (*Allen, 1983*) or point-based (*Vilain, 1986*) time logics. *Kohane, 1987* has proposed an interesting temporal knowledge representation, which includes both qualitative and quantitative relations between any arbitrary combination of time-points or time-intervals; consistency checking and temporal reasoning are performed using a form of constraints propagation.

Practical solutions have been developed for specific clinical contexts. VM (*Fagan 1984*) adopts a rule-based approach to monitor an intensive care unit: it provides predicates to query for time intervals from manifestations in the data base. ONIX (*Kahn 1986*) detects unusual time-dependent patterns in cancer chemotherapy cycles by a combined rule-based and Augmented Transition Network approach. *Tusch, 1989* proposes a time model derived from Allen's, and describes a temporal reasoning tool which allows interactive definition and refinement of concepts such as *'the interval representing increase of bilirubin overlaps an interval representing an increase of transaminases within day 4 and 14 after liver transplantation'*, and their application to a patient's data base.

All the above mentioned approaches have a serious limitation: they cannot encode *uncertainty*. In particular they do not allow an expert system to make use of prob-ability estimates about the likelihood of possible temporal evolutions. The reason why they cannot cope with uncertainty is that probabilities hardly combine in the same way as deterministic constraints do.

Yet, there is demand for *coherent probabilistic representations* of temporal know-ledge. Since these have often been criticized with regard to computational complex-ity and difficulty of obtaining the necessary probability assessments, at first glance one might perceive the idea of introducing probability as an over-complication of an intrinsically complex area, such as temporal reasoning is.

But is probability really *unnecessary* in this context ? We shall firstly point out that without it we lack a means to deal rigorously with exceptional or rare behaviours, and that neglecting uncertainty often means unacceptable weak rankings of hypo-theses. Second: when high risks or benefits are at stake, such as in medical therapy planning, the unlimited theoretical quality of inferences obtained by an axiomatic system such as probability theory can hardly be overlooked.

Are probability estimates really a *difficulty?* A large portion of medical knowledge concerning prediction of therapy outcomes and prognosis is spread over literature in the form of probability estimates, so a system that accepts these as a basis for inference should be welcomed in these classes of applications. And, most important, probability estimates provide a natural means for the system to connect with existing data bases and to improve with experience.

Finally, probabilistic methods come with a refined 'machinery' for learning from hard data. This feature is crucial in a large class of *therapy control* applications. Consider a piece of probabilistic temporal knowledge describing the expected clinical course of a hypothetical *average* patient under a given treatment regimen. As the patient is followed over time, data will gradually become available for assessing his/her *specific* response characteristics and deviations from the usual patterns. Understanding of these specific characteristics may lead to override the typical action schedule. In fact, subsequent actions must be driven by a coherent combination of what we learned about the specific patient and the general pre-existing medical knowledge. A probabilistic approach can be hardly discarded when needing the above combination of retrospective learning/ prospective inference.

Clearly, future research work is needed to evaluate the advantages outlined above in relation to well-characterized classes of temporal reasoning applications in medicine. This work should enhance our capability of addressing the right representation technique for any given application problem.

The above discussion might suggest that probabilistic knowledge representations hardly convey *qualitative* information and ultimately reduce to a collection of *numerical* estimates. Actually, we believe the opposite. A probabilistic representation must in first place convey *conceptual* (qualitative) information, far more meaningful than the numerical estimates of the probabilities involved. A qualitative relationships fundamental in knowledge representation is that of 'direct dependency'. This relationship involves statements of the kind 'X is independent of Y, given Z'. For example, specifying that the hazard of myocardial infarction is not independent of patient's age, given the time of the previous one, is more important than the involved numerical value.

Dependency information is best represented in the form of a *diagram. Bayesian belief networks* (BN's), an increasingly popular probabilistic knowledge representation, capture both the qualitative dependencies among domain concepts, and serve as a framework for specifying necessary probability estimates. They are directed graphs whose nodes represent concepts and uncertain quantities, and whose links represent direct dependencies between such concepts or quantities.

The power of BN's has two main aspects. First, thanks to their graphical nature, BN's have proven an effective tool for communicating knowledge among domain experts and users. Second, besides their descriptive role, they have an operational role: network propagation techniques serve as mechanism for performing 'reasoning' out of BN's.

Now we come to *computational* difficulties. Several propagation algorithms have been developed. Unfortunately, each of them seems to prove intractable for some practical problems. For example, there are a variety of exact algorithms for general networks, using clique join trees (*Lauritzen 1988*), conditioning (*Pearl 1986*) or arc reversal (*Shachter 1986*). All of these algorithms are exponentially sensitive to the connectedness of the network, and even the first, which appears by average to be the fastest, quickly grows intractable for medium size practical problems. This is not surprising, since the general problem is NP-hard (*Cooper 1987*). Moreover, until now exact algorithms deal with continuous variables with great difficulty, which severely hampers attempts of dealing with continuous time.

The above considerations have motivated our interest into a class of approximate methods for probability propagation, namely *Monte Carlo simulation algorithms*, hereafter called *sampling* algorithms (*Geman 1984, Henrion 1988, Pearl 1987, Chavez 1989*). They promise polynomial growth in the size of the problem. Basically, two sampling approaches have been proposed: *forward* sampling and *Markov* sampling, described in the paper. Both of them suffer from drawbacks depending on the particular problem, either in terms of computing time or of convergence rate.

This paper proposes a combination of the two schemes, called *Markov sampling with restarting* (MSR). This technique is suitable for a reasonably broad range of problem structures, including problems with multiple connectedness, extreme probabilities and quasi-deterministic relationships. Moreover, and specific to the application context of interest here, our proposed scheme allows straightforward inclusion of continuous variables representing time.

A simple clinical example, which has only illustrative purposes, will be used to unify the topics in this paper, namely to show the MSR algorithm in action on a belief network representing a piece of temporal knowledge.

Bayesian Belief Networks: A Definition

A Bayesian belief network (BN) is a *directed acyclic graph,* i.e. a structure consisting of nodes and directed arcs connecting pairs of nodes. Such a structure may be used to represent, for example, a physical system, or a patient, or a decision problem, or a statistical model. The nodes correspond one-to-one with a list of uncertain quantities of the system, or patient, or problem domain, while the edges signify the existence of direct causal influences between the linked quantities or class-property relationships.

The strength of the represented influences is expressed by conditional probability tables attached to the nodes of the BN. More precisely, for each node of the BN one has to specify the conditional probability distribution of the hosted variable given all possible configurations of values of its direct parents. For nodes with no 'parents' a prior distribution has to be specified.

An important property of BN's is that their topology captures the probabilistic notion of **conditional independence** (c.i.) between variables, i.e. the probabilistic relation 'X is independent of Y, given Z'. This means that, once Z is known, then knowing Y (resp. X) adds no useful information concerning the value of X (resp. Y). C.i. relations among variables of a BN can be derived via graphical criteria, for example the topological notion of *d-separation* introduced by *Pearl, 1986*). A **Markov blanket** of a random variable $X \in C$, where C is the set of variables in a BN, is defined as any subset $Z \subset C$ for which X is conditionally independent of all elements of $(C-Z)$ given elements of Z. For any X, there is only one minimal Markov blanket, called *Markov boundary*. This latter is formed by the following three types of neighbours of X : the direct parents of X (P_X), the direct children of X (C_X), and all direct parents of X's direct children (S_X). Intuitively, the Markov boundary $P_X \cup C_X \cup S_X$ nullifies the influence that all other variables in the BN exert on X.

The concepts above can be illustrated with the BN of the simple example shown in figure 1. Mere inspection of the figure tells, for example, that given C, A is conditionally independent of E and D but not of B. The joint distribution of A,B,C,D,E is completely and consistently specified if one provides priors $p(A), p(B), p(D)$, and conditional probability tables $p(C|A,B)$ and $p(E|C,D)$. The Markov boundary of, say, C is formed by all remaining nodes, since $P_C = (A,B)$, $C_C = \{E\}$ and $S_C = \{D\}$, while the Markov boundary of, say, D is formed by C and E. In practice, once we 'marry the parents', i.e. we join all couples of nodes with at least one common children (in our example AB and CD), we obtain a graph

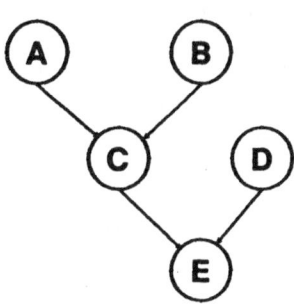

Figure 1: Simple belief network.

where each node is directly connected with all and only the nodes in its Markov boundary.

Since BN's are probabilistically precise, they can be used not only to represent generic knowledge, but statistical models, too. In fact, a BN can represent the variables involved in a model, capture the essential conditional independence structure (= which variable is relevant to which other variable) between them, and provide 'slots' for inserting the distributional specifications required by the model.

Basic Algorithms for Probability Propagation Via Sampling

In order to use BN's for 'reasoning out' inferences we must be able to propagate the impact of new evidence about some variables in the BN through the graph so that all other variables eventually will be assigned a posterior probability distribution that takes into account the available evidence. For example, with reference to figure 1, imagine that we have observed with full precision the values a and e. of variables A and E (observed nodes) respectively. Then by means of probability propagation we may want to compute, say, the marginal posterior $p(C|A = a, E = e)$. B,C,D are called *free nodes*. Propagation by sampling basically consists in counting how frequently the free variables represented in the BN take certain patterns of values in a series of simulation runs.

The length of computation of sampling algorithms is determined mainly by the degree of accuracy desired, not by the topology of the dependencies embodied in the BN, and increases only linearly with the number of nodes. They have an inherent *parallelism*: processors associated with variables may be activated concurrently provided that no two adjacent processors are activated at the same time.

The basic mechanism common to all sampling methods is the following: each free variable in the BN is viewed as a separate processor, which receives control once in each simulation cycle. Upon receiving control, the variable selects one value at random from its own conditional distribution given the current values of a predetermined set of *neighbouring variables*, and takes the sampled value. An algorithm run

consists in performing an appropriate number of cycles over the set of free variables.
A run yields a set of simulated *scenarios*, i.e. a set of complete value assignments to
the nodes of the BN. A simple way of estimating the posterior probability of a given
pattern of values on a set of free variables is as the percentage of simulated scenarios
that show that pattern. For example, after a run with m cycles, the posterior probability that, say, node Y takes value y may be estimated by k/m, where k is the number
of cycles in which Y has randomly selected the value y.
There are two well-known variants of the above sampling scheme: *forward sampling*
and *Markov sampling*.

Forward sampling

Interesting examples of 'forward' sampling, a scheme proposed by *Henrion, 1986*,
have been proposed by *Fung, 1989*, and *Shachter, 1989*. It is illustrated in figure
2(1)-(5). No initial value assignment to free nodes (B,C,D) is needed.

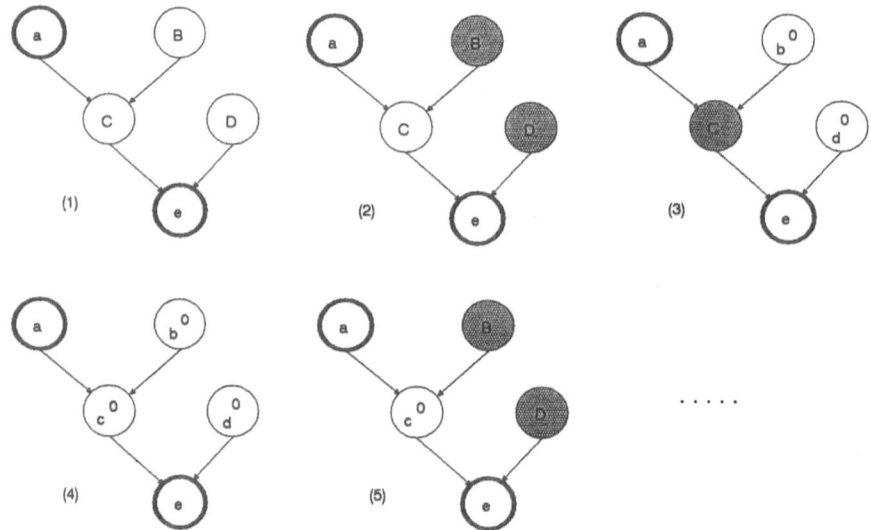

Figure 2: 'Forward' sampling on a belief network: (1) condition on variables A,E (=their values a,
e are assumed observed), (2) B samples a value b0 from p(B) and D samples a value d0
from p(D), they can do it in parallel, (3) C samples c0 from p(C| A=a, B=b0), (4) a first
scenario has been generated, (5) the second sampling cycle on variables B,C,D is started.

As described in the figure caption, a cycle consists of simulating a value for every
free node in the BN in causal order. With reference to figure 2, for example, within
each cycle node C must wait after node B for sampling. Root nodes (B, D) sample
their prior distributions. Internal nodes (C) sample from their conditional distribution given their parents. As long as nodes disregard the value of neighbours other
than their parents, they do not generally utilize the whole information available at
their respective Markov boundaries.
In figure 2, a first scenario is generated at step (4). Once generated, a scenario is
assigned a *weight*, consisting of the *likelihood* of the observed nodes given the

scenario. In the case of figure 2(4), for example, the likelihood is proportional to $p(E=e \mid c^0,d^0)$. The posterior probability of a hypothesis of interest, say $(C=c)$, can be estimated as below:

$$p(C=c \mid A=a,E=e) = (k/n)\sum_i p(A=a)p(E=e \mid c,d^i)$$

where summing is performed over the set of scenarios in which node C has selected value c, and d^i represents the value taken by D in the *i-th* scenario belonging to this set, and N is the total number of simulated scenarios.

There is a problem of efficiency: if the likelihoods turn out to be near zero, and this occurs in presence of 'rare' patterns of observation over non-root nodes, then it takes many cycles to approach the true posterior probability.

Markov sampling

Markov sampling, described by *Geman, 1984* and *Pearl, 1987*, overcomes the efficiency shortcoming suffered by forward sampling. This technique is illustrated by figure 3.

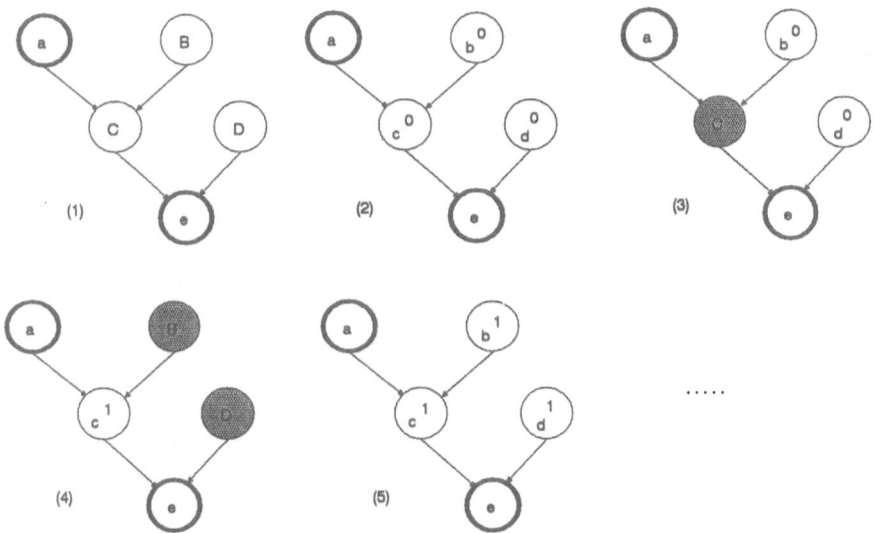

Figure 3: Markov sampling on a BN: (1) condition on variables A,E (= their values a, e are assumed known), (2) initial value assignment, (3) C samples from p(C a,b0)p(e|C,d0), (4) B and D sample from p(B)p(c1 | a,B) and p(D)p(e | c1,D), (5) first cycle terminated.

Given a BN where certain nodes have been observed (*step 1*), free nodes are first initialized to arbitrary values (*denoted by a superscript '0' at step 2*). Values of free nodes are simulated in arbitrary order and a high degree of parallelism is allowed (*steps 3,4*). Most important, each free node samples taking into account the full information on its Markov boundary.

Note, for example that at step 3 in figure 3 node C samples taking into account the current values of all the remaining nodes. More in general, the value of a generic free node Y with Markov boundary w_Y is simulated from:

$$p(y \mid w_Y) =$$

$$const\ p(y \mid P_Y)p(C_Y \mid y,R_Y)$$

Geman 1984 shows that under certain conditions (later on this) Markov sampling converges in the sense that after k cycles, for $k \to \infty$, the k-th generated scenario $(Y^k_1, Y^k_2, ... Y^k_p)$ is as if it was drawn from the 'true' joint conditional distribution, i.e. $P(Y_1, Y_2, ... Y_p \mid observed\ variables)$. In other terms, the collection of simulated scenarios tends to reflect the true distribution of the states of the network, independently of the starting scenario.

In practice, it is sensible to allow for h 'initial' cycles during which the sampling process 'warms up' and starts generating scenarios with probabilities that are reasonably independent of the initial state of the network, then further k sampling cycles are performed. Posterior probabilities are finally computed based on the last k 'post-transient' scenarios. Techniques for automatically determining the parameter h from sampling monitoring are available.

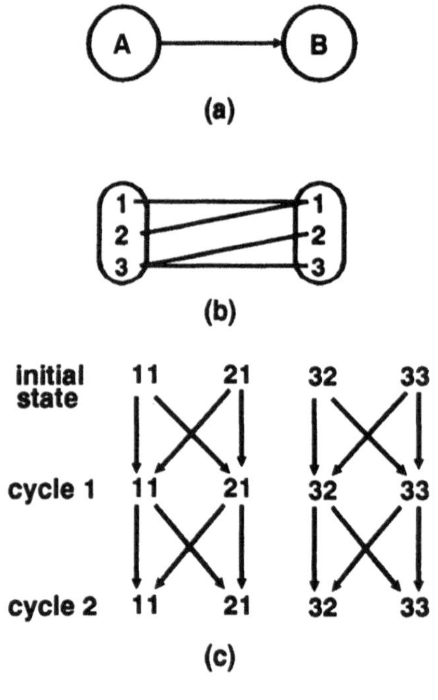

Unfortunately, even very simple BN's may not meet the condition for convergence of the Markov sampling algorithm. Consider for example the elementary two-node BN shown in figure 4(a). Figure 4(b) specifies that both nodes take three values, and each value of each node is incompatible with one or more values of the other node. For example, $(A = 1)$ is incompatible with $(B = 2)$ or $(B = 3)$, i.e. $p(B = 2\ or\ 3 \mid A = 1) = 0$. Notice that the graph in figure 4(b), formed by node values and compatibility links, is not completely connected.

This very fact suffices to destroy the convergence of the Markov sampling algorithm. The reason for this is shown in figure 4(c). The upper row represents possible initial scenarios of our two-node BN for the Markov sampling, the row just below represents possible scenarios after the first sampling cycle, and so on. The notation (ij) indicates $(A = i, B = j)$. An arrow from a scenario Q to a scenario R denotes that one cycle of the Markov sampling algorithm may lead from Q to R. The chain of scenarios generated by

Figure 4: Markov sampling does not converge on the simple two-node belief network shown in (a) because its compatibility graph, shown in (b), is not connected. (c) shows in detail why there is no convergence: whatever is the network state from which the Markov sampling starts, the sampling is constrained to a subset of the state space.

Markov sampling is indeed a Markov chain.

As figure 4(c) reveals, whatever the initial state, the sampling process on our simple net cannot generate the full set of possible scenarios, for if we start from (11) or (21) we cannot reach (32) and (33), and visa versa. Unfortunately, an essential condition for the convergence of Markov sampling is that the Markov chain of simulated scenarios be ergodic. In other terms, after a long series of sampling cycles have been performed, the chance for any particular scenario to be generated should tend to settle down to a distribution independent of the starting scenario, which does not happen on structures such as our simple net example.

It is straightforward to prove that Markov sampling would converge on the simple net in figure 4(a) *iff* the compatibility graph between nodes *A, B* (shown in figure 4(b)) were fully connected. This statement can be generalized into a theorem valid on tree-structured (= singly-connected) BN's containing only discrete variables. The theorem asserts that on such a class of BN's the Markov sampling algorithm converges *iff* there is full local connectedness (= all compatibility graphs between couples of adjacent nodes are connected).

Unfortunately, theorems on Markov sampling convergence valid on more general BN's are not available. A practical approach to this problem consists in devising more flexible sampling methods for probability propagation, which are robust to the presence of critical connectivity patterns of the type shown in the previous example, while not encountering efficiency problems typical of forward sampling.

Markov Sampling with Restarting

As an answer to this demand, we propose a combination of forward and Markov sampling, called **Markov sampling with restarting** (MSR). This method consists in periodically restarting the Markov sampling process. This means that after a certain number of Markov sampling cycles, the BN is forced onto a state independent of the current one. Such a state provides an initialization for a further batch of Markov sampling cycles, and so on. Restarting states are themselves sampled via forward sampling.

One possibility is the following: at each restart a series of forward runs is performed, and the forward-simulated state with highest likelihood is picked-up as restarting state for Markov sampling. Thanks to periodic restarting from different initial states, the overall sampling process does not get trapped in subsets of the state space (local minima). Moreover, likelihood-based selection of restarting states improves convergence, since most likely states get most chances of being sampled.

Modeling Temporal Processes

Figure 5 schematically describes how temporal processes are viewed in the following. A temporal process begins with the 'world' standing in an *initial state*. The world will sojourn in the initial state until an *event* causes it to make a transition to a *different* state. If the new state is not 'absorbing', such a pattern will replicate, since a new transition will cause a new state change, and so on. We introduce random variables $X_0, X_1, X_2,...$, where X_i represents the *i-th* visited state. Each of these

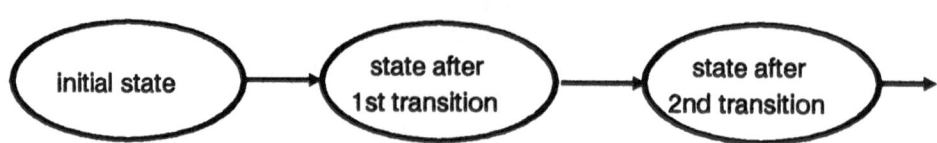

Figure 5: Our basic view of a temporal process.

variables takes a finite set of values corresponding to mutually exclusive states of the world.

In order to illustrate the concepts, we introduce now a clinical example, which is obviously not to be taken too seriously from a medical viewpoint.

A simple clinical example

Suppose that transplant on a patient may cause accidental inoculation of one of two viruses, A and B. According to the model of state progression shown in figure 6, a patient just after transplant may be, depending on chance, in one of three mutually exclusive states: *'virus A incubating'*, *'virus B incubating'* and *'no virus'*. The patient subsequently progresses to a new state that depends on the initial one. If a virus is incubating, then the patient may progress to a *'viral replication'* state, and subsequently to a state of *'fever'* caused by the replication. The patient may reach the state *'fever'* also independently of the viral process due to causes unrelated to the considered viruses.

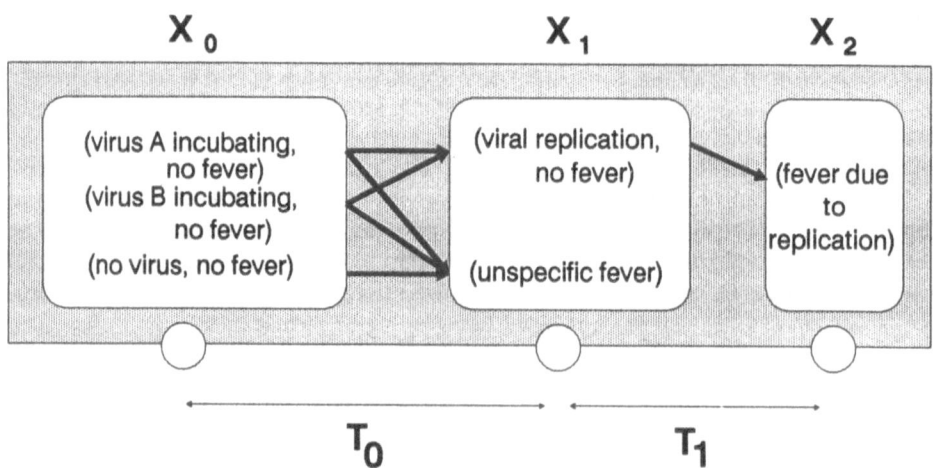

Figure 6:   'Infection' temporal process.

Individuating basic quantities involved

We may describe the process through a collection of 5 random variables:

$$(X_0, X_1, X_2, T_0, T_1)$$

X_0 represents the initial patient's state, X_1 the state after the first transition, and X_2 the state after the second transition. T_0 represents the time spent in the initial state and T_1 the time spent in the state reached via the first transition. These five variables capture the two forms of uncertainty about the process: that concerning the sequence of 'visited' states, and that concerning the time points at which changes of state occur (point process). In most applications we are concerned with both, so we shall maintain all five variables introduced above.

Specifying the conditional independence structure

Now that we have the list of quantities involved in the problem, we must provide a set of explicit judgements that some of these quantities can reasonably regarded as probabilistically independent.

The users of belief network theory have long time stressed that judgements about probabilistic independence need not necessarily involve numerical considerations, as the traditional definition of probabilistic independence, i.e. $pr(x,y) = pr(x) \, pr(y)$, seems to suggest. In fact they claim that people can often easily detect independencies based on their common sense perception. For example, I can confidently state that, once I know the time now on the television watch, information about the time on my watch is independent of information about the time on the watch of a friend, even if I am not able to provide numerical estimates of the involved probabilities.

On another side, in ordinary stochastic modelling, it is customary to select a model class and accept, with possibility of checking, all independence assumptions implied by the selected class.

Between these two views there is a common ground provided by belief networks. BN's may be used both to model judgemental knowledge elicited from a domain expert, *and* to represent the conditional independence structure of a stochastic model, as *Smith, 1988*, for example, does. This double possibility opens the door to a combined practice, by which a stochastic model is selected, the c.i. statements that form its essence are represented as a BN, and the BN is reasoned upon to confront those statements with the personal knowledge of the domain expert. The BN is at first used to make the expert understand that some.strong assumptions about the unrelatedness of individual variables are needed and test his/her acceptance of such assumptions.

Returning to our 'infection' example, a reference stochastic model for temporal processes is provided by **semi-Markov processes** (*Ross 1983*). They assume conditionally independent sojourn times, allow the dependence of the sojourn times in a state x both on x and on the state entered next, and assume independence of future states on past states, given knowledge of the present state.

A BN for the 'infection' example matching the semi-Markov specifications is shown in figure 7. Note that variable X_2 has been dropped from the BN, since, conditional on previous history, it takes only one value.

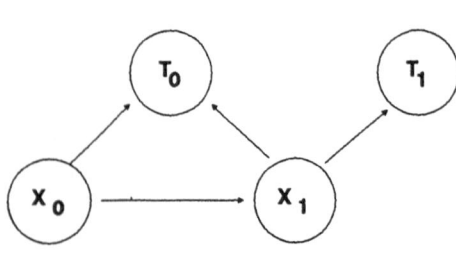

Figure 7: Belief network representing the 'infection' process as a semi-Markov process.

We can deduce individual c.i. statements by 'graphically' reasoning on the BN in figure 7. For example, each of the variables T_0 and T_1 does not belong to the other's Markov boundary. This means that, given a sequence of states, the sojourn times spent in these states are probabilistically independent. Intuitively, that statement implies, for example, that the time viral replication takes to cause clinically detectable fever does not depend on how long the virus had previously incubated.

A further feature of the c.i. structure in figure 7: the Markov boundaries of T_1 and X_0 are connected only through X_1. This means that T_1 and X_0 are conditionally independent given X_1. Intuitively, this implies, for example, that once we know that viral replication is on, knowing the type of virus is totally irrelevant to predict how long it will take for fever to show-up. In other terms, in order to predict the time of fever onset we just need to know when replication started.

Finally notice in figure 7 that T_0 depends both on X_0 and X_1. This is in accord with common knowledge, too, since it means the following: once I know the initial state, information about the subsequent state may be relevant to predict when the transition to it will occur. For example, once I know that virus A is incubating, the time at which the first transition will occur depends on whether such a transition will consist in the development of unspecific fever or in the end of incubation. Actually, the dependence of T_0 on X_0 and X_1. is very strong, in the sense that T_0 may in general 'select' a different probability distribution according to the values of X_0 and X_1. For example, T_0 might take a one-parameter exponential if $X_0 = $ 'no virus' and $X_1 = $ 'fever', while it might take a two-parameter exponential (with a virus-specific delay representing incubation latency) if $X_0 = $ 'virus A incubating' and $X_1 = $ 'viral replication'. In order to express 'dependence through distribution selection', we might adopt the device introduced by *Lehmann 1989*, namely that of introducing in the BN nodes explicitly representing the distribution type.

The notion of semi-Markov model opens the door to lots of methods for identifying the model, checking its assumptions and learning its parameters from hard data. Some statistics textbooks introduce 'strong' semi-Markov processes, where T_i is in general conditionally independent of X_{i+1}. Finally, note that **pure-Markov** processes may be viewed as strong semi-Markov processes where T_i's are distributed as one-parameter exponentials.

Specifying quantitative probabilistic information

Once the qualitative structure of the BN is well agreed-on, for the BN to provide an inference machine we need to specify appropriate quantitative probabilistic information to be inserted in it. Basically, required probabilities are priors on root nodes, and conditional (given the parents) probabilities for all remaining nodes.

Note that our example of BN includes two continuous variables representing time (T_0, T_1). Because of this, we shall now introduce some basic concepts concerning distributions of time.

The general specification for the probability density function of a continuous non-negative random variable, T, representing a time interval, is written:

$$F^T(t) = \lim_{\Delta \to 0+} \frac{pr(t \leq T < t + \Delta)}{\Delta} \qquad (1)$$

Just one of the many possible forms of (1), although the most popular, is the **two-parameter exponential distribution**:

$$F^T(t) = \lambda e^{-\lambda(t-a)} \qquad (2)$$

with $t \geq a$, and $\lambda \geq 0$. Figure 8 gives a graphical representation of this function.

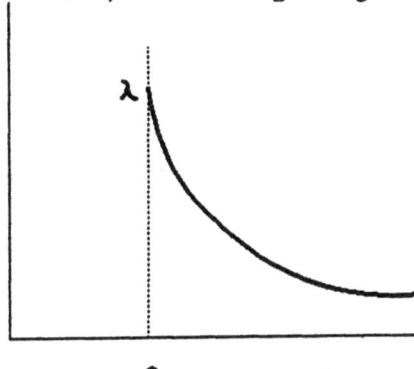

Figure 8: Two-parameter exponential density function.

Theoretical arguments suggesting this distributional form are discussed in *Cox 1984, p.18*. A strong practical reason for this choice is that the mathematics associated with this distribution is often of a simple nature. We add the consideration that parameter a in (2) enables modeling latency times often involved in the development certain symptoms, or, for example, incubation times. When latencies are not involved, it may be reasonable to take $a = 0$. The special case of (1) so obtained is called the **one-parameter** exponential distribution. A rather general distribution form is obtained by upper-truncating the two-parameter exponential at b, which may be thought of as a probabilistic counterpart of the 'temporal reasoning by intervals' proposed, for example, by *Kohane, 1987*.

The choice concerning the number of parameters to be included in the distribution should also take into account problems involved when these parameters are learned from empirical data. For one, using a distribution with only one adjustable parameter often makes the estimation very sensitive to even modest departures from the theoretical distribution in the tail of the distribution. As a matter of fact, recent work has emphasized methods that do not make stringent assumptions about distributional form, but this topic is beyond the scope of this paper.

A mathematically equivalent way of specifying the distribution of T, with special value in the present context, is the **hazard function**, defined by:

$$h^T(t) = \lim_{\Delta \to 0+} \frac{p(t \leq T < t + \Delta | t \leq T)}{\Delta} \qquad (3)$$

$F^T(t)$ and $h^T(t)$ are mathematically equivalent. For example, if $F^T(t)$ takes form (2), then $h^T(t)$ is a step function which is equal to zero for $t < a$ and constantly equal to λ for $t \geq a$.

The BN in figure 7 requires the following distributional specifications:

$$p(X_0) \tag{4}$$

$$P_{ij} = p(X_1 = j \mid X_0 = i) \tag{5}$$

$$F^0_{ij}(t) = \lim_{\Delta \to 0+} \frac{p\,(t \le T_0 < t + \Delta \mid X_0 = i, X_1 = j)}{\Delta} \tag{6}$$

$$F^1_j(t) = \lim_{\Delta \to 0+} \frac{p\,(t \le T_1 < t + \Delta \mid X_1 = j)}{\Delta} \tag{7}$$

where i denotes the value of X_0, j the value of X_1, and t a generic time. p is a vector of prior probabilities associated to initial states, P_{ij} a square matrix of probabilities, called *transition matrix*, F^0_{ij} is a square matrix of continuous density functions for T_0 with elements corresponding one-to-one to combinations of values of X_0 and X_1, and F^1_j a vector of continuous density functions for T_1 with elements corresponding one-to-one to values of X_0. Note that we might have written (6) and (7) in terms of an equivalent hazard function representation.
Assume the two-parameter exponential as general distributional form for (6) and (7), numerical information reported in figure 9 is sufficient to determine (4)-(7) completely.

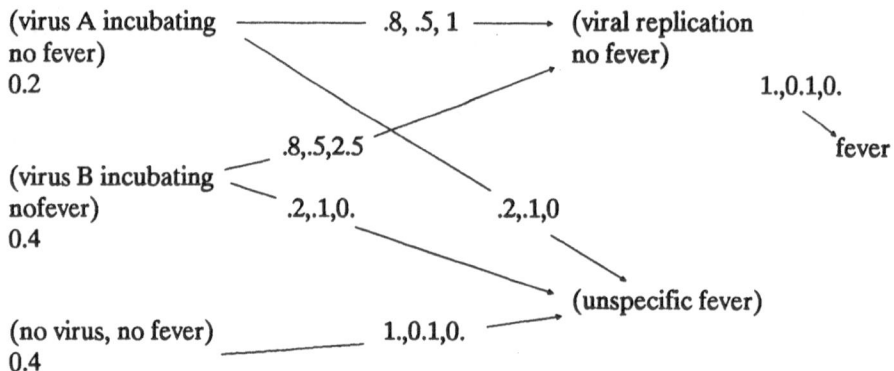

Figure 9: Fictitious parameters for our 'infection' example. The nodes of the above state-transition diagram represent states, and the edges represent transitions between these states. Each transition is assumed governed by a step-function hazard and is characterized by the following three parameters: (1) probability that the transition overcomes its competing transitions, (2) associated hazard after latency, (3) latency time. Each initial state has an associated prior.

Figure 9 is to be interpreted as follows. Probabilities (1) are reported by each of the three possible initial states. The probability (2), for each possible combination of states X_0 and X_1, is the first number in the triple associated to the arrow connecting such two states. The distribution (3), for each possible combination of states X_0 and

X_1 is an exponential with parameters λ and a corresponding to the last two numbers in the triple associated to the arrow connecting such two states.

Reasoning

A BN describing a temporal process can be used to 'reason out' posterior probabilities for specific hypotheses of interest about the process that take into account the available evidence. Reasoning is carried out by applying to the BN the probability propagation techniques discussed in section above where the BNs were defined.

The following are just three of the many possible patterns of temporal reasoning:

- *prediction* = given precise knowledge of the present state of the process and of its entry time, compute the posterior probability for specific evolutions of interest.

- *explanation* = given precise knowledge of the final state and of the time taken to reach it since entry in the initial state, compute the posterior distribution on the initial states.

- *reconstruction* = only *partial* knowledge is available concerning both initial and final states and transit time.

Technically speaking, *prediction* is straightforward, and can generally be accomplished by employing only forward sampling propagation on the BN. Therefore in the remaining part of the paper we restrict to *explanation*, using again our 'infection' example for illustration.

Consider the following problem of explanation (again, let's not take the problem too seriously from a clinical viewpoint):

three months after transplant the patient has developed fever, what causes the fever?

Here the evidence consists of two items: the final state (*fever*) and the time to reach it since the time origin (*three months*). Asking about the cause of fever is equivalent to asking what was the initial state of the patient. Therefore, it is required to compute the posterior distribution on the initial states, given the evidence. Note that the structure of this problem is typical of a large class of clinical problems in which a pathological process unfolding in time finally develops observable symptoms.

The *transit time*, defined as the time elapsed between entry into the unknown initial state and entry into the known final state, is an observed quantity in our problem. Therefore it is convenient to label it with a letter, say T, and represent it as an additional node of our BN. T functionally depends on variables T_0, T_1 and X_1:

$$T = \begin{cases} T_0 & \text{if } X_1 = \text{'unspecific fever'} \\ T_0 + T_1 & \text{if } X_1 = \text{'viral replication'} \end{cases}$$

Such functional dependencies are shown in the BN reported in figure 10(a). Node T has three parents. Therefore we need to specify the distribution of T conditional on these parents.

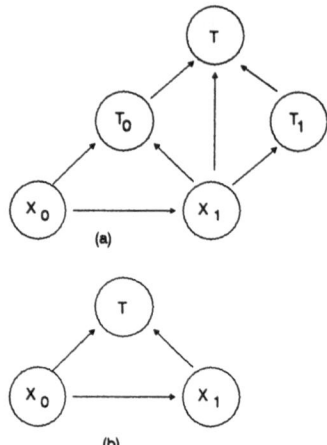

Figure 10: BN's for 'backwards' time reasoning in the 'infection' example

By definition, T *switches* distribution depending on the value of X_1. When $T = T_0$, its density $F^T(t)$ is $F^0(t)$ as in (6). When $T = T_0 + T_1$, its density is the **convolution**, denoted $F^{01}(t)$, of the densities of T_0 and T_1 (on the assumption that T_0 and T_1 are independent).

When T_0 and T_1 have identical one-parameter exponential distributions, $F^{01}(t)$ is gamma. But in general, denoting with λ_i and a_i the parameters of T_i, $i = 0, 1$, we obtain:

$$F^{01}(t) = \frac{\lambda_0 \lambda_1}{(\lambda_1 - \lambda_0)} e^{-\lambda_0(t - a_0 - a_1)} - e^{-\lambda_1(t - a_0 - a_1)} \quad (8)$$

Remember that λ_0 and a_0 are completely determined by X_0 and X_1, while λ_1 and a_1 are completely determined by X_1. In other terms, all parameters of $F^{01}(t)$ are completely determined when one has knowledge of X_0 and X_1. And remember that the same is true for $F^0(t)$. In conclusion $F^T(t)$ is completely determined by X_0 and X_1.

This enables us to 'reduce' our BN as in figure 10(b), by removing T_0 and T_1 into T. In this way, not only we have simplified the net, but, more important, we have eliminated functional constraints which would destroy the convergence of Markov sampling.

Once $p(X_0), p(X_1 \mid X_0)$ and $F^T(t)$ are specified, the BN in figure 10(b) is completely quantified, and we are ready to put the artificial 'virus identifier' into operation to provide the answer to our question about the cause of fever. Here comes the moment of applying to the BN the propagation techniques discussed above.

Consider, as an example of computational scheme, the operations carried out by node X_1 upon receiving control during Markov sampling. The task of X_1 is that of sampling $p(X_1 \mid X_0 = x_0) F^T(T = t \mid X_0 = x_0, X_1)$, where x_0 denotes current value of X_0 and t denotes current value of T. We assume $p(X_1 \mid X_0 = x_0)$ stored in node X_1, and $F^T(t)$ in node T. As a consequence, X_1 finds $p(X_1 \mid X_0 = x_0)$ within its own frame. But for what concerns $F^T(T = t \mid X_0 = x_0, X_1)$, X_1 has to send a 'message' to T requesting information.

Activated by the message, T performs the following steps:

- inspects current values of X_0 and X_1,
- selects $F^0(t)$ or $F^{01}(t)$ according as X_1 is *'unspecific fever'* or *'viral replication'*, respectively; for now assume $F^{01}(t)$ is selected;
- conditions $F^{01}(t)$ on the current values of T and X_0, which gives $F^{01}(T = t \mid X_0 = x_0, X_1)$,
- sends $F^{01}(T = t \mid X_0 = x_0, X_1)$ back to X_1.

The distribution (8) can be straightforwardly generalized to the case when the transit time T is the sum of a set of conditionally independent sojourn times T_i, $i = 0, ..., h$, each one distributed as an exponential with parameters λ_i and a_i. In this case the density of T is:

$$F^T(t) = \frac{\prod_{i=0}^{h} \lambda_i \sum_{i=0}^{h} e^{-\lambda_i \left(t - \sum_{j=0}^{h} a_j\right)}}{\prod_{j \neq l} (\lambda_l - \lambda_j)} \tag{9}$$

Formula (9) can be conveniently computed via Laplace transform, the Laplace transform of a convolution being the product of the Laplace transforms of individual factors. The nice algebraic form of (9) is a benefit of the exponential assumption.

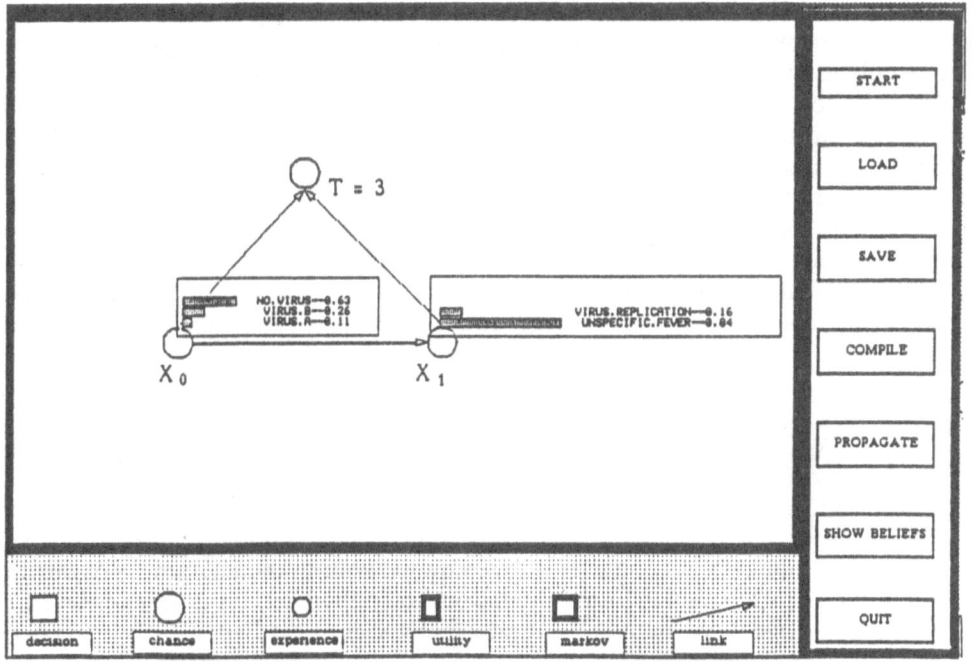

Figure 11: Running the 'infection' example on the computer.

Figure 11 gives an idea of how the simple 'infection' problem is set up using a 'Bayesian Reasoning Tool' developed by our Department. It took few minutes to draw the structure of the BN using a reference icons facility, and to insert into slots of frames representing the network nodes the probabilistic specifications discussed above and based on figure 9. Then available evidence was specified by simply clicking on node T and setting its value equal to 3 (months). At this point, a general 'probability propagation engine' (Markov sampling with restarting) was called into action. Resulting posterior probabilities were automatically visualized under the form of probability histograms by each node.

The result is that there is .63 probability that the patient got no virus, fever being due to unspecific causes, .26 probability that the patient got virus A and .11 probability that the patient got virus B.

On the same network we could have performed other types of inference. For example, if we knew for sure that the patient has got virus A, we might compute the expected time to fever as well as its median and confidence interval. We like to emphasize that these networks lend themselves to any kind of conceivable inference. In this respect they differ from rules, which force to pre-thought uni-directional inferences.

Developments

In this paper we have been constrained to a very simple application example but, obviously, this work has the perspective of complex and interesting applications. Some problems may have a structure like the one shown in figure 12. The portion of the BN with nodes X_0, X_1 and T is identical to figure 10(b), where X_0 represents pathological causes, X_1 represents clinical evolution and T the time taken to reach a known final state. Node D hosts a *decision variable*, whose values correspond to alternative therapeutic actions. The uncertain consequences of the action (node O) depend on the pathological causes and on the therapeutic action itself. Patient's conditions (node C), such as patient's age, and so on affect both the transition probabilities of the temporal process and the outcome. A *utility node U* represents preferences about the outcome. This BN can be solved to determine the action that maximizes the expected utility, conditioning on D, C and T.

There are problems where observed states are imprecise, so that the BN has to be made more complex to account for error processes. Many problems involve longer and more complicated chains of transitions. We are now evaluating the usefulness of the approach described in this paper on interesting clinical applications.

Finally, a forthcoming paper reports the results of a research by the same authors, where Petri-nets are used to generalize temporal reasoning with probabilities and to extend greatly its practical scope.

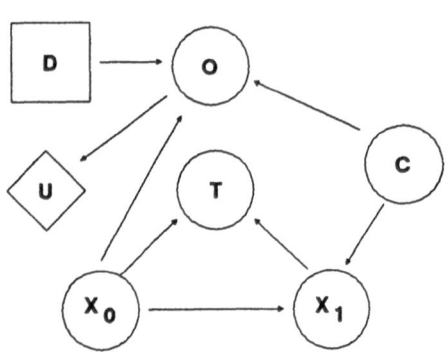

Figure 12: Example of decision problem involving temporal reasoning

Acknowledgements

The authors are indebted to J.Pearl, D.Spiegelhalter and M. Stefanelli for stimulating discussions on the topic. The author's insight into the problem was greatly helped by participation in the 1989 Edinburgh Workshop on Statistics and Expert Systems, supported by the U.K. SERC and organized by Drs. D.Hand, D.Spiegelhalter and Mr. P.R.Fisk.

References

Allen, J.F.: Maintaining knowledge about temporal intervals, Communications of the ACM, 26, No.11, 832, 1983.

Cooper, G.F.: Probabilistic Inference using Belief Networks is NP-hard, Technical Report KSL-87-27, Medical Computer Science Group, Stanford University, Ca, U.S.A, 1987.

Cox, D.R. and Oakes, D.: Analysis of Survival Data, Chapman and Hall, 1984.

Davis, R.: Personal communication, panel session at the 1985 International Joint Conference on Artificial Intelligence in Los Angeles, 1985.

Fagan, L.M. Kunz, J.C., Feigenbaum, E.A., Osborn, J.J.: Extensions to the Rule-based Formalism for a Monitoring Task. In: Buchanan, B.G., Shortliffe, E.H. (Eds.): Rule-Based Expert Systems: The MYCIN Experiments of the Stanford Heuristic Programming Project, Addison-Wesley, Reading, 397-423, 1984.

Geman, S. & Geman, D.: Stochastic relaxation, Gibbs distributions and the Bayesian restoration of images, IEEE Transactions on Pattern Analysis and Machine Intelligence, 6, 721, 1984.

Henrion, M.: Propagating uncertainty by logic sampling in Bayes' networks, Technical Report, Department of Engineering and Public Policy, Carnegie-Mellon University, 1986.

Kahn, M.G., Fagan, L.M., Shortliffe, E.H.: Context-Specific Interpretation of Patient Records for a Therapy Advice System. In: Salamon, R., Blum, B., Jørgensen, M. (eds.): MEDINFO 86, Proc. 5-th Conference on Medical Informatics, Washington, october 26-30 1986, North Holland, Amsterdam, 175-179, 1986.

Kohane, I.S.: Temporal Reasoning in Medical Expert Systems, Ph.D. Thesis, Boston University, Ma, U.S.A, 1987.

Lagakos, S.W., Sommer, C.J., Zelen, M.: Semi-Markov models for partially censored data, Biometrika, 65, 2, 311, 1978.

Lauritzen, S.L., Spiegelhalter, D.J.: Local Computations with Probabilities on Graphical Structures and their Application to Expert Systems, J.R.Statist.Soc B, 50, No.2, 157, 1988.

Lehmann, H.P.: A Decision-Analytic Model for Using Scientific Data, Proceedings of the 5-th Workshop on Uncertainty in Artificial Intelligence, august 1989, Windsor, Ontario., 208, 1989.

Pearl, J.: Evidential reasoning using stochastic simulation of causal models, Artificial Intelligence, 32, no. 2, 245, 1987.

Ross, S.M.: Stochastic Processes, Wiley & Sons, 1983.

Smith, J.Q.: Statistical Principles on Graphs, Research Report, Dept. of Statistics, University of Warwick, 1988.

Stefanelli, M.: Personal communication, Second Conference on Artificial Intelligence in Medicine, London, august 1989.

Tusch, G., Bernauer, J., Gubernatis, G., Rading, M.: Knowledge acquisition using syntactic time patterns, Proceedings Second European Conference on Artificial Intelligence in Medicine, London, august 1989.

Vilain, M. and Kautz, H.: Constraint propagation algorithms for temporal reasoning, Proceedings of the National Conference on Artificial Intelligence, AAAI, Philadelphia 1986, 377, 1986.

Decisions Based on Qualitative and Quantitative Reasoning

Steen Andreassen

Department of Medical Informatics and Image Analysis, Aalborg University, Denmark

Abstract

Causal networks can be used to reason quantitatively or qualitatively about optimal decisions. Quantitative reasoning in causal probabilistic networks requires the specification of conditional probabilities, which in a medical application reflects the doctors current knowledge about the problem at hand. It is also necessary to specify a utility function, which reflects the priorities of the patient. A small medical example is analysed quantitatively. The results of the analysis are compared with the results from a previous qualitative analysis. Based on this example it is argued that although qualitative reasoning can eliminate a range of sub-optimal decisions, the "interesting" decision must be based on a detailed quantitative analysis. The quantitative specification of a causal probabilistic network represents an unambiguous way of stating the opinion of the doctor (and of the patient). The firm theoretical foundation in probability and decision theory allows independent evaluation of the doctors' and the patients' assumption3.

Introduction

Several medical expert systems employ causality in their knowledge representation and in their inference systems, e.g. CASNET (*Weiss et al., 1978*), ABEL (*Patil, 1981*), or INTERNIST/CADUCEUS (*Pople, 1982; Banks, 1986*). This has several advantages: The inferences that can be made when causality is acknowledged is considerably more powerful that the inferences that can be made in rule- or logic based systems, despite numerous attempts to overcome these shortcomings through the invention of a "non-standard" logics (*Pearl, 1988*). Another advantage is that systems that acknowledge causality tend to model the application domain rather than

3   The research is partially funded by the ESPRIT Program of the European community under contract P599.

modelling the rules of thumb of a domain expert. This encourages the utilization of deep knowledge expressed as quantitative or qualitative models of the application domain. Theoretical and practical work on qualitative modelling (*De Kleer and Brown, 1984; Forbus, 1984; Kuipers, 1984; Long, 1985*) has shown the importance of qualitative modelling. However, through the work of Pearl (*Kim and Pearl, 1983; Pearl, 1986*), *Lauritzen and Spiegelhalter, 1988*, and *Jensen et al, 1988*, a probabilistic inference machine has been developed which makes full use of the strong inferences that are possible in systems that acknowledge causality. At the same time the work with the MUNIN expert system (*Andreassen et al., 1987, 1988*) has demonstrated that through the application of quantitative and semi-quantitative models causal probabilistic networks of non-trivial size can be constructed. It has been argued (*Andersen et al., 1987*) that since knowledge based systems with causal models represent an "understanding" of the application domain it should be possible to calculate optimal decision strategies. The purpose of this paper is to assess the validity of this assertion for systems using qualitative and quantitative reasoning. For this purpose a small fictive medical example, previously analysed qualitatively (*Wellman, 1987*) will be analysed quantitatively. It will be argued that while qualitative reasoning can be used to eliminate a number of inferior strategies the "interesting" decisions have to be based on quantitative reasoning. It will also be argued that the quantitative specification of a causal network does not represent an unrealistic faith in the quality of the available knowledge. Rather, it represents an unambiguous way of stating the current opinion of the doctor (and the patient). Due to the firm theoretical foundation in probability and decision theory the semantics of the quantitative information allows independent evaluation of each of the assumptions in the specification of the network.

The Medical Example

A doctor is suspecting that a patient may have a certain "DISEASE" (fig. 1). The doctor may affect the probability of the patient's continued illness ("DISEASE CONT.") by initiating a treatment ("TREAT"). The treatment may have some "SIDE EFFECTS". A "TEST" is available. When the test is performed a "TEST RESULT" becomes available. The test result depends on whether the patient has the disease or not. The test is likely to cause "COMPLICATIONS". These relations are expressed in the causal network in fig. 1. In this situation the doctor has the following three "interesting" choices: 1) Should he advise to initiate treatment immediately, 2) Should he advise to avoid treatment, or 3) Should he let treatment depend on the test result?

Conditional probabilities

The network in fig. 1 can be used to make predictions about the probable consequences of different test/treat decisions if quantitative information about the causal links is provided. Let us therefore assume the following: The test has a specificity of 95% (5% false positives) and a sensitivity of 80% (20% false negatives) (fig. 2A). Complications always occur (fig. 2B). The disease cures itself spontaneously in 10% of the cases (i.e. 90% continue to be ill without treatment). All but 25% are cured by the treatment. In 10% of the cases the treatment may induce the disease it is intended to cure (fig. 2C). Side effects occur in 50% of the cases (fig. 2D). Finally it is assumed that the doctor currently believes that there is a 50% a priori probability that the patient has the disease (fig. 2E).

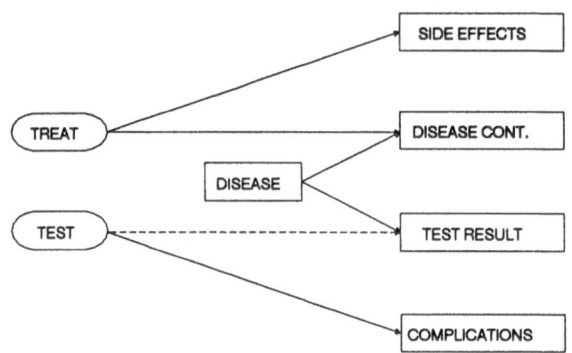

Figure 1:   A causal network for the test/treat decision. Nodes that represent decisions have
            rounded corners. The causal links are indicated by arrows. The broken arrow,
            which is not a causal link, indicates that the TEST RESULT becomes available
            when the TEST is performed.

A

P(TEST RESULT|DISEASE)	
DISEASE	¬DISEASE
80%	5%

B

P(COMPLICATIONS|TEST)	
TEST	¬TEST
100%	0%

C

P(DISEASE CONT. | DISEASE,TREAT)		
	DISEASE	¬DISEASE
TREAT	25%	10%
¬TREAT	90%	0%

D

P(SIDE EFFECTS|TREAT)	
TREAT	¬TREAT
50%	0%

E
A PRIORI: P(DISEASE) = 50%

Figure 2:   A complete specification of all probabilities in the causal probabilistic network.

With this information the causal probabilistic network can predict the consequences of all test/treat decisions. In the initial state with no treatment and no testing the network predicts a 43% chance of a positive test result (TEST RESULT) and a 45% chance of the patients continued illness (DISEASE CONT.) (fig. 3).

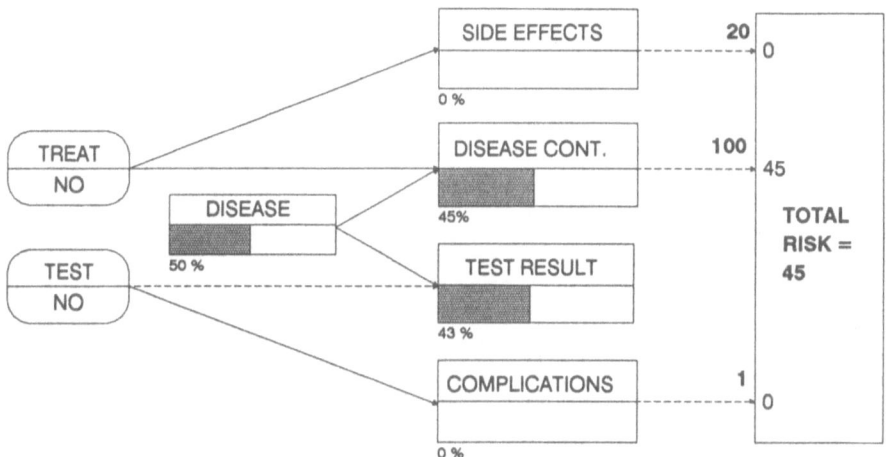

Figure 3: The no-test, no-treat strategy (¬TEST, ¬TREAT). The expected risk of this strategy is 45.

Losses and Risk

Predictions are not sufficient to make decisions. It is also necessary to specify that some situations are preferable to other situations. To do this, losses are assigned to nodes in the network: A loss of 1 is assigned to the COMPLICATIONS node, a loss of 20 to the SIDE EFFECTS node, and a loss of 100 to the DISEASE CONT. node Just as the conditional probabilities represent the doctors current knowledge the losses represent the decision makers subjective evaluation of the relative desirability of different outcomes. The patient will have to evaluate his problems due to his disease in some convenient "currency", for example "days in bed". He must then convert all inconvenience incurred to this currency. For example seen from the point of view of the patient the loss associated with COMPLICATIONS of the TEST are likely to represent the time and money spent on the test with some additional contributions from the discomfort and pain associated with the testing procedure. A loss could also be associated with the DISEASE node. This loss would account for the discomfort already suffered by the patient due to the disease. Since this obviously cannot be changed by any future decision, this loss need not be specified for the purpose of making decisions.

With these losses the expected future discomfort of the patient will be 45 ($\sum$RISK = 45), provided that testing is not performed and treatment is not initiated.

Calculating Decisions

By means of the risk function the best test/treat strategy can be determined as the strategy that gives the smallest risk. It has already been determined that the strategy of no-test and no-treatment (strategy #1 in table I) gives a risk of 45. An alternative strategy (strategy #2) of initiating treatment without testing gives a risk of 27 (fig. 4), 18 better than the no-test, no-treat strategy.

	STRATEGY			RISK	RANK
#1	¬TEST	¬TREAT		45	4
#2	¬TEST	TREAT		27	2
#3a	TEST	¬TREAT	TEST RESULT	86	
#3b	TEST	¬TREAT	¬TEST RESULT	17	
#3	TEST	¬TREAT		46	5
#4a	TEST	TREAT	TEST RESULT	35	
#4b	TEST	TREAT	¬TEST RESULT	24	
#4	TEST	TREAT		28	3
#5	TEST	TREAT	= TEST RESULT	25	1

Table I.

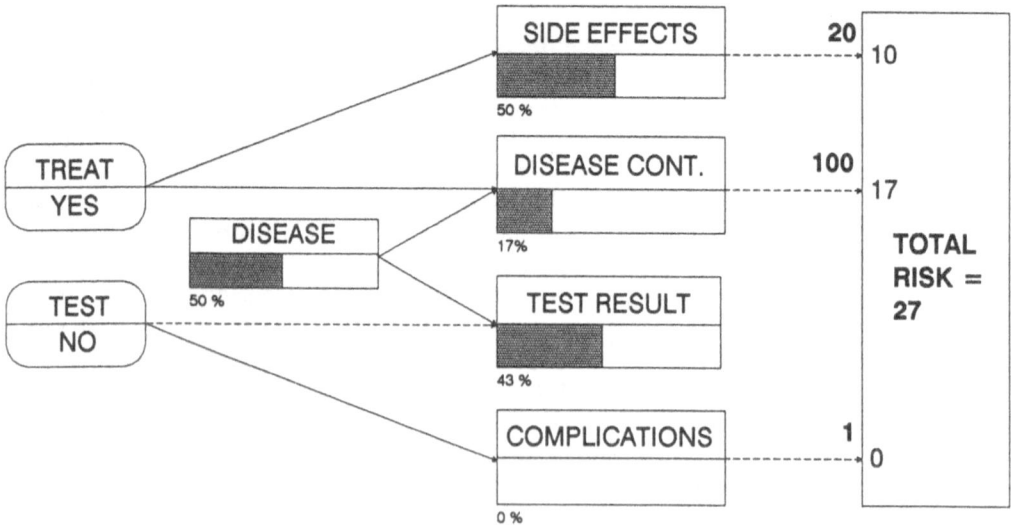

Figure 4: The no-test, treat strategy (¬TEST,TREAT). The risk of this strategy is 27

The strategy of testing without treating (strategy #3) has to be evaluated in two steps (fig. 5).

If the test result is positive, which has a probability of 43%, then the risk is 86 (strategy #3a). In the remaining 57% of the cases the test result is negative, which gives a risk of 17 (strategy #3b). The resulting risk of test, no-treat can then be calculated as 86 * 0.43 + 17 * 0.57 = 46, which is 1 worse than the no-test, no-treat strategy. This is a reassuring result, since it simply means that if it has been decided not to treat then the test and the associated complications are wasted.

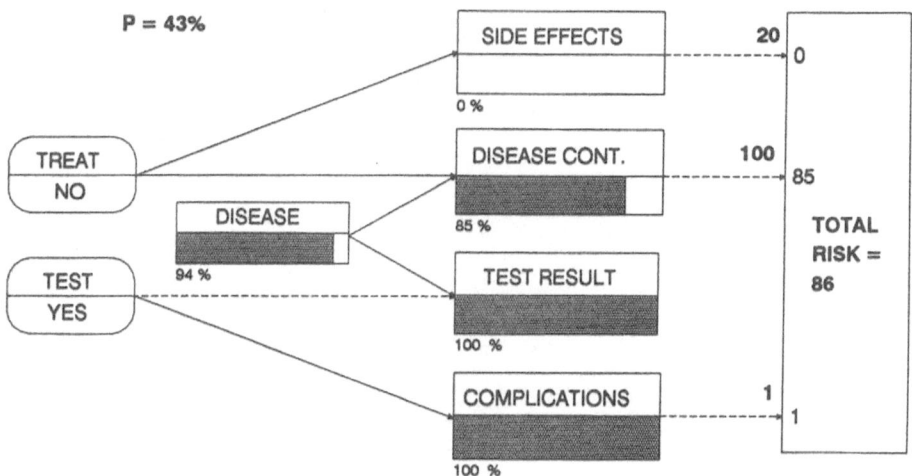

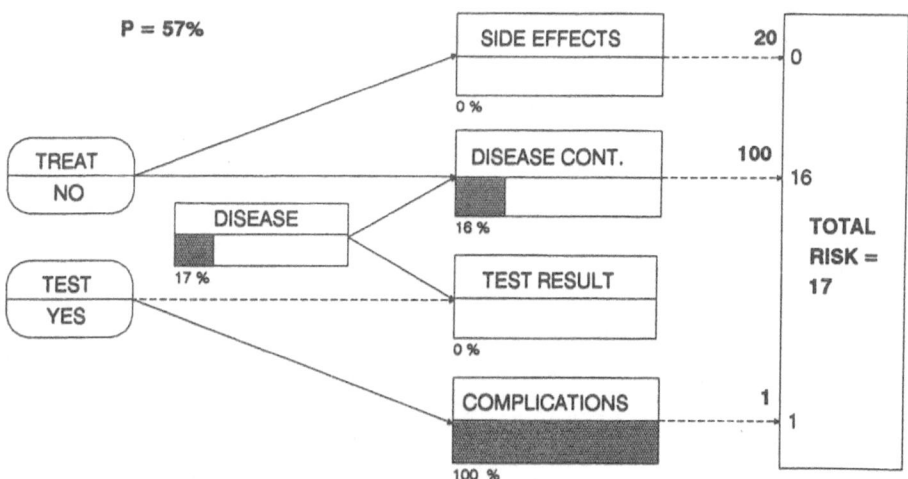

RISK(TEST,NO-TREAT)= 86*0.43 + 17*0.57 = 46

Figure 5: The test, no-treat strategy (TEST, ¬TREAT). The risk of this strategy is 46.

The test, treat strategy (strategy #4) can also be evaluated in two steps (fig. 6) with the risk of 35 and 24 for TEST RESULT positive and negative respectively (#4a and #4b). The resulting risk of the test, treat strategy is 28, which is 1 worse than the risk of the no-test, treat strategy: Again the test is wasted.

Inspection of table I reveals that if the TEST RESULT is positive, then TREAT has a lower risk (35) than ¬TREAT (86). If TEST RESULT is negative then ¬TREAT has a lower risk (17) than TREAT (24). This suggests an alternative strategy in which

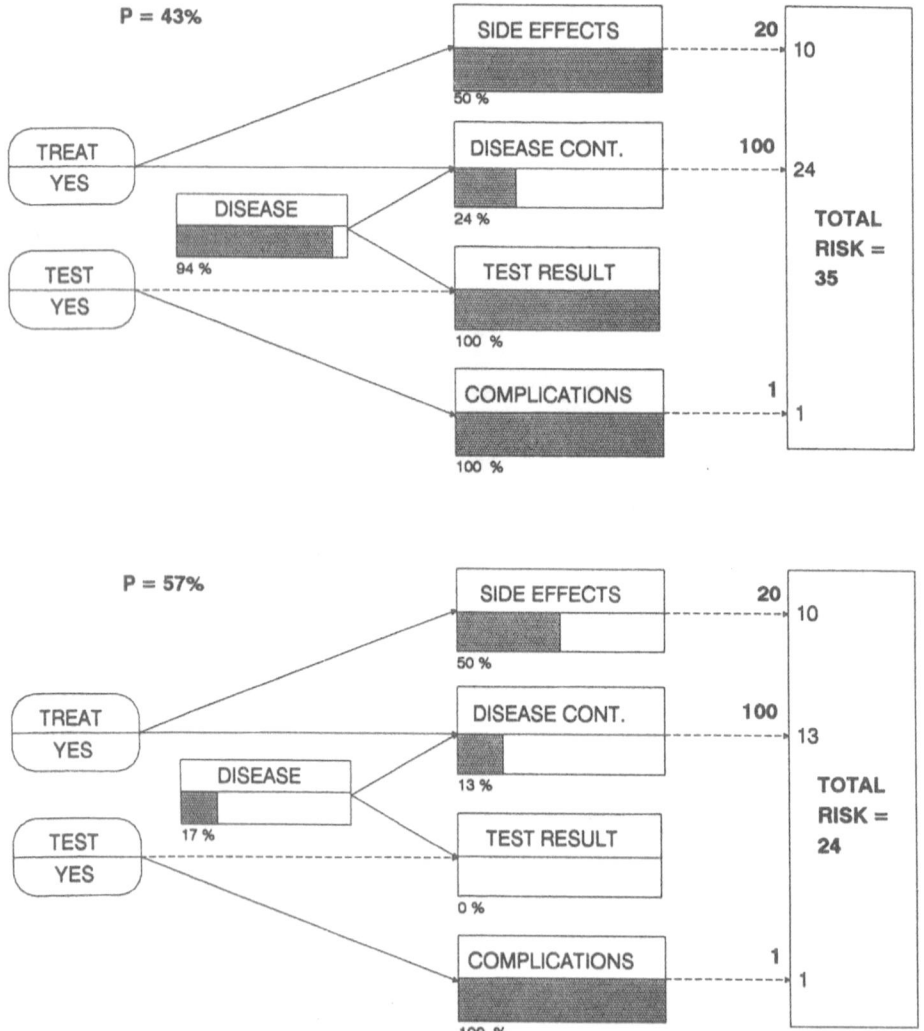

RISK(TEST,TREAT)= 35*0.43 + 24*0.57 = 28

Figure 6:   The test and treat strategy (TEST, TREAT). The risk of this strategy is 28

the TREAT decision is made dependent on the TEST RESULT in the way that TREAT = TEST RESULT, i.e. TREAT if the TEST RESULT is positive otherwise not (strategy #5). The resulting risk of this strategy is then 35 * 0.43 + 17 * 0.57 = 25. This is 2 better than the second best strategy which is ¬TEST, TREAT.

Discussion

Quantitative or qualitative reasoning

The small medical example used to illustrate how different types of decisions can be made is similar to an example used by *Wellman, 1987*. He used the formalism of influence diagrams (*Howard and Matheson, 1984*). Using qualitative probabilistic reasoning he showed that strategy #4 (TEST,TREAT) is inferior to strategy #2 (¬TEST,TREAT) and that strategy #3 (TEST,¬TREAT) is inferior to strategy #1 (¬TEST,¬TREAT). This is equivalent to concluding that testing that does not affect the TREAT decision should be avoided. However, this intuitively reasonable result does not depend on the actual structure of the network, nor does it depend on the numerical value of the losses associated with the nodes. Using the formalism of causal probabilistic networks it can be shown as a direct consequence of Bayes theorem that information that is not used to change decisions has zero value (see Appendix).

Therefore, quantitative reasoning can be used to identify and eliminate obviously inferior plans, just as it can be done by qualitative reasoning (*Wellman, 1987*). The result from the appendix makes it clear that for this purpose the quantitative reasoning is not dependent on the actual numerical values. The inferiority of some plans can be determined from the structure of the problem: In the small medical example it can be decided from the structure alone, based on qualitative or quantitative reasoning that a test that will not effect future decisions should not be done. However, for most decisions, plans with each their pro's and con's have to be weighed against each other, and for this purpose quantitative reasoning is required: In the small medical example the decision on unconditional treatment strategy #1 or 2 or a treatment dependent on the outcome of the test strategy #5 can only be made when the negative effects of the disease are help up against the side effects of the treatment and the complications of the test.

Rationality of quantitative reasoning

The knowledge required to carry out the detailed quantitative analysis of optimal decision strategies falls into two categories: conditional probabilities and risk. The validity of the quantitative reasoning depends on the correctness of these numbers. Since this correctness is difficult to guarantee in a large "real life" decision situation, what is then gained by this type of quantitative reasoning? The most important is the guaranteed rationality: If the numbers are assumed to be correct then an optimal strategy can be found. This is important since human decision makers have repeatedly been demonstrated to perform poorly when decisions with uncertainty are involved even when all the numbers are known (*Schwarz and Griffin, 1986*).

Validity of the knowledge

According to a subjectivist Bayesian view the conditional probabilities reflect the doctors current knowledge about the disease, the test, and the treatment. This knowledge may be based on the literature about the disease or on the doctor's personal clinical experience. If the doctor is poorly informed, this will not surprisingly lead to poor decisions. Specifying the knowledge in the form of conditional probabilities has two virtues: 1) It is very close to the form in which information is usually presented in the scientific literature. For example, it is a standard approach to specify the quality of a given test through its specificity and its sensitivity, which provide exactly the conditional probabilities required. 2) Although the remaining uncertainty about the exact value of the conditional probabilities is of little value to the patient, it is important for the doctor. It helps him to determine to what extent he should be willing to modify his opinion in the light of experience. The procedure for Bayesian revision of conditional probabilities is currently being developed (*Spiegelhalter and Lauritzen, 1988*).

The risks are also subjective. Ideally they should reflect the priorities of the individual patient and different patients must be expected to assign different risks to the nodes. This is important since different risks eventually lead to different decisions. For example, if the patient values the loss due to COMPLICATIONS to 5 instead of 1, then the test should never be performed: Treatment should be initiated without further testing. From an ethical point of view it is very important to keep in mind whose priorities are expressed through the losses. The losses assigned to the different nodes are different for different decision makers, e.g. the patient, the doctor, the insurance company, the hospital, or the national health authorities.

References

Andersen, S. K., Andreassen, S., Woldbye, M.: Knowledge Representations for Diagnosis and Test Planning in the Domain of Electromyography. Advances in Artificial Intelligence, ed. Du Boulay, Hogg and Steels, Elsevier, 461-472, 1987.

Andreassen, S., Jensen F.V., Andersen S.K., Falck B., Kjærulff U., Woldbye, M., Sørensen A.R., Rosenfalck A., Jensen F.: MUNIN An Expert EMG Assistant, In: Computer-Aided Surface or Needle Electromyography and Expert Systems in Diagnosis. p.p. 255-277. Desmedt, J. E. (ed.). Elsevier, 1989.

Andreassen, S., Woldbye, M., Falck, B., Andersen, S. K.: MUNIN A Causal Probabilistic Network for Interpretation of Electromyographic Findings. Proc. of 10th IJCAI 1987, 366-372, 1987.

Banks, G.: Artificial Intelligence in Medical Diagnosis. The Internist/Caduceus Approach CRR Critical Reviews in Medical Information, 1, 23-54, 1986

De Kleer, J., Brown, J.S.: A Qualitative Physics Based on Confluences. Artificial Intelligence, 24, 7-83, 1984.

Forbus, K.: Qualitative Process Theory. Artificial Intelligence, 24, 85-168, 1984.

Jensen, F.V., Olesen, K.G., Andersen, S.K.: An Algebra of Bayesian Belief Universes for Knowledge Based Systems. Institute of Electronic Systems, Aalborg University, R-88-25, 1988.

Kim, J.H. and Pearl, J.: A Computational Model for Causal and Diagnostic Reasoning in Inference Systems. Proc. IJCAI 1983, 190-193, 1983.

Kuipers, B.: Commonsense Reasoning About Causality. Artificial Intelligence, 24, 169-203, 1984.

Lauritzen, S.L. and Spiegelhalter, D.J.: Local Computations with Probabilities on Graphical Structures and Their Application to Expert Systems.R.Statis.Soc. B, 2, 157-224, 1988.

Long, W.: A Program for Management of Heart Failure. Sigart Newsletter, n.93, July 1985.

Pearl, J.: Embracing Causality in Default Reasoning, Artificial Intelligence, 35, 259-271, 1988.

Pearl, J.: Fusion, Propagation, and Structuring in Belief Networks. Artificial Intelligence, 29, 241-288, 1986.

Pople, H.E.Jr.: Heuristic Methods for Imposing Structure in Ill-structured Problems: The structuring of Medical Diagnosis. In: Artificial Intelligence in Medicine, Szolovits, P. (ed.). Westview Press, chap. 5, 1982.

Schwarz, S., Griffin, T.: Medical Thinking. The Psychology of Medical Judgment and Decision Making. Springer Verlag, 1986.

Spiegelhalter, D.J. and Lauritzen S.L. Statistical Reasoning and Learning in Knowledge-bases Represented as Causal Networks. In: Lecture Notes in Medical Informatics, Reichertz, P.L (ed.), 105-112. Springer-Verlag Berlin Heidelberg, 1988.

Weiss, S.M., Kulikowski, C.A., Amaral, S., Safir, A.: A Model-Based Method for Computer-Aided Medical Decision Making. Artificial Intelligence 11, 145-178, 1978.

Patil, R.S. Causal Representation of Patient Illness for Electrolyte and Acid-Base Diagnosis. Laboratory for Computer Science, MIT, PhD Thesis, 1981.

Wellman, M.P.: Qualitative Probabilistic Networks for Planning Under Uncertainty. In: John F. Lemmer (ed.). Uncertainty in Artificial Intelligence 2, 197-208. Elsevier Science Publishers B.V, 1987.

Appendix

New evidence leaves the risk associated with a node in a causal probabilistic network unchanged

Let A and B be two nodes in a causal probabilistic network. A has the outcomes a1, a2,...aN and B has the outcomes b1, b2,...bM. The outcomes of A have utilities associated: The risk associated with A, before node B is observed, is:

$$RISK(A) = \sum_{i=0}^{N} P(A_i)U_i$$

where U_i is the LOSS associated with outcome A_i. B is an observable node, i.e. a node that can be used to enter evidence into the network. Observing B changes the probability of Ai from $P(A_i)$ to $P(A_i \mid B_j)$, where Bj is the observed outcome of B. The risk associated with A, given Bj is:

$$RISK(A \mid B_j) = \sum_{i=0}^{N} P(A_i \mid B_j)U_i$$

The risk of A after observing B, weighhted over all outcomes Bj is:

$$\text{RISK}(A|B) = \sum_{j=1}^{M} \left[\sum_{i=1}^{N} P(A_i|B_j)U_i \right] P(B_j) \qquad (1)$$

Inserting Bayes theorem:

$$P(A_i|B_j) = \frac{P(B_j|A_i)P(A_i)}{P(B_j)}$$

into equation (1) gives:

$$\text{RISK}(A|B) = \sum_{j=1}^{M} \left[\sum_{i=1}^{N} \frac{P(B_j|A_i)P(A_i)U_i}{P(B_j)} \right] P(B_j)$$

$$= \sum_{i=1}^{N} \left[\sum_{j=1}^{M} P(B_j|A_i)P(A_i)U_i \right]$$

$$= \sum_{i=1}^{N} P(A_i)U_i \sum_{j=1}^{M} P(B_j|A_i)$$

$$= \sum_{i=1}^{N} P(A_i)U_i$$

This implies that:

$$\text{RISK}(A|B) = \text{RISK}(A) \qquad \textbf{Q.E.D.}$$

Questions from the discussion

Berzuini: How can you apply these networks in cases where you have 20 different causes for one condition? in these circumstances you have to estimate 20^{20} probabilities.

Andreassen: In the MUNIN network, used to diagnose muscle and nerve diseases we have encountered that situation. For example, we have 8 nodes representing different causes of a pathophysiological condition. Each of these nodes has 5 states, requiring the estimation of 5^9 or about 2 million conditional probabilities. Clearly, so many numbers cannot be determined form case based statistics. Instead we have

developed small pathophysiological models that account for the expected interaction between multiple diseases as described in *Andreassen at al, 1989.*
A recent medical evaluation of the MUNIN network documented that this approach allows the network to diagnose multiple diseases with a performance similar that achieved by experienced neurophysiologists.

Berzuini: How do you handle the propagation of probabilities in large networks? It seems that you need techniques like stochastic simulation to obtain a result in reasonable time.

Andreassen: The inference method is based on the work of *Lauritzen and Spiegelhalter, 1988,* which provides exact probabilities. The time required to propagate probabilities in a network with a tree-like structure (a singly-connected network) us very modest. When the network contains "loops" generating large "cliques" the propagation time increases dramatically. However, in the MUNIN network, which currently has about one thousand nodes and numerous "loops" the propagation time is about 5 seconds on a SUN 3 workstation.

Breuker: How sensitive is your method for errors in the probabilities?

Andreassen: We have tried to insert conditional probabilities collected from two different sources into the network. Our impression from this informal sensitivity analysis is that even though the actual probabilities vary considerably, their ranking seems to be fairly robust.

Wyatt: Is there any metric for assessing the correctness of a network or is that task NP-hard or NP-complete?

Andreassen: The probabilities for the nodes at the edges have to be in agreement with the experience, i.e. collected statistics, and a formal metric could probably be devised to quantify the agreement. In our own work we modify the structure and numbers in the network until we believe that a good fit is obtained between the probabilities at the edges and the available statistics. A more systematic way of incorporating experience into the network is currently developed by *Spiegelhalter and Lauritzen, 1988.*

Knowledge Representation and Data Model to Support Medical Knowledge Base Transportability.

O.B.Wigertz[1] , P.D. Clayton[2], G. Hripcsak[2] and R. Linnarsson[1]

1 Linkoping University, Linkoping, Sweden.

2 Center for Medical Informatics, Columbia Presbyterian Medical Center, New York, NY, USA.

Introduction.

A rich knowledge base is the primary source of power of any medical decision support systems even if the implementations are quite different. Since it is evident that no single decision support system will cover the entire spectrum of medical knowledge, the possibility of sharing knowledge bases between different groups and systems has been proposed. The transfer of knowledge from the system where it was built up to other decision support systems would save a lot of efforts in knowledge acquisition and probably also would increase the use of decision support systems in clinical practice.

However, there are some major problems associated with knowledge base transportability. One problem is the different forms in which knowledge is represented and that it is often hard to understand, analyse and validate for possible use in foreign environments. Another problem is to transfer the implicit knowledge from those hard coded programs, in which the knowledge base is not separated from the data base.

In this paper we will discuss the thesis that it is possible to design a data model and a representation of the medical decision-making knowledge in a sufficiently high level and modular format to ease transportability between institutions and systems. We will discuss some of the prerequisites of this uniform representation of medical terms, medical data and medical logic. The possible impact of the sharing of knowledge bases on the development and use of medical decision support systems is also considered.

Knowledge Based Programs.

In many Hospital Information Systems (HIS) today the ordering physician will receive a suggestion of the interpretation of laboratory tests together with the results. Computer programs, capable of converting numerical results into diagnostic or therapeutic information, have been developed. Many algorithms and mathematical models (Beck et al, 1987) have been applied in these programs to assist in the interpretation of laboratory results. This has increased the efficacy and clinical impact of laboratory tests. It is possible by using traditional programming techniques to transport these algorithms to other laboratory information systems.

In these programs the algorithmic logic or expertise is embedded directly in the computer instruction codes. Contrary to such implicit knowledge, the knowledge based programs have their interpretive and clinical expertise stored separated from the computer program which uses this knowledge to interpret clinical data about a patient.

There are several advantages to this knowledge base approach. A single control program, the "inference engine", can function across broad areas of medical applications if the appropriate expert rules are contained in the knowledge base. The clinical expertise and interpretive rules in the knowledge base can be reviewed, modified and expanded independent of the rest of the application. The clinician doing this is not required to have any programming capability. Any logical errors, biases or miscalculations are exposed and open for inspection by the clinician as well as by the computer scientist. By using the knowledge base approach it is also possible to improve the system by expanding and modifying the knowledge base in a modular fashion.

For the sake of efficiency it is often necessary to compromise between the two methods, but we foresee an ever increasing use of the knowledge base approach and our proposal below how to implement increased knowledge portability refer to this type of systems.

Uniform Representation Of Medical Data.

Transportability of computer programs in general and that of medical knowledge base systems in particular would certainly benefit from having a more uniform language for both the terms per se being used as well as for the decision logic.

There is currently a great lack of any precise conceptual links among related medical information in different machine readable databases. Information files about published literature, clinical record databases, biomedical databank, and knowledge bases all use different schemes for organizing and classifying the data they contain. Clinicians wishing to examine literature relevant to clinical findings retrieved from an automated medical record system or to a diagnosis suggested by an expert system are forced to turn to a different automated system and might have difficulties to make the associations.

The solution to this fundamental medical information problem might lie in the newly started endeavor to develop a Unified Medical Language System or UMLS (Lindberg and Humphreys, 1987) initiated and sponsored by the National Library of Medicine (NLM). The goal is not to impose a single medical vocabulary on all users and systems but to allow the selection of certain UMLS features to interpret questions, identify information sources by providing mappings between vocabularies of medical terms.

A Data Model.

UMLS will be built on a metathesaurus, which will link, merge and integrate MeSH and other thesauri and classification schemes such as SNOMED and ICD as well as terms and concepts from knowledge bases such as HELP, QMR and DXplain. Thus the UMLS metathesaurus will be a kind of synthesis of existing bio-medical nomenclatures (Tuttle et al, 1988).

The metathesaurus will function as a link to the bio-medical literature, and also as a link between different information sources. It is obvious that the UMLS in the future could play the role of metalanguage and act as a bridge between not only different nomenclatures but also different languages.

In the design of a medical information system, the needs of uniform representation of medical nomenclature, medical information and medical knowledge must be taken into consideration. This uniformity may be achieved through the use of a data dictionary, which is compatible with (contains mappings to) the UMLS metathesaurus.

We will briefly outline a suitable data model of a medical information system. The model is based on an infological approach (Tsichritzis and Lochovsky, 1982). The "real world" is represented in an object-oriented way. The objects in this case are all the medical actions performed in a health care unit, as well as the concepts that constitute the medical information stored in the clinical database and the knowledge base.

The model will include not only concrete objects like patients or providers, but also abstract objects like diagnoses and procedures. Time and temporal relationships between objects are important aspects that must be considered.

The medical information system, according to the model, has three main components: the clinical database, the medical knowledge base and the data dictionary. These main components are interconnected by system modules, such as interpreters, query languages, editors, database managers etc.

The medical event is the basic concept of the clinical database and represents a medical action taken by a provider on a patient at a specific time, e.g. a diagnosis, a

Clinical Information System Architecture

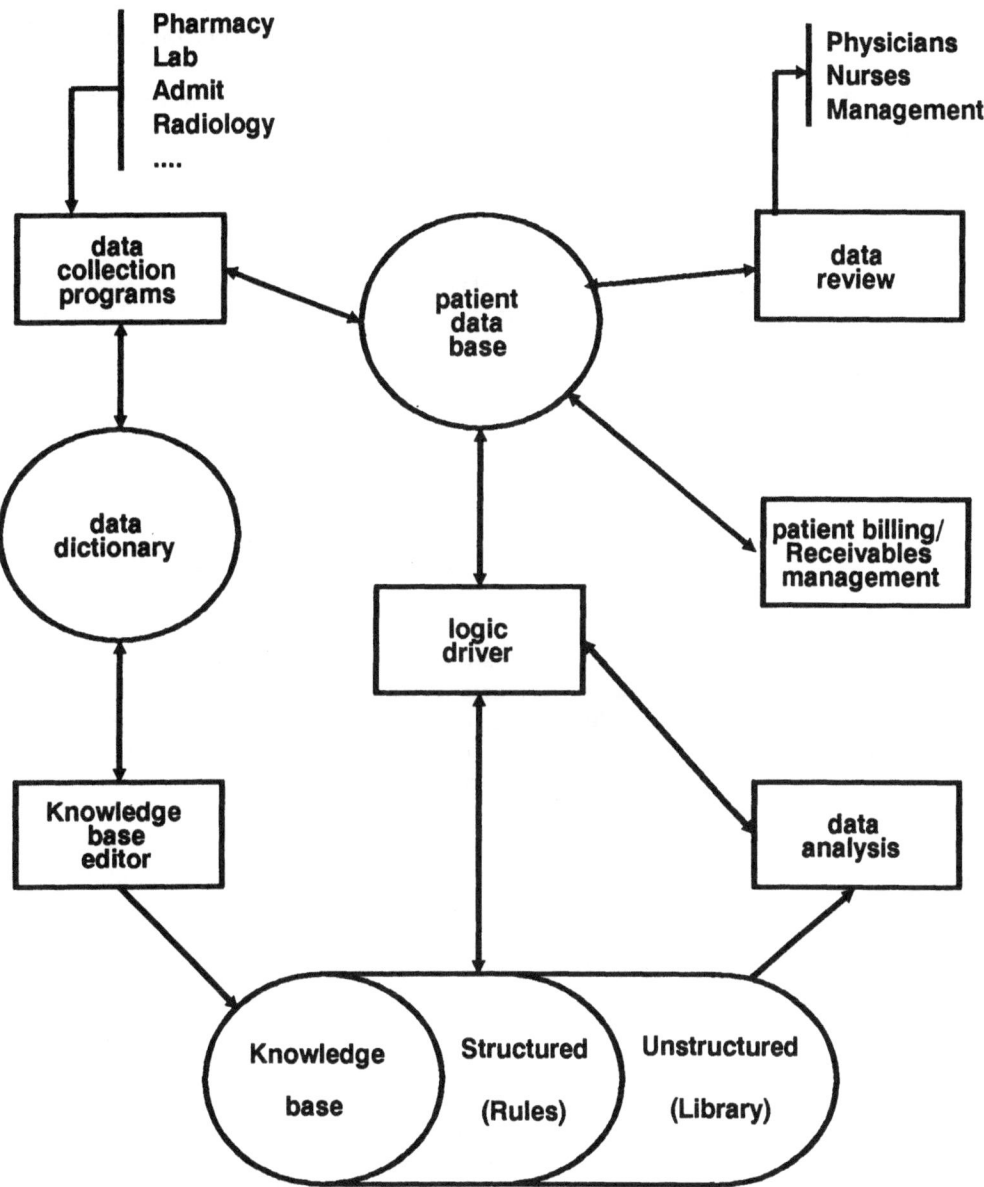

Figure 1: Clinical Information System Architecture.

drug prescription or a laboratory test. The medical event can be regarded as the instantiation in the patient database of a medical term from the data dictionary.

In the model the event is regarded as a relation between a patient, a contact and a medical term. Contact is an encounter, a telephone call or any other notation of a contact between a provider and a patient. The contact and its attributes (provider, date, site, type etc) establish the context in which the medical event takes place.

Let us look at an example. A typical event would be the prescription of digitalis to a patient visiting a health center:

```
EVENT:
          patient          (unit  number = 111111-1111)
          contact          (date = 14 July 1989,
                            site = Health Center,
                            type = scheduled visit,
                            provider = Dr  NN)
          type of event    (drug prescription)
          medical term     (Digoxin)
          attributes       (time = 2 pm,
                            problem = heart failure,
                            value = dose 0.25 mg;
                              frequency 1 daily; quantity 100)
```

The particular event is characterized by a set of properties (attributes) such as the time when it occurred and the value (numeric, textual or other). The corresponding data structure will be stored in the database as a separate unit. Consequently the entire medical record can be regarded as a collection of events, which are specified according to patient, source (provider), time and problem.

Different documents in the medical record, such as the medication list, the laboratory report or progression notes, correspond to different views of this database of events. The medical record content may be presented to the user in the traditional source oriented way with the events arranged according to source and time or it may be presented in a problem oriented way with the events arranged according to which medical problem they are linked to.

The medical terms used in a clinical database or a medical knowledge base form a subset of the entire medical nomenclature. Unfortunately, none of the existing classification schemes of medical terminology has yet been generally accepted. The dictionary, therefore, has to be organized with regard to different taxonomies (ICD, SNOMED, MeSH etc), i.e. each medical term in the dictionary may be mapped to several classifications.

Medical taxonomies all have in common a basic hierarchical structure with two or more axes, thus reflecting the hierarchical structure of matter and nature (Blois,

1984). One of these axes is represented by the level of description or semantic content of the term. Another dimension is part of the body or organ system.

In the model described the data dictionary terms are thought to be organized hierarchically in a rather flat hierarchical structure with two levels. The top level has 10 categories:

1. Anatomy,
2. Organisms,
3. Medical and social history,
4. Symptoms and signs,
5. Physical examination,
6. Laboratory and other diagnostic procedures,
7. Diagnosis,
8. Medication,
9. Therapeutic procedures,
10. Health care.

The second level differs between categories. The categories 1-10 above correspond roughly to the categories A-F and N of MeSH. Categories 3-9 above correspond to the main logical parts of the medical record. The structure described above is the basic medical term hierarchy, which places each term at one and only one location. The needs of the clinical database and the relations to common classification schemes are the main aspects that have been taken into consideration when choosing this structure.

An important characteristic of the model is that an unlimited amount of hierarchies may be included and each term may be located in several different hierarchies, such as MeSH, SNOMED, ICD-9 or any application specific hierarchy.

A Uniform Representation of Medical Knowledge.

For the knowledge base decision support system there is also a need for the development of a uniform, high-level (ASCII) syntax for representing medical expertise used in decision-making that can be used by a wide variety of contributors (Wigertz et al, 1987). Such a syntax could be distributed via a widely available high level editor that could also be run on a variety of personal computers. This syntax would aim to unify major segments of the currently available capability for automated medical decision making. Whereas the current thrust of UMLS is to produce mappings between vocabularies of medical terms, a corresponding Medical Logic Module (MLM) Standard would help to manipulate the medical terms and that will use procedurally oriented modular program code.

Recently a group of experts met to have a workshop at Arden Homestead, N.Y., a Columbia University retreat, to discuss a proposal for a uniform medical logic module standard (Clayton et al, 1989). An example of such a logic module is shown in Fig. 2.

A Medical Logic Module (MLM) is made of a list of slots. A slot contains a slot name that identifies the slot (e.g., "version:"), a slot body that contains the data for the slot (e.g., "1.01"), and a terminating semi-colon.

Slots are grouped into three categories. The first two categories help to maintain a knowledge base of MLMs. The first category, "maintenance:", contains slots that are not related to the medical knowledge in the MLM (e.g., title, version, date). The second category, "library:", contains slots that are related to the medical knowledge in the MLM (e.g., keywords, citations). The third category, "knowledge:", contains the actual medical knowledge of the MLM.

The depicted MLM is identified as being data-driven in the "type:" slot. The "evoke:" slot tells when the MLM should be fired. In this case it will be fired when an absolute neutrophile count is stored in the patient database. The "logic:" slot determines whether an action needs to be performed. Here an action is performed when the patient is taking Trimethoprim/Sulfamethoxazole and the neutrophile count is below 1000 and falling. The "action:" slot contains the MLMs action. In this case it is a message to the physician.

There needs also to be developed a working editor which will accommodate several existing decision making models. Such an editor should produce ASCII coded output, as shown in Fig. 2, which would be suitable both for direct scrutiny by medical personnel who are not required to have programming skills and for translation to one of the supported systems.

Quality Control

The evaluation and validation of the transferable knowledge base are difficult and very important issues. It will be necessary to assess the quality and performance of each MLM and to compare the resulting action, e g the differential diagnosis lists or the medication alerts generated by different modules.

Each author must assume his/hers responsibility for the validity of the contributed module by providing appropriate scholarly references to justify the logical criteria. The contributor should also specify the actual status of the MLM, whether it has been newly developed or has been used and tested in clinical practice.

Empirical validation of the knowledge base will be possible in institutions with patient databases. The MLM could be tested retrospectively against the database in terms of sensitivity and specificity. The problems of false negatives remains an issue, but some databases may be developed in which gold standards are available.

maintenance:
    title: Agranulocytosis and Trimethoprim/Sulfamethoxazole;
    filename: anctms;
    version: 1.01;
    institution: CPMC;
    author: George Hripcsak;
    specialist: ;
    date: 7/20/1989; 8/7/1989;
    validation: research;
    format: USA;
library:
    purpose: To display the Arden Homestead MLM Standard;
    keywords: granulocytopenia;
            agranulocytosis;
            trimethoprim;
            sulfamethoxazole;
    citations:
    1. Anti-infective drug use in relation to the risk
    of agranulocytosis and aplastic anemia. A report
    from the International Agranulocytosis and Aplastic
    Anemia Study. Archives of Internal Medicine, May
    1989, 149(5):1036-40.
    links: CTIM .34.56.78;
         MeSH agranulocytosis/ci and sulfamethoxazole/ae;
knowledge:
    type: data-driven;
    data:
    anc := last 2 of(
     select absolute_neutrophile_count from pt_db
) between now and 1 week before now;
    last_anc := last(anc);
    previous_anc := first(anc);
    bactrim := exist(
     select current_meds from pt_db
     where
      current_meds = trimethoprim_sulfamethoxazole);
    evoke: on storage of anc;
    logic:
    IF bactrim and (last_anc 1000) and (last_anc previous_anc)
     THEN conclude(true);
    action:
    send "Caution: patient's relative granulocytopenia may be
        exacerbated by trimethoprim/sulfamethoxazole."
     to user;

Figure 2: Sample Medical Logic Module.

Discussion.

With the help of a broadly available editor individual users would enter their expertise into the medical knowledge base in the ASCII level representation. This format would also require eventual maps or links to a particular system's native data dictionary. For example the word "fever" in a particular module of decision logic must be mapped into the way information about "fever" is stored in the system in which the logic module will be used. This mapping process would be facilitated by the introduction of the UMLS metathesaurus and also by the adoption of a more uniform data model for the clinical database.

A machine processable representation of medical knowledge could also be a suitable format for library collections just as the knowledge today is stored in books and journal articles. Multiple authors could contribute to and criticize the contents of the knowledge base, libraries could better manage the knowledge, and efforts for validating and evaluating the quality of the knowledge base could be coordinated. Commercial vendors would be expected to support the standard and thereby broaden the base of users and contributors.

The maintenance of the knowledge base is an important issue. To make the maintenance possible each MLM must include some management slots which identify the author, the date it was created, statistics describing prior use and testing, the level of validation reached by the module, references to the medical literature supporting the decision logic, etc. In addition, some classification scheme for knowledge modules must be developed, e.g. a hierarchical organization of the types of medical decisions made. In this way a user can formulate queries about MLM's in an appropriate query language, for example a request to see the most recent MLMs pertaining to heart disease which have passed a given level of validation.

The practice of knowledge base management is in its infancy although individuals have started to address the issues. How do you know that by putting one new MLM in the knowledge base, you won't invalidate the results of other previously tested logic? This problem is especially difficult in the production rule oriented systems and required special programs to be written within the MYCIN system (Suwa et al, 1982). The problem is solved to some extent by the modular nature of the MLMs as opposed to the control issues involved in a production system.

A crucial issue involves the question whether the modular format with combinations of procedural and declarative knowledge that this unified representation would imply would be sufficiently flexible to accommodate enough of the knowledge from existing and developing medical decision-making systems. This approach is obviously insufficient to accommodate the current work on casual networks, but the corpus of currently applicable knowledge appears sufficient to justify the modular approach as an evolutionary step of indefinite duration.

It is also important to ascertain whether individual authors and institutions are willing to share freely their knowledge bases. They might be reluctant to make it too easy to copy specific medical knowledge although no commercial system should ever be used in which the medical knowledge is not transparent, understandable and open for user validation and evaluation. In addition, established institutions might not find the uniform concept worthwhile enough to adapt their current editors to fit the evolving syntax.

Perhaps the largest current obstacle to the distribution of knowledge bases is the liability which may be associated with giving advice to potentially thousands of users. Based upon the experience by the users of the HELP system in Salt Lake City, Utah, USA and the Regenstrief System in Indianapolis, Indiana, USA it was the general consensus of the users that the reminders generated by the system reduced rather than increased the liability for the user. Hence from the user's and institution's point of view, it appears that one must balance the risk between using an imperfect source of assistance versus using nothing at all. We assume that many will choose the imperfect source of assistance and face their attendant risk in order to reduce the overall liability which an institution may face.

In spite of these potential obstacles for sharing expert system knowledge, we think that the alternatives are even more distressing. In essence each laboratory would continue to independently develop its own knowledge base and the ability of non-development sites to acquire medical knowledge would be limited by the capabilities of the particular system which they have purchased.

On the other hand cooperation and the ability to share medical decision support knowledge would greatly promote the development of the field.

References.

Beck JR, Meier FA, Rawnsley HM. Mathematical approaches to the analysis of laboratory data. Prog. Clin. Pathology 1981, 8:67-100.

Blois MS. Information and Medicine. Berkeley and Los Angeles: University of California Press, 1984.

Clayton PD, TA Pryor, OB Wigertz and G Hripcsak. "Issues and structures for sharing knowledge among decision-making systems: The 1989 Arden Homestead Retreat."

Lindberg DAB, Humphreys BL. Toward a Unified Medical Language. Proc MIE 87, Rome Sept. 1987, Vol I, pp 23-31.

Suwa M, Scott AC, Shortliffe EH. Completeness and Consistency in a Rule Based System, AI Magazine, 3:16-21 (Autumn), 1982.

Tsichritzis DC, Lochovsky FH. Data Models. Englewood Cliffs: Prentice-Hall 1982.

Tuttle MS, Blois MS, Erlbaum MS, Nelson SJ, Sherertz DD. Toward a bio-medical thesaurus: building the foundation of the UMLS. Proc Twelfth Ann Symp Computer Applications in Medical Care, Washington, D.C., November 1988. New York: IEEE, 1988:191-5.

Wigertz OB, Clayton PD, Haug PJ, Pryor TA. Design of Knowledge Based Systems for Multiple Use, Truth Maintenance and Knowledge Transfer. Proc MIE 87, Rome Sept. 1987, Vol II, pp 986-991.

Questions from the discussion:

De Vries Robbé: Do you have suggestions how to come to a
common language?

Wigertz: A proposal for a Medical Logic Module Standard will be discussed at an
expert meeting at Columbia University in New York, (Arden Homestead) next
coming June. It is expected that this format will be tested in real experiments to
transfer knowledge, to represent different declarative and procedural knowledge
and to what extent the resulting logic models using this standard will be easily
readable and writeable for application area specialists.

De Vries Robbé: How do you think that the different reasoning strategies, like causal
nets, production systems and abductive reasoning systems fit into one common
knowledge representation?

Wigertz: Hopefully this standard will cover a great deal of different reasoning
strategies particularity logics leading to reminders, alerts etc. Other forms of
reasoning might have to use other representation schemes, but hopefully these
could then be linked with MLMs as subroutines and therefore work well together
in more complex systems.

Breuker: You are proposing a kind of Esperanto for knowledge representation. In
the AI community, this will never work, because each one has its own view on the
problem. Do you think that an Esperanto for knowledge representation can be
achieved in the medical community?

Wigertz: We do hope so and particularly our planned efforts will be able to shed
more light on this question. Do we really differ substantially in reasoning
strategies or is it more a difference in used semantics?

Reliable and reusable tools for medical knowledge based systems

John Fox, Andrzej Glowinski, Mike O'Neil [1]

Imperial Cancer Research Fund LaboratoriesLondon WC2A 3PX

Abstract

The scope for reusing medical knowledge bases across applications is discussed. The construction of knowledge based systems is currently often an ad hoc process, in which knowledge representations and problem solving techniques are freely mixed. This provides flexibility but works against both reusability of knowledge and reliability of designs. A set of standard tools, methods and knowledge bases is required which provides the necessary flexibility based around principles of simplicity, uniformity, maintainability etc. The Oxford System of Medicine exemplifies an approach to reusability in which knowledge bases are decomposed into domain-specific collections of facts, generalised inference schemas, and generalised task control procedures.

Introduction

Work in medical knowledge based systems is growing substantially, though not as rapidly as the interest in the field might suggest. Many clinical researchers informaticians and biomedical engineers who are new to the field but would like to investigate the value of expert systems and other AI methods face considerable obstacles in developing applications. Apart from lack of experience and expertise with the underlying technologies, there is also a shortage of appropriate tools. Although many tools are now available, the biomedical community has specialised requirements. Designers' options are rather limited. They can opt to use a "generic" tool, but medical applications are technically demanding and generic packages may be too restrictive, or lack the specific features that are required for clinical application, or be discouragingly obscure, complicated and/or difficult to master. Alternatively designers can (and still disconcertingly often do) start with some AI or conventional programming language which means they will frequently have to reimplement, or reinvent, standard AI techniques.

---

1   We would like to acknowledge the fire-fighting, life-saving and murk-clearing role played by Saki Hajnal throughout the Oxford System of Medicine project. Colin Gordon has also made many technical and conceptual contributions. We gratefully acknowledge their help.

It is also generally recognised that development of a knowledge base is a heavy consumer of resources. Consequently, we want to be able to reuse components wherever possible. This has proved difficult to achieve (*Hayes-Roth, 1983; Buchanan and Smith, 1988*). Some causes of this problem are recognised and can again be linked to the use of heterogeneous representations.

It would seem desirable to have software which has state-of-the-art expert system capabilities but also provides support for biomedical applications, offering a range of high-level, reusable components which are appropriate for clinical applications. In this paper we shall discuss the goal and potential benefits of a set of reusable knowledge engineering tools for biomedical applications, although space does not allow a full discussion of the wider issues involved. Some of these reusable components may be based around the idea of "generic tasks" in data interpretation (see recent reviews by *Chandrasekaran, 1988, Keravnou and Washbrook, 1989*), but the idea of reusable tools is of course more general. Conventional software tools for building clinical user-interfaces, standardised bodies of knowledge about diseases, drugs etc, and generic methods for reasoning about diagnostic strategies are just a few examples of areas where medically-oriented functions could be designed for reusability.

Reusability of knowledge

It has also been hoped that knowledge from one application might be reused in other applications in the same general domain, though few practical demonstrations of this have been reported. The originators of early expert systems saw potential for reusing components of specific systems on different applications. EMYCIN pioneered reusability in generalising the diagnostic components of the MYCIN package. In practice the scope for reusing expert systems components has not met expectations. While shells of the EMYCIN variety can be used for applications of a single generic type (eg diagnosis) it is now widely thought that they are often too inflexible for tasks which are not easily cast in this form (eg *Alvey 1983*).

A common response to such inflexibility has been to extend the core problem solver in various ways. One method is to combine several problem solvers in a single shell. KnowledgeCraft provides both Prolog and OPS5 interpreters, for example (*Laurent, 1986*). Many packages provide a range of representational tools - for building semantic nets, frame systems, rule sets etc and facilities for incorporating conventional code into the application are normally provided.

This pattern of combining many techniques is commonplace. Even versions of MYCIN used a mixed approach, using inference rules and an associated numerical procedure for calculating certainty factors; frames and a range of datatypes for representing application parameters; attached LISP procedures for calculating drug dosages, and so forth.

On the surface an *ad hoc* approach appears to permit the designer great flexibility. Nevertheless, there is reason to be concerned, particularly in applications which are "safety critical" such as medical applications. Good engineering in any field demands a constant effort to achieve clarity, precision, reliability of design and predictability of behaviour. Heterogeneity tends to work against all of these. This has implications for reliability, soundness and reusability.

Reliability.

- It may be difficult to predict interactions between components which are implemented with different mechanisms.
- It is more difficult to understand and maintain systems over time if a number of formalisms and implementation styles are adopted.

Soundness

- Most knowledge based systems are designed for decision support in which the decision procedure is the central (and possibly safety-critical) component. If the decision mechanisms are distributed over a number of representations or procedures then it may be impossible to establish the procedure's properties (*Fox, 1989*).
- Formal specification of a programme's intended functionality, and demonstration that an implementation reliably satisfies the specification, are more difficult to achieve with heterogeneous designs.
- Evaluations and comparisons of systems are made more difficult where different mechanisms and representations are used. This particularly so where study of individual components is attempted (*O'Neil et al 1990*).

Reusability

- The intended use of knowledge can be implicit in the representation (eg *Clancey, 1981*). The more varied the representations the more likely it is that extraneous assumptions about when the representation is appropriate will be inadvertently incorporated.
- Communities who wish to design compatible systems need technical standards to guide design. Heterogeneity is the enemy of standards.

We advocate an approach to the design of a toolset which uses well understood techniques from classical first-order logic and other generic methods. These are clearly separated from methods which, though still quite general, are domain specific, and the domain facts themselves. Some of these ideas have been developed within an application designed to provide physicians with a wide range of information handling aids, *The Oxford System of Medicine*. We shall first give a brief outline of facilities currently in the OSM (more detail is provided by *Glowinski et al 1989*), then illustrate the general design approach in which the system's knowledge is clearly decomposed into specific medical knowledge and general strategic knowledge.

The Oxford System of Medicine (OSM)

The OSM has been designed as an integrated system to assist general physicians in retrieving information which is relevant to a wide range of clinical problems, and to assist in carrying out diagnosis, investigation, referral, management and many of the other decisions that routinely face the general practitioner. The OSM provides a mixed-initiative interface with the user able to volunteer data, specify a decision, request information from the database, case reviews, explanations, etc at any time. This provides the user with considerable discretion in using the system, and consistent functionality though it may range over the whole of the medical knowledge base and carry out many tasks.

Figure 1 illustrates some of the facilities of a recent version of the OSM. Core interactions with the current OSM are by means of a browser which ranges over the fact base. This can be used for a range of simple database functions on facts, text files, images etc. The browser can treat the database of facts as a network of frame-like objects, or as a flat semantic network, assembling different views of the knowledge base as required. Facilities for decision support are invoked as required, to provide diagnosis, treatment etc. During any task a consistent range of user-interface functions is available on demand, including dynamic menus and checklists, explanations, patient summaries and reviews, recommendations.

All OSM procedures use a uniform method of access to the knowledge base, and in effect have access to all types of declarative knowledge, whether case data, medical knowledge, task knowledge, control knowledge etc. Explanations, for example, are provided by using case-specific facts (the patient history; current decision options; justifications for those options), relevant medical facts (such as "causes of weight loss include cancer") and facts about the current decision task (eg facts which specify the types of information that are relevant for a task, as in "causes of symptoms are relevant to diagnosis"). More details of the functionality of the system are provided by *Glowinski et al, 1989*, and the decision procedure by *O'Neil et al 1989*. The concept of a symbolic decision procedure and its general role in expert systems are discussed in *Fox et al, 1988*, giving special attention to safety critical issues in *Fox, 1990* and to formalising the underlying decision theory in *Fox et al, 1990*. The design has also been independently reviewed by *Keravnou and Washbrook, 1989*, in the context of a discussion of second generation expert systems and the role of generic tasks.

The version of the system discussed here uses a logic language, Props2.5 (*Fox et al 1987*)[2]. This provides a variety of logic-oriented facilities for knowledge engineering, notably a well-defined scheme for integrating goal-driven and data-driven reasoning; truth-maintenance on dynamic data; data-structures and control constructs

---

2   Development effort has recently moved to a version of the OSM which is implemented in Prolog and runs on a PC. This implementation reflects a demand for efficiency, but the design principles described here have been largely adhered to in the new system.

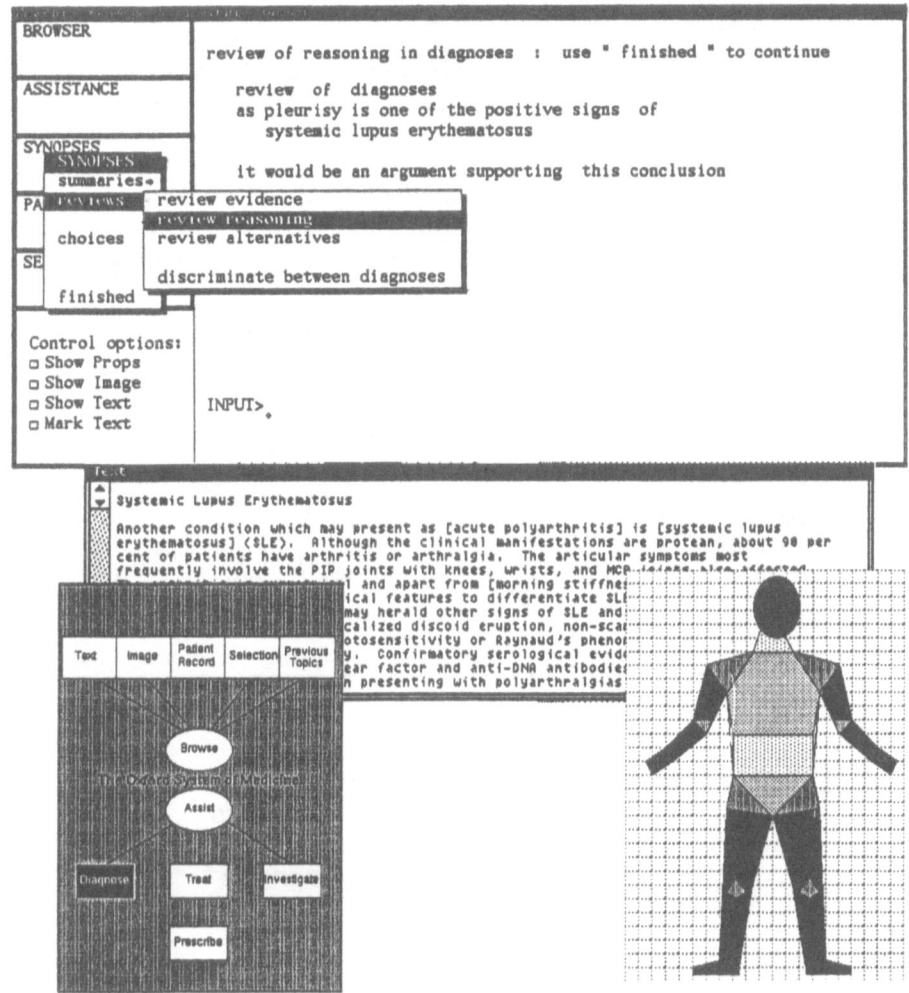

Figure 1: Some of the facilities of a recent version of the OSM. The figure shows the main window (top), with its control panel and pull down menus(top left). Related text appears in another window (centre), with two images which allow a degree of interaction - here help with diagnosis has been requested, followed by an explanation of pleurisy. The body map could be used to indicate the site of the symptoms, using the mouse.

specialised for meta-level reasoning. The user interface or "facade" permits input to Props2 via mouse and keyboard, and configuration of menus, text windows and image canvases as well as dynamically constructed textual and graphical interfaces.

Knowledge engineering in Props2

Figure 2 is a schematic view of the OSM architecture. This illustrates that all system functionality (knowledge base management, decision procedure, user-interface, task control etc) is separated from the specifics of particular medical tasks (diagnosis, treatment, investigation and prescribing) and medical details (such as relationships among, causes and symptoms of particular diseases; costs, formulations and side-effects of particular drugs etc). This is achieved by implementing all system functions as first-order procedures which interrogate a database of simple

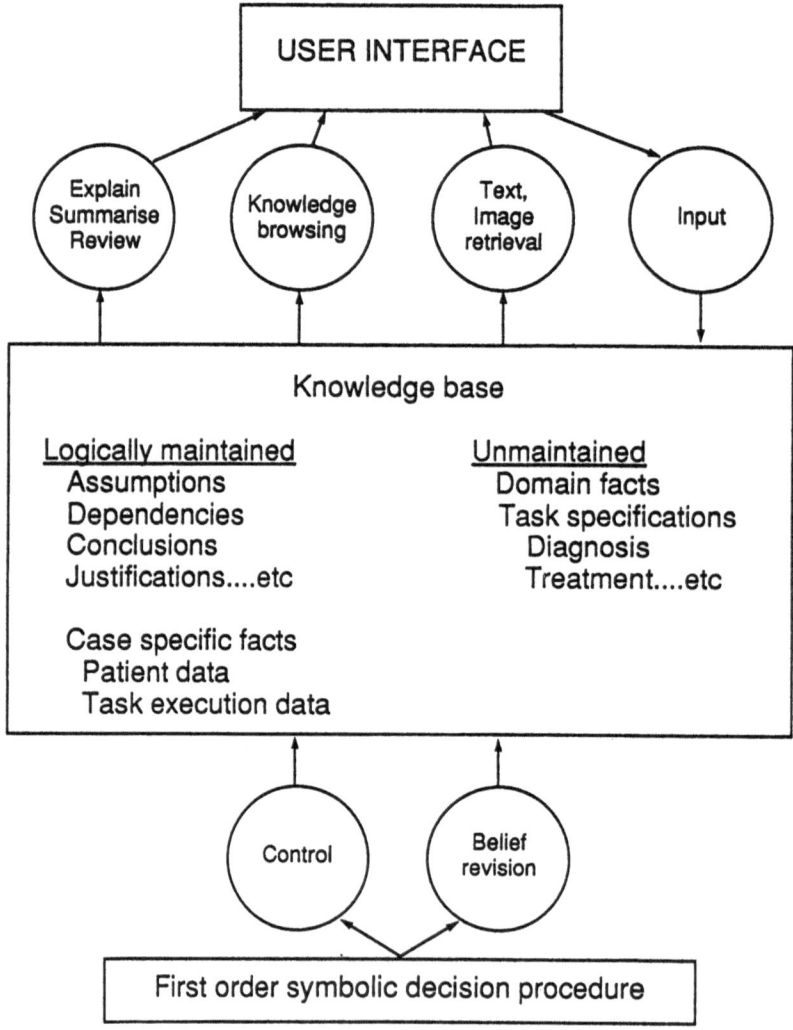

Figure 2: Schematic view of the OSM architecture. Functionality of the system (decison procedure, task control, user interface etc) is separated from tasks and specific medical facts.

facts, and generate a dynamic data base of case-specific facts. Abstraction of functions from knowledge has been long-advocated, particularly in the logic programming community, but not widely exploited in the design of medical knowledge based systems. The abstraction is at the heart of our belief that it is possible to design reliable, maintainable and reusable tools for medical knowledge based systems.

OSM facts are expressed as an unordered collection of sentences. Facts can be independently asserted or retracted from the knowledge base, but are always unique (duplicates are automatically removed by Props2):

> complaints of patient 1 on 23-4-89 include nausea.
>
> subclasses of drugs include analgesics.
>
> steps of diagnosis include refine problem.

Most facts are static, in the sense they are read but not modified by the system, and can be held on an external database management system for retrieval as required (*Gordon and Hajnal, 1989*). Case data, in contrast, are held in immediate memory, because Props2 maintains information about how data were obtained or derived, using a justification based truth maintenance system (JTMS). The JTMS overheads preclude storage in a remote, static database. In principle all facts could be maintained by the JTMS but it is only necessary to carry this overhead for the dynamic parts.

The OSM fact base is intended to be able to grow without limit and yet permit efficient knowledge retrieval and simple maintenance. Current versions of the OSM only include about 10 thousand items of medical knowledge but our goal is to support a very large fact base (say 10 million items). So far, extensions to the medical content of the fact base have proved technically easy, though future revisions in the core representation may be required. All the basic functions of the OSM have been defined in a uniform, generic, rule-based form in which rules can range over the whole fact base. The rule form turns out to be quite compact; the full set of decision making, information retrieval and user interface capabilities of the OSM are captured by less than 100 rules. These are of two types; classical inference rules, and simpler "triggered" rules. Loosely speaking inference rules maintain the set of "beliefs" which are consistent with the clinical case data, while trigger rules cause "actions" to be carried out.

Inference rules can be invoked in a data-directed or goal-directed way. In the following example the rule can spontaneously make an inference when a symptom appears or be used to establish symptoms in response to a query concerning possible diagnoses.

> if complaints of Patient on Date include Symptom
>   and causes of Symptom include Cause
> then possible diagnoses of Patient on Date include Cause.

Rules are "generic" in the sense that they use logical variables (indicated by capitalised atoms) which acquire values at run-time and variables are constrained to be consistently bound[3]. Rules are interpreted as universally quantified; ie will generate the full set of interpretations when data-driven or the full set of solutions when goal-driven. (Note the example has been selected to introduce Props2 syntax and is not taken from the OSM.)

Triggered rules have the same form as inference rules but are intended to satisfy a requirement for event-driven rather than inference-oriented computation. They can only be used in forward (data-driven) mode and the consequences of execution are not maintained by the JTMS.

Reusable logical procedures

Perhaps the fundamental role of the inference component of medical knowledge based systems is to provide assistance in making decisions. We have argued elsewhere (*Fox 1990, Fox et al 1990*) that this decision procedure should be "an explicit representation of the knowledge required to define, organise and make a decision, and is a logical *abstraction* from the qualitative and quantitative knowledge that is required for any specific application. A symbolic decision procedure may include a specification of when and how the procedure is to be executed." J-L Renaud-Salis has reimplemented the SENEX breast cancer protocol advice system (*Renaud-Salis, 1987*) within the OSM decision strategy and believes that it should offer a generic framework for many other cancer protocols (*personal communication, 1989*). The framework has also been adapted for use in a system for biomedical image interpretation.

To date we have explored the reusability of monotonic and non-monotonic reasoning in decision making. We shall only give sufficient examples here to illustrate the notion of reusable inferences as more extensive descriptions are given elsewhere (*Fox et al, 1988, Fox, 1989*, and *O'Neil et al, 1989*).

Monotonic deduction.

So far most medical expert systems have exploited monotonic inference in a propositional logic, since general principles of medical reasoning are hard to find and much medical knowledge has been thought to consist of collections of special case rules. On the contrary, we think that it is possible to identify "deductive cliches" which can be expressed as first-order inference rules. The diagnosis rule given above for example abstracts a general inference rule about symptoms and causality from specific details of medicine. Consequently the same rule can be used in an indefinite number of diagnostic situations. In the OSM we have taken abstraction further, in order to generalise over *decision tasks* and different kinds of *logical argument* as well

---

3   The handling of logical variables uses the unification mechanism of Prolog, in which Props2 is implemented.

as the medical details of a specific decision. The following rule captures a general strategy for reasoning, which is generalised across different types of decision task and the different types of argument which are relevant to those decisions:

> if observations of Patient on Date include Observation
> > and supporting arguments in Decision include Attribute
> > and provable arguments of Option include Attribute of Observation
>
> then confirmed supporting arguments of Decision of Option include Attribute of Observation

Which may be instantiated (informally) to the following argument

> "if we observe that Fred Smith has weight loss, and we know that causal information can be used to support a diagnosis, then any disease which could cause the weight loss is supported in this case".

In fact the rule yields case-specific facts of the following form:

> confirmed supporting arguments of cancer include possible cause of weight loss

This rule uses a form of causal reasoning but is more general than that. In fact such rules are sufficiently generalised that they can be reused across a range of decisions, in a variety of medical contexts, and we believe they can exploit an indefinite number of medical theories. The example above represents one of the five components of the OSM decision procedure, each of which can be expressed in one or a small number of such rules. The example rule plays the same role in diagnosis, treatment and investigation decisions, and can participate in all such decisions simultaneously. More details of logical reasoning for decision making are given in *Fox et al, 1990* and *O'Neil et al 1989*.

Non-monotonic deduction.

Inference in the OSM is principally achieved by forward chaining. This characteristic aids implementation of spontaneous (non-deterministic) problem solving and mixed initiative user interfaces. However since the system is constantly generating new facts during this process, some of which may subsequently prove to be mistaken, a JTMS permits retraction of all conclusions and their dependencies if and when this occurs.

A non-monotonic cliche that generalises over diagnostic, treatment and investigation-selection decisions illustrates how context-specific inferences (about which we may change our minds) can be linked to the standard dynamic form.

> if confirmed Arguments of Option include Argument of Observation
> > and context is Decision of Problem of Patient on Date
> > and eliminated Decision of Patient do not include Option
>
> then possible Decision of Patient include Option.

Which says:

> "if there is at least one reason to consider a particular decision (a diagnosis, treatment or investigation) and no reason to exclude it at a particular time, then that diagnosis, treatment or investigation should be considered as a *possible* option" *at that time*.

This rule maintains the set of all decision options during decision making, dynamically and automatically. If at any time the system concludes that an option is eliminated the mechanism automatically retracts the possibility, and all inferences which logically depend upon it, and regenerates the dynamic knowledge base in a form that is consistent with the revised set of possible options (see box below).

Some remarks on abduction and induction

There is growing discussion presently on the use of non-classical modes of reasoning in knowledge based systems, notably abduction (the process of generating hypotheses) and induction (the process of creating generalisations). It seems to us however that the terms are increasingly being used in ways that are misleading, and facing them clearly is important for the reusability issue. For example many expert systems contain propositional inference rules of the form:

> if weight loss is present & age of patient is elderly
> then possible diagnoses include cancer.

and

> if possible diagnoses include gastric cancer
> then possible diagnoses include cancer.

The first type of rule is sometimes called abductive (because it introduces a hypothesis) and the second an induction (because it introduces a generalisation). Abduction and induction are of logical interest because, following C S Peirce, they have been considered to involve inference processes which cannot be supported by conventional deduction. There are at least two reasons for the difficulty. First, hypothesis formation is about constructing hypotheses and induction about discovering generalisations. Rules like those above embody known facts; they create nothing. In fact the inference mechanism they require is entirely deductive and non-classical inference modes are not required. Second, as Peirce emphasised, abduction and induction are essentially "fallible" in his language or "non-monotonic" in ours. Classical deduction is monotonic, which is to say that conclusions drawn are held to be valid for all time; non-monotonic reasoning is theoretically problematic from the classical point of view. However the special case rules above raise no such difficulties. Since they embody predetermined implications and generalisations then they introduce hypotheses and generalisations, but deductively.

The main deductive components developed for the OSM, which we believe will be reusable in other applications include:

Decision making:
 proposing decision options (diagnoses, treatments, investigations, etc)
 arguing the pros and cons of decision options
 logical and quantitative evaluation of decision options
 assembly of related options into graph-like structures

Knowledge management
 non-monotonic frame editor
 integrity checks during editing
 multiple inheritance

Reusable procedural tools

This section discusses some simple reusable components developed as part of the OSM architecture, such as user interface managers and other action-oriented processes, such as those indicated at the top of figure 2. These are distinct from logical processes in the following sense; logical computations deal with the derivation and maintenance of consistent *beliefs* while triggered computations are more concerned with taking *actions*. Action-oriented computations are naturally ephemeral, that is their purpose is to *have an effect at some point in time* rather than to acquire new facts or beliefs. Consequently we need not incur logical overheads such as consistency or truth maintenance[4]. We achieve this capability in Props2 by declaring that some classes of pattern or sentence should not be treated as facts or beliefs, but rather as events or "triggers". When a trigger clause in a rule matches an input, and all other conditions of the rule are at that moment satisfied in the database then the consequent side of the rule is executed. At the end of execution the triggering data are lost.

We can illustrate the use of action-oriented processing by considering the control of decision making and user interaction in the OSM. Three types of process are

---

4 Triggered rules have the same surface form as logical inference rules but we have found it useful to observe an additional convention to reflect the typical message-passing role. The trigger antecedent uses a standard form consisting of a message and the source of the message:
   Source | Message.
   For example if the message comes from a user interface channel then the Source indicates which one (eg "graphics window" or "text window"). The message may name a menu item (see below) or embody a more complicated message, such as "mouse left at x-44 y-55". The Source management software may be foreign code and/or hardware specific but all such programmes are constrained to communicate with the standard components using messages of the standard form. We do not suggest that this is the only standard message format that could be used, nor even that it is the most desirable. It is used merely because it is simple enough to illustrate the approach.

distinguished, asynchronous processing; synchronous processing and task processing.

Asynchronous processing.
All rules can be data driven and can operate asynchronously. In effect any rule, whether an inference rule or a triggered rule, can and typically does operate in a data-driven mode. In principle all asynchronous rules can fire in parallel.

Synchronised processing.
Decision making and other processes require sequential execution, either because processes compete for use of restricted resources (such as the user interface) or because one process may be constrained to begin only after some other process has been completed. Triggered rules can be used to schedule processes that require synchronisation.

Task processing.
The symbolic control procedure of the OSM is decomposed into a set of abstract rules and specific facts about particular tasks (*Glowinski et al 1989, Fox et al 1990*). The term "task" is widely used in AI, though without standard meaning. We use the term here to mean a synchronous process which has explicit initiation and termination conditions, and whose execution can be modified as the process runs.

These explicit conditions form a specification, which may be roughly divided into two parts. The first, used by scheduling mechanisms, is concerned with running the task. This includes its decomposition into simpler subtasks, and constraints that may affect both the task and each individual subcomponent. The order in which these subcomponent processes are to be executed, although predefined in outline, may be altered as a result of the changing conditions as a task progresses.

For a process to be carried out, a number of preconditions may have to be satisfied. There may be a requirement that all the necessary information be available (eg conditional probabilities for a Bayesian calculation, as discussed in *Fox et al, 1988*). Execution may be initiated by way of an external signal, such as a request from the user, or if a particular set of criteria are satisfied. For instance, detailed assessment of specific risk factors could be started as a result of suspicions raised by automatic monitoring of a patient record. Termination conditions may be similarly defined. Hence, if further processing is incapable of providing a solution, or making the decision becomes inappropriate, execution of the process may be automatically halted.

In addition to scheduling the individual components it is necessary to provide information as to how each component is to be executed within the confines of a particular task. This part of the specification essentially deals with the way these processes interact with other components of the system, such as the database of medical facts, the patient record, etc. Included in this part of the specification will be the criteria upon which a decision is based - for instance, an instantiation for the second line of the rule example given in the section on monotonic deduction:

... and supporting arguments in Decision include Attribute

instantiates to

... supporting arguments in diagnosis include causes

This statement does not relate to a particular diagnosis or cause, but provides the decision making process with the template required to interrogate the database for medical facts relevant to the current problem. In addition, the circumstances in which these criteria apply can be explicitly stated, for instance minor side effects of a drug can be disregarded in life threatening situations.

This form of task specification has a number of important consequences. Specifications may be dynamically altered during the course of processing, allowing changes both to the way in which the task is carried out and the criteria used during execution. Alternative strategies may be adopted if the initial approach fails (eg. selecting other methods of assessment in the face of incomplete data sets, as mentioned above).

It has proved possible to implement most of the basic building-blocks required for task management in the OSM using a combination of deductive and triggered rules. Typically the implementations require only a small number of rules which, if this is confirmed in other applications, has significant benefits for maintainability. Among the general (and reusable) facilities we have implemented in this way are

- context management mechanisms - keeping track of what is happening in a task
- data entry - interpretation of input in light of the current context
- a frame-oriented browsing utility
- text retrieval mechanism - sensitive to the context of the retrieval request
- dynamic menu building and display
- process scheduler (see above)

In addition, task specifications are small collections of facts, containing general information rather than case specific data. Again, this promises simpler maintenance and reusability: for instance, the specification of a decision can be used as a template for editing and checking the database of medical facts.

Reusable databases

All generalised procedures require domain specific knowledge for application. In medicine the facts about diseases, symptoms and so on may be the major components in terms of scale and in terms of development cost. It is highly desirable that these fact bases should be standardised in form and content, and also be reusable.

The principle fact sets that we have investigated deal with:

- drugs (based on information from a standard formulary: British National Formulary);

- disease taxonomy (based on a standard classification: ICD 9);
- procedures/investigations (based on national/international classifications: ICPM; OPCS4)
- illustrative fragments of investigation and treatment taxonomies (locally developed)
- anatomy knowledge (local)
- symptoms and signs, their causes and associations (local)
- indications and contraindications of investigations and treatments (local)
- lexicons of medical terms compiled from these diverse sources

We have explored a range of areas in which it would be valuable to have well developed fact databases. We do not know how general, and hence reusable, these collections of facts are but it seems that some of the principle obstacles to reuse like heterogeneous and idiosyncratic knowledge representations, and the confounding of problem-solving and task control information with domain-specific knowledge have been significantly reduced.

Conclusions

To summarise, we are interested in the potential for reusing knowledge on different applications. The OSM project has allowed us to investigate a style in which factual information and strategic knowledge are sharply separated into an extensional database of facts and a set of generalised inference rules and procedures. In general our conclusion is that this decomposition is highly simplifying in a number of ways which are central to achieving reliability and reusability. To summarise

(a) Task models are succinct, aiding clear definition and formalisation.

(b) The strategy base can be kept small thereby simplifying maintenance of the medical knowledge base.

(c) Storage of medical facts (about drugs, diseases, investigations etc) can take advantage of database management technology.

(d) Task specifications can be used to guide the acquisition of new knowledge and in automated integrity and consistency checking.

(e) The extensional knowledge based can be given additional uses by defining new tasks.

New applications are developed by designing new rule sets which use the medical knowledge base in some new way. No doubt it will prove impossible to avoid specific tailoring of knowledge bases entirely, but our belief is that maintenance and development will be much simplified by this approach.

References

Alvey, P A: The problems of designing a medical expert system, in Proceedings of Expert Systems 83, Churchill College, Cambridge, 1983.

Buchanan B G, Smith R G: Fundamentals of expert systems, Ann Rev. Comput. Sci., 3, pp. 23-58, 1988.

Chandrasekaran, B: Generic tasks as building blocks for knowledge based systems: the diagnosis and routine design examples, Knowledge Engineering Review, 3, pp. 183-210, 1988.

Clancey, W J: NEOMYCIN: Reconfiguring a rule-based expert system for application to teaching, Proc. Seventh International Conference on Artificial Intelligence, pp. 829-836. Vancouver, 1981.

Fox, J: Symbolic procedures for knowledge based systems, in H Adeli (ed) The handbook of knowledge engineering, New York: McGraw-Hill 1989.

Fox, J: Automated reasoning for safety critical decisions, Phil. Trans. Roy. Soc. (in press), 1990.

Fox J, Clarke D A, Glowinski A J, O'Neil M: Using predicate logic to integrate qualitative reasoning and classical decision theory, IEEE Transactions, Systems, Man and Cybernetics (in press).

Fox J, Duncan T, Frost D: The Props 2 Primer, Imperial Cancer Research Fund Technical Report, London, 1987.

Fox J, O'Neil M, Glowinski A J, Clarke D A: Decision making as a logical process, in B Kelly and A Rector (eds) Research and Development in Expert Systems V, Cambridge, Cambridge University Press, 1988.

Glowinski A J, O'Neil M, Fox J: Design of a generic information system and it application to primary care, in J Hunter (ed) Proceedings of 2nd European Conference on AI in Medicine. Berlin: Springer Verlag, 1989.

Gordon C, Hajnal S: OSMDBASE: a database package for the Oxford System of Medicine, Imperial Cancer Research Fund Technical Report, London, 1989.

Hayes-Roth F, Waterman D, Lenat D (eds): Building Expert Systems, Reading, Mass.: Addison Wesley, 1983.

Keravnou E, Washbrook J: What is a deep expert system?, Knowledge Engineering Review (in press), 1989.

Laurent: Comparative evaluation of three expert system tools: KEE, Knowledge-Craft, Art, Knowledge Engineering Review, 1, pp. 18-29, 1986.

O'Neil M, Glowinski A J, Fox J: A symbolic theory of decision-making applied to several medical tasks", in J Hunter (ed) Proceedings of 2nd European Conference on AI in Medicine. Berlin: Springer Verlag, 1989.

O'Neil M, Glowinski A J, Fox J: Evaluating and validating very large knowledge based systems, Medical Informatics (in press), 1990.

Renaud-Salis J-L, Bonichon F, Durand M, Avril A, Lagarde C, Serre J P, Mendiboure P: The Senex system: A microcomputer-based expert system built by oncologists for breast cancer management", in J Fox, M Fieschi, R Engelbrecht (eds) European Conference on AI in Medicine. Berlin: Springer Verlag, 1987.

The MEDES Subshell: Towards an Open Architecture for Decision Support Systems

Pieter F. de Vries Robbé, Pieter E. Zanstra, Wim P.A. Beckers

University Hospital Groningen, Dept. of Medical Information and Decision Science, Groningen, The Netherlands

Abstract

A knowledge based system concept is presented which enables the construction of decision support systems tailored for a specific application. This concept comprises three layers, a basic low level inference engine, a so-called subshell, and the knowledge base. The function of the subshell is to provide on the one hand a data model of representing (scientific) knowledge, and on the other hand to implement a high level reasoning model. The significance of the subshell concept is to further separate reasoning algorithms from knowledge representation. As the structure for knowledge representation and the reasoning mechanisms are explicitly defined in the subshell a very open and flexible system is created.

Introduction to MEDES

Based on an extensive investigation of existing medical expert systems it was concluded that these systems were lacking facilities for adequately substantiating their conclusions (*de Vries, and de Vries Robbé, 1985*). In order to be acceptable for the user, a conclusion should be explained in terms of knowledge rather than visualise the steps along which that conclusion was reached.

In contrast to expert systems, which apparently were built from the viewpoint of performing a limited task in a specific domain (e.g. *Hupp et al, 1986, Kingsland et al, 1983*), MEDES is primarily based on a thorough investigation of information needs of medical decision making in general. The ultimate goal of our research is to supply medical professionals with a tool which enables their decision making to be based rather on logic than on association. As such the research presented here is a further development along the lines also presented by for example *Miller et al, 1982 and Davis, 1983*. Central to the MEDES concept is that the user of the system should be the centre of control, having various ways to exploit the knowledge base. The first version of the system has become available in the spring of 1988.

In preliminary experiments MEDES not only appeared to be useful for developing a support system for daily routine operation in a PA lab, it also serves as a very versatile testbed for experimentation on knowledge representation schemata, and the related medical reasoning procedures. These experiments also revealed that medical professionals outside our research group only needed little training and support to build systems for their domain, thus reducing the role of the hard to get knowledge engineer.

Global System Design

Though the primary task of the MEDES project was the design of a structure for medical decision support, a more general basic system for representing and reasoning about knowledge has been developed. The knowledge representation strongly resembles that of a semantic network, with the limitation that only a specific set of well defined types of relations are allowed. This limitation in the types of relations is of practical rather than of a principal nature, as for every relation type it's role in the reasoning process must be explicitly declared.

Only binary relations between two nodes are employed at this moment. In MEDES the relation is the basic piece of knowledge, whereas the nodes merely serve as identifiers for the concepts about which reasoning takes place. The whole knowledge base can be considered as a connected graph. Every concept (node) is connected to others by one or more relations (links) of different type. The nodes themselves are not explicitly typed. The type of a node is determined at inference time depending on the role it plays. For instance 'increased blood pressure' can act as a value as well as a variable. It depends on the type of links activated in the inference process, which of the two interpretations holds true.

The general knowledge processor features basic building blocks for constructing knowledge representation schemata as well as a collection of primitive inference functions on the knowledge graph for the declaration of types of queries. Basically the inference is finding those paths in the knowledge graph which conform to criteria specified in the query to the system.

The link types which are available for representing knowledge are declared in a so-called subshell. This part of the system also contains the specification of the high level reasoning process. The MEDES system as a whole consists of three layers:

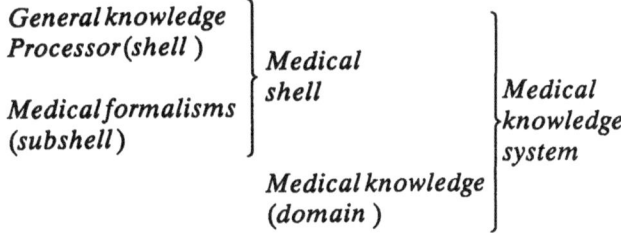

Figure 1: MEDES is built upon a general knowledge processor. In the subshell the structure and semantics of types of knowledge are user definable. The shell together with the medical formalisms make up a shell specific for the field of medicine. This shell can subsequently be filled with medical knowledge.

Knowledge Representation

The focus of our research on knowledge representation is the semantic level rather than the syntactic aspects. A set of about twenty link types for representing medical knowledge has been devised. The types in use are for instance those dealing with nosological representation (has feature, is a kind of), for representing (patho)physiological processes (causes, is value of), epidemiological data (correlates with, is followed by), but also for instance structural knowledge (is a part of, has location). The actual semantics of the link types is determined by the way they are utilized in the (medical) reasoning process. As will be shown below, this utilization is explicitly defined in the queries.

It must be realized that in MEDES different types of links are specified in the subshell. So they are open to user alteration. When the types of links are changed, the high level reasoning (queries) must be changed accordingly. Though we do have a practical set of link types for medicine, this set is not to be considered fixed.

For the domain expert the interpretation of link types needs to be described. For example the causal link (CS) mentioned in figure 2 could be described as follows: The link is directed from cause to effect, the interpretation is that the cause may render the effect. A causal link implicitly means there is in time a 'followed-by' (FB) link. There also is implicitly a 'correlation' (CI) link. In addition we also describe those link types that are not allowed in parallel to the causal link. Examples of these are characterization links (HF) and influence links (FL). When there are more then one incoming or one outgoing causal link from a node these have a logical OR interpretation.

In general, the domain expert should use the richest link type when entering knowledge. This is beneficial, as in the inference e.g. the causal link may then also be used to be part of a chain of 'followed-by' links.

The link not only has an indication of its type, but it is also possible to further specify the link by defining attributes. Next to Links and Nodes, the Attribute is the only basic building block for MEDES. In the MEDES subshell one is free to define any kind of attribute. However in our opinion the use of the attribute must be restricted to those pieces of knowledge that do not have a meaning on their own. So certain links may have one or more frequency attributes, but the attribute should e.g. never be used to connect 'high blood pressure' to 'blood pressure'. Also the Nodes can have a type indication, and attributes. The links between nodes are however in our opinion the basic elements of knowledge representation

Now consider the relation 'A causes B'. We may indicate how often B is found given the existence of A (HFREQ), but it may very well be the case that the frequency the other way around (TFREQ) does not have the same value. This problem can be solved by either using two links of opposite type, or by using two frequency attributes. The latter solution offers a more coherent approach. The definition in MEDES of such a causal relationship is given in figure 2.

As can be seen from this definition, all the elements in the knowledge base have type declaration. On the right hand side of figure 2 the description of one of the frequency attributes is depicted, including all permissible values. Once declared this TFREQ attribute can be used in the definition of other link types as well. Using such enumeration attributes facilitates a more consistent way of handling attributes. Here

Name : CS
Type: LINK
Text: CAUSES
Attributes:
    hfreq: HFREQ
    tfreq: TFREQ
    time: TIME
    synchr: SYNCHR

Name: TFREQ
Type: ATTR
Possible values:
    Never
    Sometimes
    Commonly
    Mostly
    Always

Figure 2: Link type 'causes' has been declared on the left hand side of the figure. On the right, one of the attribures (TFREQ) of the CS link is further specified.

the attribute values were arbitrarily chosen on a five point scale. Other scales can be used equally well. As of yet no calculus is available in MEDES for operations on combinations of such attributes. They are currently merely used as criterion to stop a low level inference on a link meeting that criterion.

Only few knowledge representation systems have such a strict knowledge type declaration, nevertheless we feel there are convincingly strong arguments to implement this declaration of types. Amongst others these are:

- The typing mechanism forces the domain expert to organize his knowledge base properly. Typing provides for a structuring tool.
- Typing opens the possibility of consistency checking of a knowledge base.
- The typing mechanism speeds up the inference process by dividing the universe, which reduces the search space.
- Provided proper inference mechanisms, one is sure that all the stored knowledge is in the reach of the user.

Reasoning

From our investigations it appeared that practising physicians are not intuitively appealed by the various decision analytic techniques. Their problem mainly is to have the right knowledge in the right time at their disposal, in order to be aware of all the possibly existing patient problems. From there in a cyclic process of examinations, diagnosing and therapy, the problems will be dealt with. This means there are various kinds of information needs. Support may be given for differential diagnosis, but also for therapy and prognosis, or things like possible findings when there is a suspicion for a certain disease. It is clear that different types of knowledge can play a role in answering these queries.

A dependency such as 'diagnosis of' may be inferred on a nosological basis by searching the relevant 'has feature' paths, or on a pathophysiological basis by searching along 'causal' links. The actual query 'diagnosis of' uses more different types of links. An example is given in figure 3. The procedure shown there not only searches for a single diagnosis explaining all findings, but also shows those diagnoses explaining some of the findings. The two letter combinations between [] indicate the different link types involved in this particular implementation of the query.

```
InputNodes ('Findings',LIST OF NODES,List_1)
Connections (List_1,[CI,CS,HF,DB,KO],[CI],List_2)
GetMarkedItems ([node common],List_2)
ReverseList (List_2)
OutputNodes ('Differential diagnosis',List_2)
```

Figure 3:   Example of the declaration of a simple diagnostic query: 'Differential diagnosis, all combinations'

For understanding the queries in MEDES one must realize that the procedure is basically to instantiate a patient specific sub-graph from the whole knowledge graph. In the first line of figure 3, the system will prompt for 'Findings' of the patient which are stored in List_1 by the primitive 'InputNodes'. In the next primitive 'Connections' starting with the nodes in List_1, all incoming links of type CI (correlation), CS (causes), HF (has feature), DB (defined by), and KO (is a kind of), as well as all outgoing links of type CI are instantiated. This recursive procedure that searches the whole knowledge graph, is central to the query. The Connections primitive also marks certain items. There are three kinds of markings: a) The input nodes (nodes); b) All nodes that can be reached along two or more paths from a single input node (self); c) Nodes that can be reached from two or more input nodes (common).
From List_2 GetMarkedItems selects only those items marked as node or as common. The resulting sub-graph is again written in List_2. ReverseList reverses the order of the resulting sub-graph. The OutputNodes primitive displays first the common node(s) explaining the patient findings, then a graph leading to those findings is displayed

Though in the query definition operations are performed on lists, in fact these are structured lists, and should hence conceptually be viewed as sub-graphs. In addition to the primitives used in the above query definition, there are several more that operate on the instantiated sub-graph. Amongst these are primitives that deal with intersection, difference and unification of lists.

Examples of Reasoning Strategies in the Medical Domain

Though most current medical expert systems give diagnostic support, the design of a routine for diagnosis is not trivial. There are several diagnostic strategies. Therefore we can distinguish various options for the construction of a so called differential diagnosis. A differential diagnosis is a set of diseases which are to be considered as possibly present in a patient in who some findings are present. The sort of differential diagnosis a physician is interested in is dependent on the stage of his diagnostic of therapeutic task. At the time of this writing we have implemented the construction of the following differential diagnostic sets:

● **diseases explaining all findings**

This kind of differential diagnosis is to be seen as following a rule which is learned to young beginning physicians: Consider if possible one disease which covers all symptoms instead of considering diseases for every symptom. The reason for this rule is that one disease is more probable than a combination of diseases. This is generally true if you assume that every disease is likely probable. You could see this as committing the base rate fallacy, but you could see it as a practical heuristic rule as well.

● **diseases explaining subsets of findings**

This kind of differential diagnosis is wanted if completeness is required and every disease which covers one or more findings has to be considered. A physician is interested in this set if he has no idea what to think about a patient with some findings. In general this list is rather large and consequently is of limited use.

● **diseases at least to explain any finding**

This kind of differential diagnostic set is required as a stage in the construction of all covering combinations of diseases. It consists of those diseases which have to be considered at least to cover all the findings. There are some findings which are called pathognomonical findings which can only be covered by one single explanation. These findings are used to construct this kind of differential diagnosis.

● **primary and secondary diseases**

This kind of diagnosis is required if a physician is interested in a special type of diagnosis. An orthopedic surgeon is primarily interested in bone-diseases and not in lung pathology. So he will consider the diseases in his field as primary diagnoses. However, to get a covering combination he has sometimes to consider lung diseases too.

● **common classes of the possible diseases**

This kind of diagnosis is required if there are diseases which cover each some symptoms but not all. To get suggestions for e.g. further examinations, a common disease class is an important cue e.g. both diseases belong to a same organic system the lung, or the immune system or happen to occur on the same localisation.

These different differential diagnostic options are required by physicians for their task. So in MEDES a differentiated support for differential diagnosis has been constructed.

A full description of the definition of all developed queries is beyond the scope of this paper. However, it can be seen that the primitive inference functions are so powerful that the declaration of a 'differential diagnosis' query only takes a few lines of code. Typical subshells will contain a number of different queries, not only regarding differential diagnosis.

From the above it can be seen that the subshell makes a typical medical shell from a general knowledge processor. The open structure renders it possible to provide for specific tasks to be handled by the system. Apart from the diagnosis query mentioned above also queries for screening, therapy, prognosis, examination strategy etc have been defined.

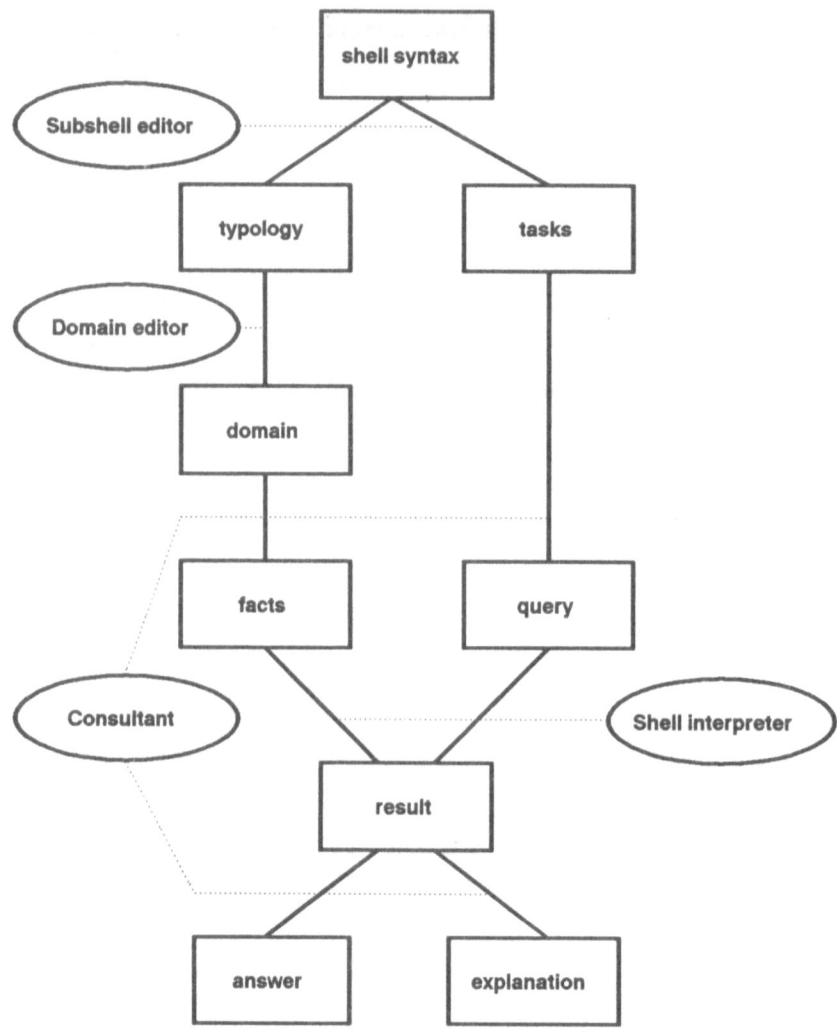

Figure 4:   MEDES conceptual structure.

Types of Users

Three different types of users result from the structure presented here. The modes of use and their place in the system is shown in figure 4. Primarily there is the end-user, the practising physician who can utilize the system for patient related advise, but also browse through the knowledge as if using a textbook.

For building systems we discern two types of users. First there is the domain expert, who can be any knowledgeable (medical) professional entering the knowledge of his domain in the system. The second is what we call the expert in 'formal medicine'. The latter must have a deep insight on a meta level in medical knowledge and reasoning. He is responsible for defining in the subshell the different types of relations (typology) for representing knowledge and the reasoning algorithms (tasks).

Using the knowledge base editor, the domain expert can make various knowledge bases which are defined on one single subshell. It also is equally well possible to design more than one subshell for a certain knowledge base structure. With this respect we envisage next to the obvious consultation subshells, the construction of a subshell specifically designed to perform consistency checking. For this one might think of queries which e.g. first search for missing epidemiological data, and that subsequently generate a query to a literature retrieval system.

Though the subshell can readily be changed, we think that in time a certain saturation in the need for new types of relations develops. The same holds true for the types of queries to be asked from the system albeit at a later moment.

This contrasts with domain knowledge which has to be continually extended, but also existing knowledge collections have to be adapted to recent scientific developments. To cope with the enormous problems arising from the maintenance of large knowledge bases, there is a need for a well defined standard for knowledge representation.

Conclusions

The subshell concept presented here facilitates building of well structured knowledge bases. Knowledge represented according to this paradigm is open for various methods of reasoning, thus rendering an effective tool for designing decision support. The explicit definition of data structures and reasoning processes is a major contribution of the MEDES project.

Considering the architecture which makes it easier to implement medical reasoning procedures these tool facilities enable the design of different reasoning strategies. The uniqueness of the MEDES concept opens the possibility to comfortable comparison of different reasoning strategies on basis of the same data.

References

Davis, R. (1983) Diagnosis via causal reasoning: Paths of Interaction and the Locality principle. Proc. AAAI 1983

Hupp, J.A., Cimino, J.J., Hoffer, E.P., Lowe, H.J. & Octo Barnett, G.(1986) DXplain A computer based diagnostic Knowledge base. Proc Medinfo 1986 117-121

Kingsland, L.C. Lindberg, D.A.B. & Sharp, G.C. (1983) AI/RHEUM A consultant System for Rheumatology. J. med. Syst. 7, 221-227

Miller, R.A., Pople, H.E., Myers, J.D. (1982) An Experimental Computer-based Diagnostic Consultant for General Internal Medicine. New Engl J Med 307, 468-476

Vries, de P.H. & Vries Robbé, de P.F. (1985) An overview of medical expert systems, Meth. Inform. Med. 24, 57-64.

Questions from the discussion

Breuker: By using the 'tested-by' links you hard-wire the testing in the knowledge representation for the generation of hypothesis. In our experience this doesn't work. Wouldn't you prefer to have the system reasoning about the tests to be performed?

De Vries Robbé: The system does! In fact in MEDES everything in the knowledge base is hardwired. However we do not also implicitly hardwire things like inheritance mechanisms as in frame based systems. As MEDES enables us to define different types of links, it is on the subshell level where by defining the queries the 'hard' effects of hardwiring the knowledge base are determined. Returning to your question: in the presented example the tests are hard-wired to the diseases, but in our knowledge graph the entities diseases and tests are also connected by links of other types. These other links are crucial to the flexibility which is regained by the query mechanism. For the selection of the most appropriate test we can search for additional qualities of the test; e.g. burden to the patient, costs, availability, etc. It is just a matter of query definition. It is very well possible to define a query that proposes to test another entity to prove a hypothesis if a certain test is not available.

Groth: One of your design ideas was 'knowledge acquisition by domain experts'. Have you been able to prove that MEDES is suitable for this type of knowledge acquisition?

De Vries Robbé: There are two aspects in your question: 'How well can a person describe his field of knowledge', and 'Is such knowledge adequately transferable to a system'. We must compare this to writing textbooks in medicine. In my opinion a person who is capable of writing a handbook of medicine should also be able to write a knowledge base. So the level of abstraction in which we handle medical knowledge should determine the level of abstraction of the system. We haven't done any specific tests to show that yet. We did hand out the system to several practising physicians. They received about half a day product training. While making their knowledge bases, they needed another day or so consulting us. It took them a few weeks to complete the domains, and some were to our surprise even quite comfortable with defining knowledge structures and medical reasoning procedures.

McNair: When domain experts can enter knowledge you need tools for assuring the consistency of the knowledge in the system. Do you have implemented such tools?

De Vries Robbé: A full semantic consistency checking of knowledge based systems is still a long way to go. In a companion project on concept identification in knowledge graphs, we had some success in knowledge bases with only a few types of links. In order to represent the richness of medical knowledge we need far more types, which makes such consistency checking very difficult. We defined several queries to browse through the knowledge. So, the domain expert can view the knowledge he just entered from different perspectives. On the entry level the syntax-driven domain editor guarantees syntactic consistency, and gives support to avoid double definitions.

APPLICATIONS
Management of the chronically ill

Evaluating Expert Critiques.

Issues for the Development of Computer-Based Critiquing in Primary Care [*]

Johan van der Lei[1], R. Frans Westerman[2],

Wilfried M. Boon[1].

[1] Department of Medical Informatics, Faculty of Medicine, Erasmus University, Rotterdam, The Netherlands.

[2] Department of Medicine, Free University Hospital, Amsterdam, The Netherlands.

Abstract

A number of workers in Artificial Intelligence have argued that, for some medical domains, critiquing the users decisions is an appropriate approach. Others have stressed the importance of integrating decision-support systems with existing information systems. Little research, however, has been directed to the issues of what consists a relevant critique and whether such a critique could be generated using data obtained from automated medical records. We therefore performed a study in which a general practitioner (GP) was asked to provide us with the computer-based medical records of five patients with hypertension. A printout of these medical records was submitted to an internist who had a recognized interest and experience in the treatment of hypertension. The internist was asked to comment on the treatment of the hypertension as documented in the medical records. Subsequently the comments of the internist were submitted to a panel of three GPs; these GPs were asked to judge the relevance of the comments. Finally the comments of the internist were shared with the GP who had treated the patient.

The internist generated 48 comments. When the GPs were asked to judge the comments of the internist, over 50 percent of these comments were judged relevant - but there was little consensus among the GPs regarding which comments were the

---

[*] This paper is an extended version of a paper that appeared in MEDINFO 89 under the title "Critiquing Expert Critiques".

relevant ones. The GPs were asked to state why a given comment was not relevant. Over 90 percent of their reasons fell into the following three groups: (a) the GP disagreed with the advice, (b) the GP agreed with the principle but he would prefer to modify the recommendation to suit his practice setting or (c) the GP felt that the advice had no consequence for the decision he had to make, although he did not disagree with the underlying principle. The treating physician judged over 50 percent of the internist's comments relevant. The predominant reason given by a treating physician for judging a comment to be irrelevant or less relevant was a misunderstanding of his intentions and/or reasoning by the critiquing physician.

Introduction

A number of workers in Artificial Intelligence in Medicine have argued that, for some medical domains, critiquing the decisions of a physician could be an appropriate approach (*Miller 1985, Miller 1986*). In this critiquing model, the physician submits his intended decisions to the program. The program evaluates these decisions and expresses agreement or suggests alternatives.

Others have stressed the importance of integrating consultation systems with routine data management functions within a medical office or institution. When decision-support systems are integrated with data-management systems, providing decision support can be viewed as a byproduct of the data-management activities (*Shortliffe 1987, McDonald et al 1984, Warner 1978, Pryor et al 1983*). Attempts have been made to combine the critiquing approach with data-management systems resulting in systems which, from the viewpoint of the physician, act as automated medical records, but 'behind the scenes' the decisions of the physician are evaluated and, if necessary, reasoned alternatives are suggested (*Evans et al 1986, Langlotz et al 1983*).

Little research, however, has been directed to the issues of what consists a relevant critique and whether such a critique could be generated using data obtained from automated medical records. We therefore performed a study in which a general practitioner (GP) was asked to provide us with computer-based medical records. A printout of these medical records was submitted to an internist, who was asked to critique the treatment as documented in the medical records. Subsequently the critique of the internist was submitted to a panel of GPs and to the GP who had treated the patient. These GPs were asked to judge the relevance of the critique.

Material and methods

We selected the system ELIAS, a system for the GP, as a source of medical data. ELIAS supports a fully automated medical record (*Westerhof et al 1987*): GPs using ELIAS no longer maintain paper records. Hypertension was selected as a medical domain because it is a common disorder treated both by physicians working in primary care and by hospital physicians. We had access to an internist with a recognized interest in the treatment of hypertension in primary care. One of the GP's was asked to provide us with the computer-based medical records of five patients with hypertension: patients he considered to be average patients, i.e. neither the easy cases, nor the most complex cases. The ELIAS system was introduced in the practice of this GP in Spring of 1985; the selection of patients took place in Spring of 1987. We thus had access to the computer-based medical record of the previous two years. The number of visits per patient to the GP during these two years ranged from four to 40. Although the blood pressure was recorded at almost all visits, not all visits were related to hypertension: one patient was also treated for infection of the respiratory tract, another suffered an exacerbation of a depression, and a third developed a myocardial infarction.

The study consisted of three stages: During the first stage a printout of the computer-based medical record was submitted to the internist. The internist was not associated with the GP who made the medical records available. In 'thinking aloud' sessions, the internist was asked to review the treatment of the hypertension as documented in the medical record. His free-flowing critiques were subsequently divided into discrete 'comments'. Each comment was considered to be an individual remark - an entity that was directed to a specific action (or the absence of an action) described in the medical record. If the internist would state: "I would not treat this patient with medication A but with B, but if you insist on treating with A, then the dosage is too high", this remark would be considered as two separate comments. The comments recorded by the investigator were handed back to the internist for review and approval.

A major restriction that we imposed on the critiquing process was that the critiquing physician have only the medical record at his disposal. When the critiquing physician was in doubt about the contents of the medical record (e.g., the exact meaning of a given diagnosis), then the treating physician was not available for clarification. This restriction stemmed from our desire to develop critiquing systems that rely on operational information systems as their source of data.

The second stage of the study involved submitting the comments of the internist to three GPs who acted as a panel judging the relevance of these comments. The GPs were aware of the fact that these critiques were generated by an internist who worked in a large clinic. The GPs were not associated with the internist or with the treating GP. Each of the three GPs was asked individually to rate each comment of the internist as either 'relevant', 'irrelevant' or 'partially relevant'. If the GP did not consider a comment relevant, he was asked to state why.

The third stage of the study involved sharing the critique of the internist with the same GP who made the medical records available. The GP was also asked to rate each individual comment of the internist as either 'relevant', 'irrelevant' or 'partially relevant'. If the GP did not consider a comment relevant, he was asked to state why.

Results

The internist generated in total 48 comments. The comments ranged from recommendations for minor adjustments in the dosages of given drugs to suggestions for major revisions of the therapy plan. The investigators assigned each comment to one of three groups. The first group involved comments dealing with the detection of the cause of the hypertension and assessing the severity of the hypertension: designated as diagnostic comments. The second group involved comments dealing with the selection of the optimal treatment for the patient: designated as selection comments. The third group involved comments dealing with the execution of the treatment, the prescribed dosage, the precautions which should be taken, the side effect to monitor: designated as execution comments. Of the 48 comments, 18 were diagnostic comments, 13 were selection comments, and 17 were execution comments.

In the second stage of the study these comments were submitted to the three GPs individually. The results are shown in Table 1: GPa judged 15 comments as either irrelevant or only partially relevant, GPb judged 21 comments as either irrelevant or

	GPa	GPb	GPc
comment is relevant	33	27	25
comment is partly relevant	4	12	4
comment is irrelevant	11	9	19

Table 1:   GP's judgment concerning the relevance of the internist's comments.

only partially relevant,and GPc judged 23 comments as either irrelevant or only partially relevant.
One needs an impression of the inter-observer variability: Was there a consensus among the GPs as to what comments were the relevant ones? When a comment received the verdict 'relevant' from two out of the three GPs and the third GP judged the comment 'relevant' or 'partially relevant', we labeled that comment 'accepted'. When two out of three judged the comment 'irrelevant' and the third judged it as 'irrelevant' or 'partially relevant', we labeled the comment 'rejected'. All other comments (e.g. one GP judged the comment 'relevant' whereas the other two judged it 'irrelevant') were labeled 'scattered'. The results are shown in Table 2: 18 comments of the internist fell in the category 'accepted', 26 in the category 'scattered', and four in the category 'rejected'. Of the 17 execution comments 12 were accepted, whereas of the 18 diagnostic comments only three were accepted.

When the GP's judged a comment to be irrelevant or only partially relevant, they justified their disagreement in several ways:
- The GP disagreed with the medical reasoning as presented by the internist.
- The GP stated that the comment had no consequences; the GP did not disagree with the underlying principle, but he felt that the comment was irrelevant to the decision he had to make.

	accepted	scattered	rejected
diagnostic comments	3 (17%)	14	1
selection comments	3 (23%)	7	3
execution comments	12 (71%)	5	0

Table 2: GPs judgement on internist's comments related to diagnosis, selection of treatment, execution of treatment.

- The GP agreed with the internist in principle, but the GP wanted to modify the recommendation to suit his own practice setting.
- The GP stated that the comment was based on an incomplete understanding or misunderstanding of the intentions and/or reasoning of the treating physician.
- The reasoning could not be assigned to any of the previous groups for miscellaneous reasons.

The most frequent reasons for not judging a comment to be relevant were (a) agreeing with the underlying principle yet applying it somewhat differently, (b) disagreeing with the medical reasoning as presented by the internist and (c) stating that the comment of the internist had no consequences for the treatment (Table 3).

In the third stage of the study the GP who treated the patients was asked to judge the comments of the internist: He judged 25 comments relevant, 11 comments partially relevant, and 12 comments irrelevant. In seven cases, the GP disagreed with the medical reasoning, in three cases the GP agreed with the principle but wanted to modify the recommendation to suit his own practice setting, and in two cases the GP felt that the comment had no consequences for the treatment under consideration. But the predominant reason (on 10 occasions) given by the treating physician for judging a comment to be irrelevant or less relevant was a misunderstanding or incomplete understanding of his intentions and/or reasoning by the critiquing internist.

Discussion

When humans interact with their environment they form models of themselves and of the environment with which they are interacting. Such internal models are known as mental models. These mental models provide predictive and explanatory power for understanding the interaction with the environment. Similarly, the physician forms a mental model of the patient whom he is treating. When another physician is asked to critique this treatment, he has to reconstruct the intentions and reasoning of the treating physician. The critiquing physician has to formulate a model of the treating physician's mental model (Figure 1). Such a model of a mental

	DA	NC	BA	MU	MIS
diagnostic comments	7	9	11	2	1
selection comments	11	7	1	0	2
execution comments	0	0	7	0	1

Table 3:   Reasons given by GPs stated for judging internists' comments as irrelevant
            or only partially relevant:Reasons given by GPs stated for judging internists'
            comments as irrelevant or only partially relevant:
            DA: disagreement with the medical reasoning,
            NC: the comment has no consequences,
            BA: basic agreement with the principles stated in the comment, but wanting
            to modify the recommendation,
            DA: disagreement with the medical reasoning,
            NC: the comment has no consequences,
            BA: basic agreement with the principles stated in the comment, but wanting
            to modify the recommendation,
            MU: the internist misunderstands the treating physician,
            MIS: miscellaneous.

model is known as a conceptual model (*Gentner and Stevens 1983*). In the medical record, one encounters both data describing the patient's state (e.g., the results of laboratory tests) and data describing the mental model of the treating physician (e.g., a description of treatment goals). The creation of such a conceptual model of the treating physician lies at the heart of a critique: The recognition of the intentions (the treatment objectives) of the physician in combination with the actions undertaken to achieve these treatment objectives (*Miller 1985*).

In the domain of hypertension, the printout of the computer-based medical record seems to contain enough information for a human observer to generate considerable advice. The ability to generate critique indicates that some conceptual model can be formulated by the critiquing physician. The ability to generate critique, however, does not prove the validity of the underlying conceptual model: The predominant reason that the treating physician believed a comment to be irrelevant was a misunderstanding of his intentions by the critiquing physician.

One might argue that the working situation of the GP and the methods which the GP uses to manage this situation differ from those of the clinician (*Pendleton and Hasler 1983, Bentsen 1984, Perlman et al 1976, Fry 1980*). Consequently, the internist is limited in his ability to deduce the intentions of the GP. However, if the difference between a GP and an internist would account for the inability of the internist to understand the GP, then one would expect that other GPs, just like the treating GP,

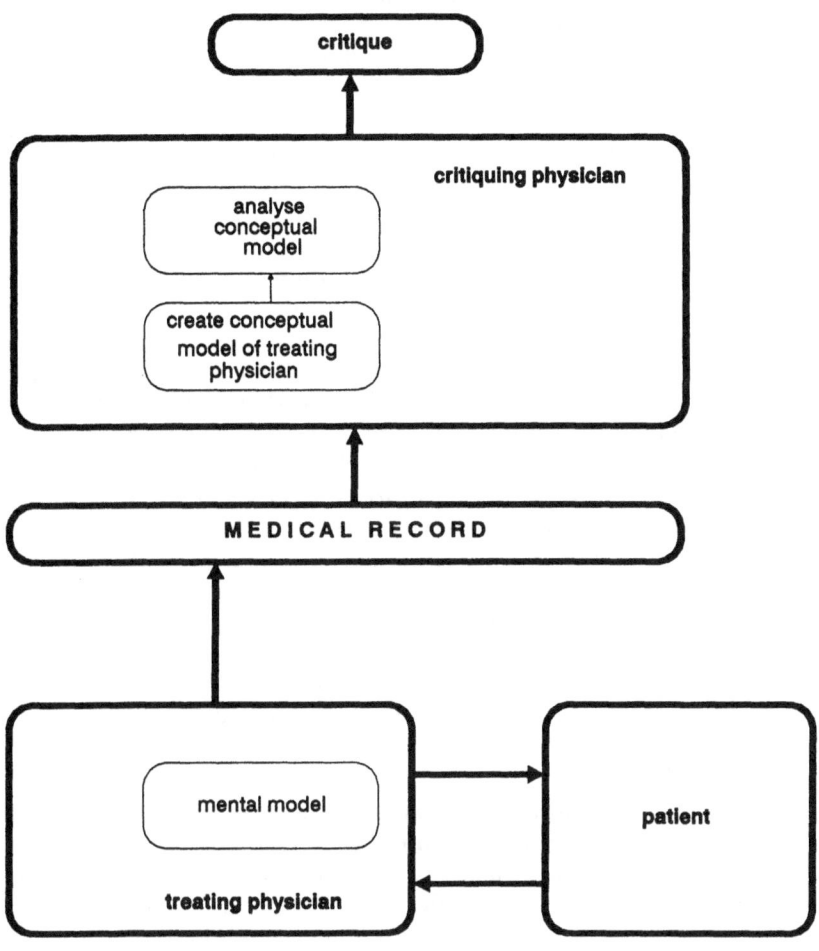

Figure 1: The treating physician develops a mental model of the patient he treats and his role in that treatment. In the medical record, data describing both the condition of the patient and the intentions of the treating physician are recorded. The critiquing physician formulates a conceptual model of the intentions of the treating physician.

would be able to identify these misunderstandings. Yet, the panel of three GP's failed to detect a misunderstanding of the intentions of the treating physician by the internist as a cause of the generation of irrelevant critique.

A significant cause of the failure of the critiquing physician to accurately detect the intentions of the treating physician could be traced to the manner in which the

automated medical record was kept. The medical record of the GP is primarily a
record of the actions he/she performed; it is a "what did I do" record, not a "why did
I do it" record. A particular prescription is not always labeled "for the treatment of
hypertension". Diagnostic tests are not always labeled "to exclude disease X". The
underlying reasoning has to be reconstructed. (Similar observations prompted Weed
(*Weed 1971*) to the development of his Problem Oriented Medical Record.) Moreover, not all actions or decisions of the GP are mentioned in the medical record.
Missing data may lead to an incorrect interpretation of other data and subsequently
lead to a conceptual model that, when used to generate a critique, produces 'irrelevant' advice. The word 'irrelevant' used in this context denotes a situation where the
treating physician identifies the critiquing physician's incorrect assumptions, recognizes the consequences of these incorrect assumptions for the conceptual model of
the internist, and subsequently disregards the advice.

A conceptual model that captures the intentions of the treating physician does not
guarantee that a critique generated on the basis of that conceptual model will be
judged relevant by other physicians. Clinical practice is not solely based on scientific
facts and evidence. Both training and practice setting have an effect on medical
decision-making (*Palchik et al 1987, Petersdorf 1978, Goldenberg et al 1979, Weil and
Schleiter 1981*). When a physician receives a critique, he will not only verify the
conceptual model underlying that critique, but will also evaluate whether, in his
practice setting and with his training, the critique is relevant. The three main reasons
the GPs gave for judging a comment less than relevant were: (a) the GP disagreed
with the advice, (b) the GP agreed with the principle but he would prefer to modify
the recommendation to suit his practice setting or (c) the GP felt that the advice had
no consequence for the decision he had to make. We will consider these three
reasons in turn (Figure 2).

- The GP judges the advice of the internist to be less relevant or irrelevant because
  he <u>disagrees with the medical reasoning</u>. The GP recognizes the inferences of
  the internist and disagrees with those inferences. The resulting advice is subsequently judged irrelevant. The GP does not disagree with the conceptual model
  that the internist constructed of the treating physician's behaviour based on data
  in the medical record; if the GP disagrees with the conceptual model of the
  internist, he would argue that the internist misunderstands the intentions of the
  treating physician.

  An example, in the case of a 48 year old male with blood pressures as high as
  190/100 mm Hg, the internist argued that because of the age of the patient and
  the severity of the hypertension renal-artery stenosis should be considered. The
  GP responded that, although he agreed with the observation that the patient was
  young and was suffering from a severe hypertension, he disagreed with the need
  to investigate the possibility of a renal-artery stenosis. He would only consider
  this diagnosis only if the patient would not respond to therapy. Since the patient
  was responding to therapy a stenosis was, in his opinion, highly unlikely.

- Another situation arises when the GP states that the advice of the internist has
  <u>no consequences</u> for the treatment of the patient. The GP does not disagree with
  the inferences made by the internist, but states that the comment has no effect

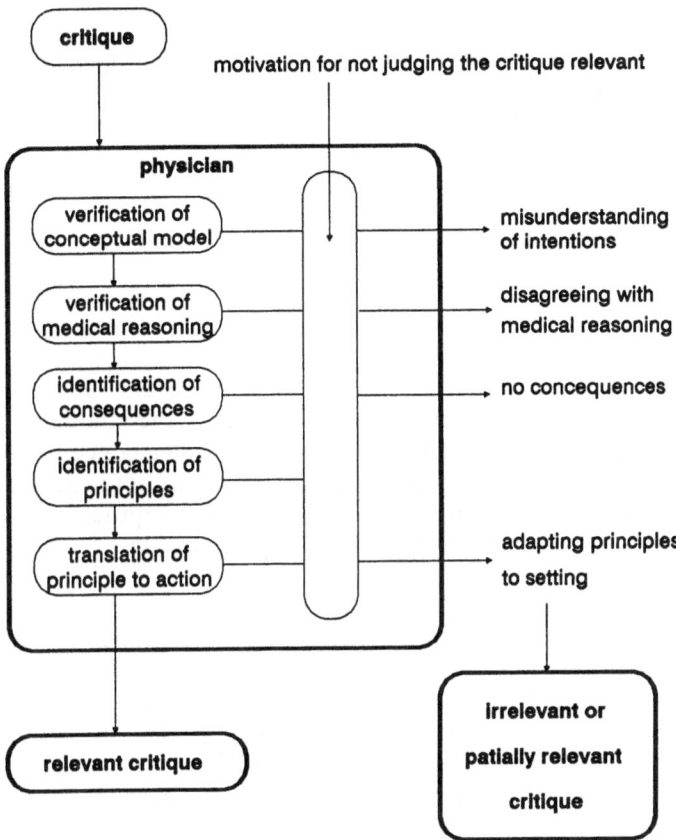

Figure 2:   The physician receiving the critique may have a variety of reasons for judging the critique irrelevant or only partially relevant. For an analysis of these reasons see text.

on his decision making. In the majority of these comments, the internist was recommending the collection of additional data (e.g., laboratory tests) without stating how, once obtained, the data would influence the treatment. The response of the GP was, typically, that no matter what the outcome of these test, he would treat the patient in the same manner.

● When reviewing the advice of the internist, the GP may be able to distinguish treatment principles from the translation of these principles into actions. The GP may agree with the fact that the principles should be applied but may disagree with the actions that the internist recommends. The opinion of the GP differs from that of the internist when viewed at the level of specific actions to be taken, yet the opinions are congruent at the more abstract level of treatment principles.

When comparing the judgments of the three GPs, one observes a lack of consensus on whether the advice is relevant. The comments dealing with the execution of the anti-hypertensive treatment were better received by the majority of the GPs than the comments dealing with diagnosis or the selection of treatment. The predominant reason for judging the comments dealing with the execution of the therapy as irrelevant or only partially relevant did not involve the treatment principles stated in the comments, but involved the translation of those principles to actions; the GP wanted to modify the recommendations of the internist to suit his practice setting. In the areas of diagnosis and the selection of treatment, comments are seldom rejected by all GPs, but the GPs judge the relevance of the comments differently.

Conclusions

The automated medical records did contain enough information for a human observer to generate substantial critiques. Both the treating physician and the panel of GPs judged more than half of the critiques as relevant. Generating a critique will often involve discussing the actions of a physician in the context of a conceptual model of that physician. However the need to create such a conceptual model of the treating physicians was not anticipated in the design or use of the automated medical record. Subsequently, the ability to generate these conceptual models is limited. Errors in an observer's conceptual model will often invalidate his critiques.

In our study, critiques dealing with the execution of a treatment are judged more frequently relevant than those dealing with a diagnosis or the selection of a treatment. Critiques dealing with the execution of treatment are often adapted by the GP to suit his setting. In this process of modifying the recommendation, the GP separates the treatment principle from the translation of that principle into action. Multiple translations of the same treatment principle into different actions are possible. Apart from critiques dealing with the execution of a treatment, there is little consensus among the GPs on what constitutes a relevant critique.

Issues for the development of computer-based monitoring in primary care

The wish to develop systems which produce critique as a byproduct of medical data-management activities adds several major research issues to the already non-trivial task of developing a stand-alone critiquing system. In our opinion, two issues will be of prime concern: the development of methods which will make the intentions of the treating physician explicit, and further research to establish a better understanding of what constitutes a relevant critique.

The issue of making the intentions of the physician explicit can be addressed from two perspectives: the medical record and the critiquing system. Including the intentions of the physician in the medical record in a structured manner would allow the critiquing system to evaluate the actions of the physician in the context of those intentions. Though attempts to automate traditional medical records have met with some success (*McDonald and Tierney 1988*), attempts to modify the content and structure of the medical record, for example the Problem Oriented Medical Record (*Weed 1971*), have met considerable resistance and only limited success. Yet in order to further develop critiquing systems, the explicit recording of the intentions of the physician would be of great value.

Any critiquing system that relies for data-input on automated medical records relies, explicit or implicit, on a model or approximation of the physician's intentions. If treatment protocols are available, then critiquing systems can be developed by monitoring, based on the automated medical record, adherence to that protocol. In settings where well-defined treatment protocols are available (e.g. in oncology), the feasibility of this approach has been demonstrated (*Langlotz et al 1983*). This approach hinges on the assumption it is the physician's intention to follow the protocol. The system does not need to reason about the intentions of the physician - the protocol is used as a **substitute**. Ultimately, the only critique of the system is that the physician does not follow the specified protocol. An alternative approach involves the definition of such clear and well-defined criteria that, for a population meeting those criteria, there is little room for doubt as to what are the intentions of the physician. By defining stringent criteria one **restricts** the population for which the advice is generated. Thus one can escape the problem of reasoning about the physician's intentions: In the restricted population the physician's intentions are, ideally, clear. This process of defining criteria in order to restrict the population for which the advice will be generated, often involves a number of iterations in which the number of 'false-positive' warnings is evaluated, followed by an attempt to further refine the criteria. In hospitals where substantial portions of the medical record have been automated, the feasibility of this approach has been demonstrated (*McDonald et al 1984, Pryor et al 1983*).
In contrast to (or possibly complementary to) modifying the medical record one could consider developing critiquing systems which will **reason** about the intentions of the physician. Our current work is aimed at developing systems which will reason about what the physicians' intentions could have been and subsequently couch the critique in terms that reflect those possible intentions.

When critiquing systems are integrated with automated medical records the identification of **relevant critique** becomes of prime concern. Physicians do not request critique but receive it whenever monitored patient data warrant it. Therefore one has to avoid generating excessive amount of critique which is subsequently judged irrelevant. Too much 'irrelevant critique' may not only create antagonistic responses, but may also blunt the usefulness of those critiques that have greater clinical significance. The notion of a 'correct critique' should not be confused with that of a 'relevant critique': a correct critique may be irrelevant. In our study, disagreement with the medical reasoning was not the dominant reason for judging a critique as irrelevant. The lack of consensus on what constitutes a relevant critique poses significant problems. Additional research is required to create a better understanding as to what type, and the reasons why, a critique is likely to be judged relevant.

Acknowledgements

The support of the Nederlandse Hartstichting (Dutch Heart Foundation, grant no. 88.236) is gratefully acknowledged.

References

Bentsen BG. Fundamentals of general practice. Scand J Primary Health Care 1984;2:11-7.

Evans RS, Larsen RA, Burke JP, et al. Computer surveillance of hospital acquired infections and antibiotics. JAMA 1986;256:1007-11.

Fry J. ed.Primary Care. London: Heinemann, 1980.

Gentner D, Stevens AL, eds. Mental Models. London: Lawrence Erlbaum Associates, 1983.

Goldenberg DL, Pozen JL, Cohen AS. The effect of primary-care pathway on internal medicine residents' career plans. Ann Intern Med 1979;91:271-4.

Langlotz CP, Shortliffe EH Adapting a consultation system to critique user plans. Int J Man-Machine Stud 1983;19:479-96.

McDonald CJ, Hui SL, Smith DM, et al. Reminders to physicians from an introspective computer medical record. Ann Intern Med 1984;100:130-8.

McDonald CJ, Tierney WM. Computer-stored medical records: Their future use in medical practice. JAMA 1988;259:3433-40.

Miller PL. Goal-directed critiquing by computer: ventilator management. Comp Biomed Res 1985;18:422-38.

Miller PL. Expert Critiquing Systems: Practice-Based Medical Consultation by Computer. New York: Springer Verlag, 1986.

Palchik NS, Dielman TE, Woolloscroft JO, et al. Practice preferences of primary care and traditional internal medicine house officers. Med Educ 1987;21:441-9.

Pendleton D, Hasler J. Doctor-Patient Communication. London: Academic Press, 1983.

Petersdorf RG. The doctor's dilemma. N Eng J Med 1978;299:628-34.

Perlman LV, Graham T, Christy W. Primary care internal medicine residencies: definitions, problems and opportunities. Arch Int Med 1976;136:111-3.

Pryor RA, Gardner RM, Clayton PD, et al. The HELP system. J Med Syst 1983;7:87-102.

Shortliffe EH. Computer programs to support clinical decision making. JAMA 1987;258:61-6.

Warner HR. Computer-Assisted Medical Decision Making. New York: Academic Press Inc, 1978.

Weil PA, Schleiter MK. National study of internal medicine manpower: VI. Factors predicting preferences of residents for careers in primary care or subspeciality care and clinical practice or academic medicine. Ann Intern Med 1981;94:691-703.

Weed L. Medical Records, Medical Education and Patient Care. Cleveland: Case Western Reserve University Press, 1971.

Westerhof HP, Boon WM, Cromme PVM, et al. ELIAS: Support of the Dutch General Practitioner. In: Reichertz PL, Engelbrecht R, Picollo U, eds. Present Status of Computer Support in Ambulatory Care. New York: Springer Verlag, 1987, 1-10.

Knowledge Acquisition for a Decision Support System for Anti-epileptic Drug Surveillance

R.P.A.M. Smeets[1], J.L. Talmon[2], P.J.M. van der Lugt[1], R.A.J. Schijven[2]

1 Dept. of Neurology, University of Limburg, Maastricht, The Netherlands.

2 Dept. of Medical Informatics and Statistics, University of Limburg, Maastricht, The Netherlands.

Abstract

This article describes techniques for knowledge elicitation. An interpretation model for the analysis of expertise used for the initiation of drug treatment of epilepsy patients is presented. A prototype for intake advice as developed with this methodology is described.

Introduction

Epilepsy is a chronic dysfunction of the electrical activity of the brain. The symptoms which may occur range from mild changes in the level of consciousness to the development of seizures with increased muscle activity.

Treatment of epilepsy consists mainly of prescription of anti-epileptic drugs. The intention is to relieve the patient from his symptoms and achieve a complete suppression of the seizures. The choice of a drug is based on the type of epilepsy and the seizure type. In case the effectiveness of the drug is not sufficient another drug may be tried.

Although monotherapy is generally accepted, polypharmacy - the prescription of more than one drug - may be tried in case monotherapy proves to be ineffective (*Shorvon et al 1978, Goodridge et al 1983, Overweg 1984*). The selection of drug dosage is based on the principle of reaching a maximal effect with a minimal drug dosage. In practice the daily dosage of the drug(s) is increased in case the clinical findings suggest that the current dosage does not control seizures effectively.

One of the problems of anti-epileptic drug treatment is the development of side-effects such as drowsiness and headache due to toxic concentration levels of the drug in the blood. Although the neurologist will try to prevent the induction of drug side-effects by monitoring the blood level of the drug, the occurrence of intoxication can not always be prevented because of interindividual differences in pharmacokinetics of drugs.

A second problem in the management of epilepsy patients is the multiple use of information. Information about symptoms, complaints and compliance presented by the patient may be used when treatment is initiated. The same information is used later when assessing the efficacy of the treatment. This reinterpretation of information may induce inconsistency in use of information.
Besides this, seizures may occur intermittently with periods without seizures followed by periods of increased seizure frequency. The intervals between visits may change considerably. This may cause inconsistency in the interpretation of information.

A third problem for the neurologist is the registration of information. Incompleteness of the information caused by insufficient registration or by consultation of different neurologists during the patient's period of illness may reduce the effectiveness of treatment of epilepsy.

Effective drug treatment is essential for the patient. A successful treatment reduces the number of seizures and thereby the fear and uncertainty the patient experiences. Furthermore, it may increase the chance of a good long-term prognosis in case seizures are controlled at an early stage. Also a reduction of the medical and social complications may be expected (*Shorvon et al 1982, Goodridge et al 1983*).

Effective treatment of epilepsy is supported by systematic drug treatment and accurate registration of data. Therefore we decided to develop a decision support system. We formalized the knowledge for treatment of epilepsy used by an expert. Part of the knowledge is implemented in a prototype knowledge based system.

Method

The development of a knowledge based system can take place by rapid prototyping or by structured design. Prototyping may present a solution when it is difficult for the expert to verbalize knowledge. In this methodology, the expert is confronted with an incomplete system. It's performance can be criticized and improvement and extension of knowledge to be incorporated may be suggested. Furthermore, it may be used to identify domain problems more clearly. Prototyping may not present an overview of the knowledge used by the expert. It will tend to focus on details. This may cause the system to become incomplete. Furthermore, the system will be developed by confronting the expert with an insufficiently performing prototype. Although there will be an improvement in performance over time the expert might lose interest in presenting more knowledge because of constant changes in the knowledge base and the representation of the formulated knowledge. The medical expert might see the process as the treatment of symptoms without really curing the disease. Besides this the use of specific cases for the development of the system may cause incompleteness and redundancies in the knowledge. The iterative approach may

cause the knowledge base to become inconsistent (*Hayes et al 1983, Waterman 1986, Heng 1987, Dijk et al 1987*).
We think that obtaining an overview on the knowledge before implementation is essential for preventing at least parts of these problems. Therefore we chose KADS as a structured methodology for the development of our system (*Breuker et al 1984, 1987, 1989*). In KADS a systematic analysis of the domain knowledge is made first. The elicited knowledge is structured by means of interpretation models, which show the reasoning process in a general way. These models provide a framework for further detailed elicitation and analysis. They can be used for showing the expert the elicited knowledge.
Furthermore, they facilitate discussion on the structure, completeness and usefulness of knowledge before implementation starts. KADS presents a conceptual model in which the expertise is described at four different levels.

Knowledge Elicitation Techniques

Techniques for knowledge elicitation can generally be divided into two groups: indirect and direct techniques (*Reitman Olsen et al 1987*). Indirect techniques are, among others, card sorting, multi-dimensional scaling, cluster analysis, general weighted networks and
repertory grids. The use of these techniques is based on the assumption that the semantically related concepts are represented closer in memory than semantically unrelated concepts. Another basic assumption is that the relatedness of the concepts can be expressed by a distance value (*Cooke et al 1987*). These techniques can be useful when no clear view on the structure of concepts in the domain of expertise is present. Furthermore, they may also be used to assess globally the correctness of the structure of the knowledge as elicited. The expert has to present the strength of the relation by a numerical or symbolic value. The techniques can be used for elicitation of knowledge from different experts due to the standardized elicitation and analysis procedure. However, how to interpret the results of the analysis is unclear.
Techniques such as multi-dimensional scaling presents the relations between concepts in a n-dimensional space on a two dimensional display. The expert has to interpret the dimensions on which the concepts are mapped without actually knowing whether a meaningful dimension exists. The links in networks, derived by general weighted network techniques such as pathfinder, may also be interpreted by the expert. The cluster analysis technique is a straightforward technique in which the assumption is that a concept belongs to a cluster of concepts or not. The expert may be confronted with concepts that do not make sense when trying to relate them to a cluster. Repertory grid also assumes the existence of a bi-polar dimension for rating all the concepts (*Cooke et al 1986, Cooke et al 1987, Wright et al 1987*). The algorithms used for joining the concepts can lead to different hierarchical structures and networks. All techniques suffer from the fact that there must be an initial set of concepts for the rating procedure. How these concepts should be obtained is not expressed by the methodology. In case the initial set is not complete there may be severe bias in the judgement of the distances. Apart from the card sort technique all of them require the use of a matrix in which all possible combinations of concepts are presented. Filling in this matrix is a tiresome procedure. Reducing this work by

presenting only half of the matrix assumes that the distance between concept A and B equals the distance between B and A. Besides this the expert may not see the necessity of such an exercise. Hence, he may not be willing to participate.

Direct techniques consist of techniques such as focussed interview, structured interview, introspection, dialogues, protocol analysis, interruption analysis and questionnaires. The main assumption of direct techniques is that knowledge is verbalisable. Furthermore, there is the assumption that knowledge can be obtained through introspection. These techniques are not designed for elicitation of a specific type of knowledge. Thus they are flexible to unforeseeable information which may be presented by the expert. Furthermore, they do not make any assumptions on the representation of knowledge in memory. Making use of interview techniques enables the expert to express his knowledge in a familiar way in a sequence he thinks best. Observations of patient-physician dialogues enable the analysis of when decisions are made. By means of thinking aloud techniques a normal task involvement is recorded. Analysis of these protocols provide information on goals, methods and inferences (*Breuker et al 1984, Hoffman 1987*). Disadvantages of these techniques are that much depends on the observer's skills for interviewing the expert. Furthermore, direct techniques are as time consuming as indirect techniques. The interviewer has to transcribe the recorded information and subsequently analyse it.

Elicitation Techniques	Elicited Knowledge
multi-dimensional scaling	global structure of concepts
cluster analysis	hierarchical organization of concepts
general weighted networks	local relations between concepts
ordered trees from recall	organization of concepts and attributes
card sorting	organization of concepts and attributes
repertory grid	attributes of concepts
focussed interview	global description concepts, tasks and strategy
structured interview	detailed description of concepts and attributes, tasks and strategy 'why and how'
dialogues	tasks and strategy
introspection	classes of concepts, tasks, strategy and 'how'
protocol analysis	concepts, inferences, tasks, 'how'
review	refinement elicited knowledge

Table 1:   Elicitation techniques and the main type of elicited knowledge.

Research on expertise is difficult due to the complexity of expert knowledge and because a standard for identifying expertise is lacking. Ascribing expertise to a person is mainly based on aspects such as recommendations of supervisors, teachers or patients and the number of years of clinical experience. The expert in our project is a neurologist who works in a general hospital. He has been a medical practitioner for 20 years. Furthermore, he treats about 400 epilepsy patients a year. This means that he sees about two patients suffering from epilepsy a day. He is specially interested in the standardization of drug treatment.

The techniques we used for knowledge elicitation so far were direct techniques. The use of elicitation techniques was based on the four different layers of knowledge present in a conceptual model. This means that we needed information about the domain concepts, tasks and strategies for treatment.

An overview is needed of the problems and the different concepts used by the expert. Therefore we started with a global technique, the focussed interview. The expert was asked to present as much knowledge about the domain as possible without going too much into detail. The obtained information from these interviews consists of the concepts which may be involved for problem solving. Furthermore, information about the types of problems in the domain is presented.

Secondly we used the structured interview technique. The concepts which were presented in the focussed interviews were analysed more deeply. This took place by questioning the expert about a specific concept. Furthermore, the expert was asked to describe concepts more detailed in order to obtain a structure of concepts.

Thirdly we used introspection. A case was presented and the expert was asked to explain how he would treat the patient. This technique revealed information about the global strategy for patient treatment. Besides this the different tasks during the problem solving process may become clear.

Fourthly the dialogue technique was used. We observed that it is difficult for the expert to explain the tasks while solving an artificial problem. Therefore we decided to confront the expert with a real patient and observe the process. Although questions about the how and why of the problem solving were not possible during these on-the-job-recordings, identification of the different steps in the process was possible. Furthermore a short interview on why specific information was needed took place after the patient left.

The review technique was used for assessment of the developed structures of concepts, the evaluation of the task structures and the strategy. In this process the use of models made it possible to show the expert which part of his knowledge was discussed and had to be refined.

Results

Interview techniques and dialogue/on-the-job recordings were used to obtain information about the problems a physician encounters during the treatment of an epilepsy patient. These problems consisted of selection and monitoring the anti-epileptic drugs, registration of patient data, incomplete formulation of motivation for selection of drugs and establishment of intake advice.

Based on this analysis the following system requirements were established:

1 The system must provide advice about anti-epileptic drug treatment.

2 The system must enhance the registration of patient data.

3 The system must provide the reasons for a specific anti-epileptic drug treatment.

4 If possible the system must support the education of students and resident neurologist so that the introduction of a standardized drug treatment is augmented.

The creation of a conceptual model which consists of four levels of the expert's knowledge is the goal of the KADS methodology. The first level in this model is the strategic level for the description of the general approach for solving the problem and the alternatives. At the task level the different tasks can be described. These descriptions consist of goals and control statements. The control statements contain the order in which inferences, described at the lower inference level take place. At the inference level two structures are present knowledge sources and metaclasses. Inferences are described by knowledge sources; concepts are described by metaclasses. The domain level contains the declarative domain knowledge, the concepts and rules.

We used information from the interviews and the introspection technique to develop the strategic level for drug treatment of chronic diseases, such as epilepsy. The strategy consists of establishing a diagnosis, initiating a treatment, monitoring the effect of the treatment and the reduction and the therapy (fig. 1).

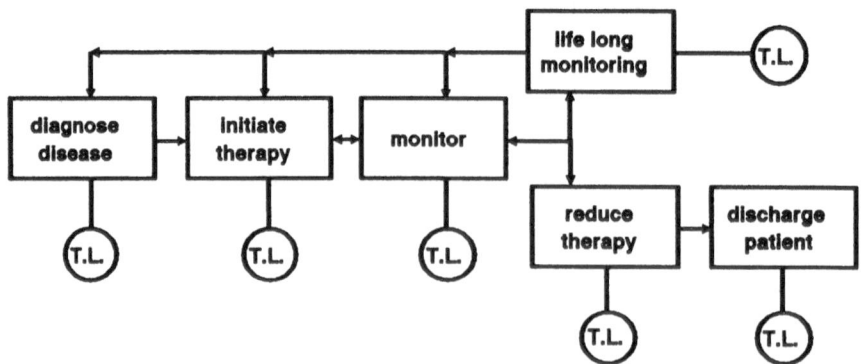

Figure 1:   The global strategy for drug treatment of chronic diseases with reference to the task level (TL).

The monitoring of the treatment may induce the establishment of a new therapy because the current therapy does not work. Furthermore it may lead to the establishment of a new diagnosis. One can think of the ineffectiveness of treatment which causes the physician to review the diagnosis or to obtain a second opinion. Another possibility is the withdrawal of a treatment because of successfully curing the patient. In case the treatment may not be completely successful the patient may enter the phase in which a change in treatment is not necessary but follow-up may be indicated because of possible side-effects. The use of this global strategy picture for a chronic disease may be specified to the domain of epilepsy.

The strategy followed can be described by first:
  a) try to make the patient free from seizures by prescribing anti-epileptic drugs.
  b1) if the patient has been free from seizures for two years reduce the therapy
  c1) and discharge the patient from further follow-up.
Secondly the strategy can be:
  b2) if the patient is not free from seizures, treat the most disabling type of seizures and/or
  c2) check the patient's diagnosis.

The elicitation process so far was focussed on that part of the strategy in which the initialization of the therapy takes place.
To analyse the knowledge for this part of the problem solving we had to develop an interpretation model because the presented models did not fit the domain. In this process we used the interview techniques and the introspection technique to develop an initial model. This model was further refined by information obtained from introspection, dialogues and review.

The main aspects to arrive at the final intake advice are described by an interpretation model (fig. 2). This model consists of metaclasses and knowledge sources. The metaclasses contain the domain concepts. They are represented by rectangles. A metaclass stands for a series of instances. The knowledge sources, represented by ellipses, are functions which transform an input metaclass into an output metaclass. The interpretation model describes the expertise at a higher level of abstraction. Thus, the usefulness of the interpretation model is not restricted for analysing expertise in the domain of epilepsy but should be of equal value for analysing the expertise in the domain of drug treatment of other diseases. By using the interpretation model the elicited expertise can be analysed through the description of more specific tasks and the inferences (*Smeets et al 1989*).

The order in which the knowledge sources are used is described at the task level. The first compound task is the identification of the disease. This means that the disease concept is obtained from the metaclass CASE DESCRIPTION. This metaclass contains all information about the patient such as age, weight, diagnosis, co-medication, reported drug side-effects and laboratory results. In this case the concept epilepsy is described by the epilepsy type and the seizure type. The concept is placed in the metaclass DISEASE DESCRIPTION.

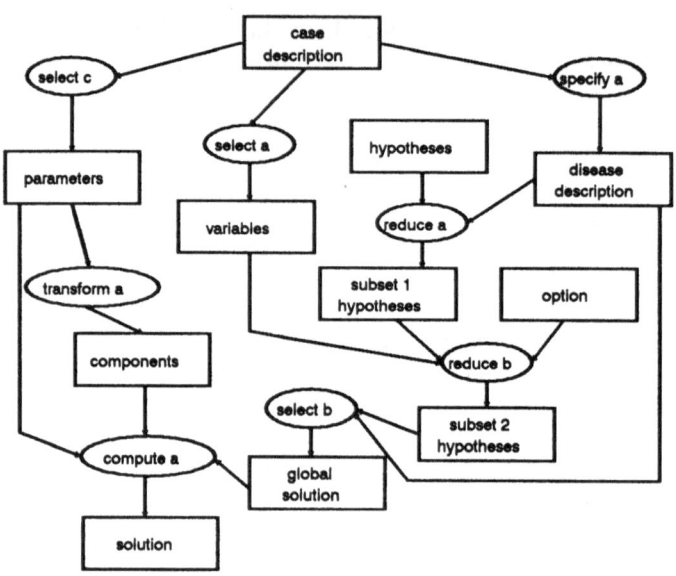

Figure 2:   Interpretation model for initiation of drug therapy.

In the second compound task this concept is needed to establish the identification of possible appropriate drugs, present in the metaclass SUBSET 1 HYPOTHESES from the anti-epileptic drugs in metaclass HYPOTHESES.

The third compound task is the identification of the appropriate anti-epileptic drug. In this process the expert decreases the set of drugs which are described in the metaclass SUBSET 1 HYPOTHESES. This identification process takes place using the metaclass VARIABLES which contains concepts selected from the CASE DE-SCRIPTION of the patient such as age, drug side-effects and no-successful drugs. The metaclass SUBSET 2 HYPOTHESES contains those drugs which may be pres-cribed. Although the number of anti-epileptic drugs decreases it is still possible that more than one drug is appropriate. Thus, the expert selects one drug, described in the metaclass GLOBAL SOLUTION.

In the fourth compound task the computation of the intake advice takes place. Information from the metaclass GLOBAL SOLUTION is used, such as the selected anti-epileptic drug and administration dose of tablets. Furthermore, concepts se-lected from the CASE DESCRIPTION such as the age and weight and laboratory results, present in the metaclass PARAMETERS are used. Some of these concepts such as the liver and kidney functions are transformed into the concept metabolism, present in the metaclass COMPONENTS. All three metaclasses, GLOBAL SOLU-TION, COMPONENTS and PARAMETERS are used to compute the intake advice consisting of the drug, daily intake dose, dosage of tablets, number of tablets, intake schemes. All this information is present in the metaclass SOLUTION.

The Prototype

Although prototyping may seem contradictory with the KADS approach, the development of a prototype provides insight in the functioning of the described system. Therefore we consider it a useful completion in the validation of a described model.

The prototype is developed by means of the frame-based tool KEE on an EXPLORER 1. The system consists of three components. The component called MEDICATION consists of the declarative knowledge and rules. The declarative knowledge is represented by frames. These can be divided into general frames and more specific frames. The general frames are use to describe global concepts such as anti-epileptic drugs and complaints. The more specific frames are instances of the global frames. Instances inherit their structure from the more general frames.

The rules are grouped into rule sets. In this way the activation of the rules is limited to those rule needed for a specific purpose. The sets consist of rules for specification of the seizure type, specification of subsets of hypotheses and selection of specific drugs and establishment of metabolism.

The second part is the MEDICATION-IMAGES component, which consists of procedural knowledge for determination of tasks, activation of rules and creation of displays. Furthermore, procedures for explanations about the how and why aspects of decisions are present. Besides this there are procedures for checking the data base for patients and creation of frames.

The third part is a data base for frames for patients. The prototype works by a generate and test strategy. This means that the creation of a subset of anti-epileptic drugs takes place first. Secondly this subset is reduced by testing the set against the selected constraining variables. The intake advice consists of the brandname of the drug, the dosage of the tablets, the intake schemes and the number of tablets. Furthermore, advice is given on the laboratory examinations and the date of the next visit.

The evaluation of the prototype so far was informal. We used a static evaluation to check the representation of declarative knowledge. Frames were checked on completeness of attributes. Furthermore, the constraints of attributes were checked on legal, illegal and contradictory values. The inheritance of attributes was evaluated by graphic displays. Knowledge rules and procedural knowledge were tested on an ad hoc basis.

Conclusion

KADS is a valuable methodology for the analysis of expertise. The use of interpretation models facilitates the knowledge elicitation process. With these models the interviewer can show the expert what part of the expertise will be analysed. The description of concepts by their roles in the problem solving process may induce difficulties in communication with the expert. Therefore, more detailed descriptions of the concepts in the metaclasses may be necessary. Although KADS does not provide an interpretation model for each generic task the use of the conceptual modelling language provides the possibility to create or refine interpretation models. The models enhance the insight in the elicited knowledge. Still there may be a need for evaluation of the conceptual model. The development of a prototype system provides the possibility to validate the conceptual model.

Summary

The effectiveness of anti-epileptic drug treatment is crucial for a patient suffering from epilepsy. Providing the physician with a decision support system may enhance the effectiveness of the treatment. Thus we formalised an expert's knowledge on drug treatment. The knowledge elicitation process took place by direct techniques. The elicitation process focused on the initialisation of the anti-epileptic drug treatment. KADS enhanced the insight in the problem solving process of the expert by the development of interpretation models. The prototype system we developed so far can give an intake advice on anti-epileptic drugs.

Literature

Breuker J., Wielinga B. Model-driven knowledge acquisition, interpretation models. Deliverable Task A1 Esprit Project 1098, Dept. Social Science Informatics, University of Amsterdam, 1984.

Breuker J., Wielinga B. Use of models in the interpretation of verbal data. In: Knowledge elicitation for expert systems, a handbook (Kidd A. ed.) Plenum Press, New York, 1987.

Breuker J., Winkels, R. The use of the KADS methodology in designing an intelligent teaching system for diagnosis in physiotherapy. This volume, pp 1-26, 1989.

Cooke N.M., McDonald J.E. A formal methodology for acquiring and representing expert knowledge. Proc. of the IEEE, 74, no. 10, 1986, 1422-1430.

Cooke N.M., McDonald J.E. The application of psychological scaling techniques to knowledge elicitation for knowledge-based systems. Int. J. Man-Machine Studies, 1987, 26, 533-550.

Dijk van J.E.M. Hilgevoord F.G. Jacques M.T. Otten G.A.M. Sittig A.C. Talmon J.L. Drie methoden voor kennisverwerving. Kennissystemen, 1987, 3, 20-32. (in Dutch)

Goodridge D.M.G., Shorvon S.D. Epileptic seizures in a population of 6000, demography, diagnosis and classification, and role of hospital services. British Medical Journal, 1983, 287, 641-647.

Hayes Roth F., Waterman D.A. Constructing an expert system. In: Building Expert Systems, Addison Wesley, 1983, pp 127-168.

Heng M.S.H. Why evolutionary development of expert systems appears to work. Future Generations Computer Systems, 1987, 3, 103-109.

Hoffman R.R. The problem of extracting knowledge from experts from the perspective of experimental psychology. A.I. Mag. 1987, summer, 53-67.

Overweg J. Epilepsie; prognose en behandeling. Ned. Tijdschr. Geneeskd. 1984, 128, 1710-1716. (in Dutch)

Reitman Olsen J., Rueter H.H. Extracting expertise from experts: methods for knowledge acquisition. Expert Systems, 1987, 4, 152-168.

Shorvon S.D., Chadwick D., Galbraith A.W., Reynolds E.H. One drug for epilepsy. British medical Journal, 1978, 1, 474-476.

Shorvon S.D., Reynolds E.H. Early prognosis of epilepsy. British Medical Journal, 1982, 285, 1699-1701.

Smeets R.P.A.M., Talmon J.L., Lugt van der P.J.M., Schijven R.A.J. The development of a knowledge system for surveillance of anti-epileptic medication. In: Proc. of AIME 1989, Springer-Verlag, 1989, 14-23.

Waterman D.A. Building an expert system, in A guide to expert systems, Addisson-Wesley, 1986.

Wright G., Ayton P. Eliciting and modelling expert knowledge. Decision Support Systems, 1987, 3, 13-26.

DIACONS - Diabetes Consultant: Goals and Status

Rolf Engelbrecht[1], Jutta Schneider[1], Klaus Piwernetz[2]

1 Institut für Medizinische Informatik und Systemforschung (MEDIS) Gesellschaft für Strahlen- und Umweltforschung (GSF), Neuherberg, West Germany

2 Diabeteszentrum Krankenhaus München Bogenhausen, München, West Germany

Introduction

The main application of computers in health care systems concentrated on hospitals, the reason being that in early days they were, from an economical point of view, the minimum size of organizational unit required to yield some efficiency. With this restriction the influence of the computer technology on the development in medical informatics was significant. So it is recommended to explain the history, the status, and the future of hospital information systems with respect to the information technology and a look to the communication and information structure in health care delivery and finally with respect to medicine itself.

Due to specialization in different medical disciplines usually more than one physician is responsible for the patient including physicians in the different service units and laboratories. Therefore, communication is a fundamental process in medicine, which still relies on telephone, paper, and personal contact for information transfer and authentication.

The application of new techniques , therapies, drugs, etc. in the medical practice remains a continuous research project. Requirements result coming from the demands of quality of care and cost containment.

Medical Informatics plays an important role in the domains briefly characterized above and could be regarded as:

- the support of well understood routine tasks in broad application areas of prevention, diagnostic, therapy, education, and research in medicine in an effective and cheap way;
- the provision of information, advice, expertise, and knowledge in multiple situations and environments to enhance the quality of care and local problem handling;
- the provision of local and regional communication facilities to obtain patient data, information etc. at various localities accurately and without delay ;
- the provision of epidemiological and economical aggregated data for managerial decisions and health care resources planning.

In general, the goals of the project DIACONS as part of a hospital information and communication system correspond with the requirements mentioned above.

It is a challenge for medical informatics to give assistance by the use of tools to enhance the quality of care by reducing costs at the same time. Peterson stated in his opening speech at Medinfo 86, that about 30 percent of all hospital costs are spent on information processing, and studies showed that 50 percent of the physicians' workload is documentation and information handling.

The best way to give assistance in this situation is to bring information processing to the workplace of the user and to deal with new techniques of medical informatics including that of artificial intelligence (AI), especially expert systems.

Medical expert systems can be described as computer software products with a medical knowledge base that are designed to assist physicians and medical personnel in diagnosis, therapy, patient management and related tasks in medical care. The use of medical expert systems is assumed to produce tremendous changes in today's health care system.

DIACONS Diabetes Consultant

The project DIACONS is an approach to assist medical professionals and patients in the field of Diabetes mellitus with techniques and methods of medical informatics and artificial intelligence. Partners in the project are the MEDIS-Institute, the teaching hospital Bogenhausen, Munich, and, during an initial phase, IBM Germany.

The aims of the DIACONS project are the support of diagnosis and therapy, quality assurance, cost containment and education. Side effects are the gathering of data for other routine use and epidemiological purposes including knowledge elicitation. This will be done by knowledge based support of medical documentation, modules for interactive diagnostic and therapeutic consultation and education for doctors, nurses, students and patients. The first prototypes to reach these goals are under development, resp. are used in daily routine.

The sensitive areas in the care of patients with diabetes are the monitoring and tuning of the metabolism, the lack of knowledge and treatment experience of physicians and general practitioners not specialized in Diabetes, and self education and training of patients and their relatives.

In order to reach the targets as defined above, three major problems are to be tackled and this is done through the following services:

● DIADOC medical documentation including watchdog-functions
● DIAMON monitor for long-term care
● DIAED   education.

DIADOC supports medical documentation which plays an important role especially in chronic diseases. Watchdog-functions are used for static tolerance verification and trend forecasting (for example monitoring of blood glucose values, i.e. recognizing trends and, if necessary, warning of too high or too low blood glucose values). DIADOC must also be seen as a diagnostic aid and an information basis for therapeutic decisions.

DIAMON offers individual therapy plans, monitors adequacy of therapy and accuracy of time intervals between check-ups, along with quality of metabolic control. It also includes self-monitoring by the patient, a key element in the therapy of diabetes, since it improves both quality and safety of treatment.

DIAED helps educating patients and clinical staff through computerized training programs and thus substantially increases the patients' knowledge about diabetes. In addition, it contributes to the reduction of workload for clinical personnel and it may even be used for continuing medical education, features that set new standards in time and cost efficiency.

All three components are developed separately with respect to later integration.

The basis of the system is a ward oriented network of personal computers backboned by a mainframe. The different knowledge based modules can run either on the PCs or on the data base oriented mainframe computer.

Of great importance is the distribution of processing power and data. The principle is that the data should be processed where they are stored. On the mainframe computer there is the central data base containing the administrative patient data, the medical patient data like patient's history, anamnesis, and current treatment, and data images from subsystems like the laboratory subsystems. The knowledge bases are the essential parts for the processing of medical records and giving therapeutical advice.

The concept includes local processing facilities like blood glucose measurement units and application programs for generating reports from the medical records.

DIADOC - Diabetes Documentation Assistance

The medical treatment is based on the diagnosis, the patient history and previous experiences made during the patient's treatment. Data of all these events are stored normally in the patient's medical record which is a central point in each information system in medicine. DIADOC has to fulfill the followings tasks:

- data entry with full syntactic and semantic checks
- storing of medical records
- watchdog functions to serve as an alert for physicians or nurse in case of any possible complications concerning the patient
- nursing assistance through patient care related information
- retrieval assistance based on medical knowledge and previous reports available, resp. the content of the reports.

To achieve these goals a prototype (*Engelbrecht et al, 1987a*) has been developed containing

- 28 menus
- 20 screen forms, resp. relations, with a total of 700 data items
- 68 print forms or reports.

This has been the basis for the data base design, which has been done for ADABAS on the mainframe computer and dBase III on the network database server.

The data are first gathered in the ward-oriented PC-database, and for long term medical documentation and hospital wide communication the relevant information is stored in the mainframe medical database which is the reference database during the project separated from the hospital administrative database. The data base manipulation language is decided to be SQL in all environments.

The SQL-type data base interface (DBI) was tested in the SMA (Scholz-Medis-Arzneimittelinformationssystem) (*Engelbrecht et al, 1987b*) and has shown its flexibility using different DBMS such as Btrieve and INFORMIX. In this project it will be used for the ADABAS mainframe medical data base and it is planned to install SQL on the network DB-server, e.g. DB2 or dBase IV.

All data are checked by watchdogs before updating the database. There are several types or functions of watchdogs starting like the check for out of range data or initiating alert actions. In combination with simulation techniques even a normal value may lead to an action when looking at the patient history or the physiological model, a dangerous situation may occur for the patient. In a first prototype watchdogs are built to check the data obtained from the ward laboratory.

DIAMON - Monitor for long-term care

The aim of treatment of diabetes patients is to attain near-normoglycemia. This is done by specific therapy elements which could be assembled to therapy schemes. Single elements are e.g. insulin, oral antidiabetic agents, slow down absorptioner, diet, additional drugs, education monitoring and self monitoring. The therapy scheme is typical for a class of patients and has to be adapted to the individual patient. In addition, the therapy, as in all living and feedback systems, has to monitored and constantly be readapted.

A prototype for the selection and adaptation of the suitable therapy element insulin has been built in a first version. Since it is easy for the medical professionals to explain their reasoning by rules and most parts of the knowledge about diabetes therapy can be expressed in rules, we decided to use ESE/VM as an expert system shell for implementing the prototype DIAMON. ESE uses the MYCIN paradigm with certainty factors and is produced by the project partner IBM.

Knowledge can be structured hierarchically in units called 'focus control blocks' (FCBs). This form of representation corresponds to the known 'object-attribute-value relationship'. An FCB contains control information used in solving problems. This information, like forward-/backward chaining, is specified as properties that determine the control flow desired for a given unit of work. Complex problems can usually be subdivided into smaller components, each of them can be processed by its own FCB (Fig. 1). We use FCBs among other things for the different classifications needed to determine the adequate therapy. For instance, we use one FCB for classifying the type of diabetes, another for checking the contraindications.

The expert system (DIAMON) retrieves the patient's data directly from the database as far as available, otherwise from terminal input. Once it has determined the two diagnostic components, namely the type of diabetes and the quality of metabolic control, and taken into account case history, late complications, specific circumstances, etc., the system checks the indications, offers up to 3 adequate insulin schemes and points at possibly existing contraindications. More information on this prototype is available in *Schneider et al, 1988, 1989*.

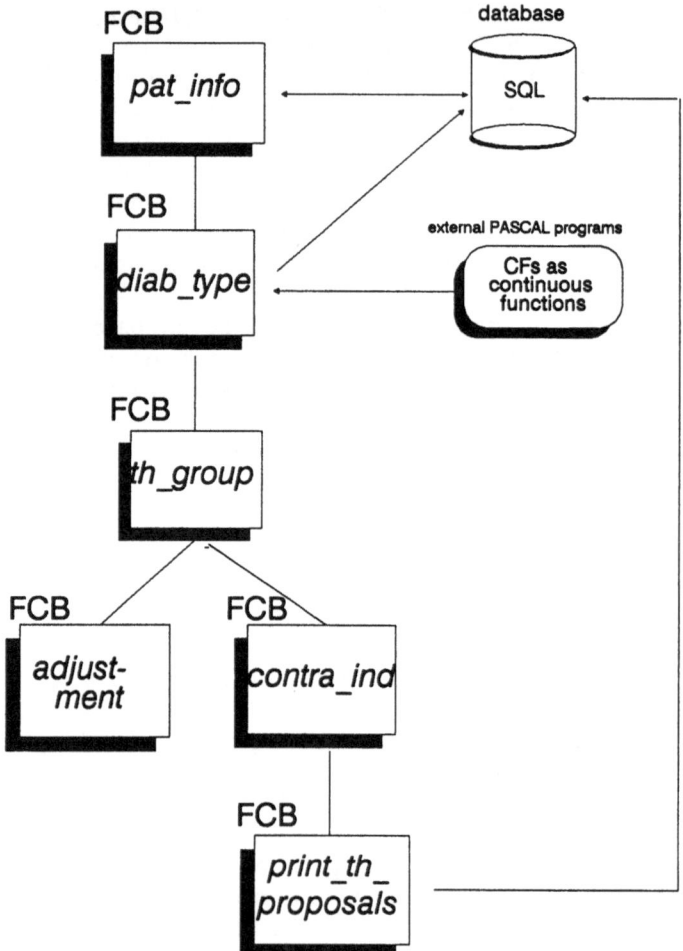

Figure 1:   FCB- Hierarchy in DIAMON
            pat_info: patient information
            diab_type: diagnosis Diabetes type
            th_group: classification therapeutical group (schema)
            adjustment: adjustment of therapy
            contra_ind: checking for contraindications
            print_th_proposals: printing and storing of therapy proposals

One of the major reasons to select ESE as a tool was the ability of accessing patient data from a data base. SQL/DS is integrated into ESE and for this prototype data were loaded from the hospital based PCs into the mainframe, where the current available version of ESE is running. A runtime version on a PC is announced and will be used as soon as available for practical use and evaluation. In the meantime DIAMON is evaluated with typical testcases and usable via a leased line from the hospital to our development environment.

As soon as the PC-runtime version of ESE is available it has to be to decided whether the extended prototype has to be used in the mainframe version via leased line or on PC.

DIAMON is one basis for the AIM project EURODIABETA and will be extended and integrated in a European model for computer assistance in chronic disease. Enhancements in this context are

- the inclusion of additional therapy schemes for type II diabetics;
- full integration of the data base including the extension of the update function to store earlier consultations;
- a module for rule based dosage calculation based on a mathematical model and previous data;
- continuous monitoring and adapting the chosen therapy using XTOOL as a complex shell, developed by SIEMENS, one of the EURODIABETA partners. This approach requires time oriented reasoning.

For later implementation in the hospital environment a second prototype is under development which uses the shell MED2 for diagnostic expert systems developed by Puppe and coworkers. MED2 runs on the Macintosh during the development phase especially when the knowledge acquisition tool CLASSIKA is used, and is able to produce runtime versions for PCs under MS-DOS. The supported data base management system will be dBase and it is planned to access the ADABAS medical data base in later versions.

DIAED Education

The success in the treatment of diabetes is based on the active cooperation by the patient and the medical staff. Therefore it is necessary to instruct the patient about the causes, characteristics and consequences of his disease and in a second step to train him in the different therapy elements which are discussed before. Some of these elements could be subject to a computer assisted education and training program.

In the scope of the DIACONS project several modules for patient education have been developed dealing with basic knowledge about diabetes and risks, such as hypoglycemia, car driving and diabetes, and diet. In these examples the authoring system SEF-PC and STORYBOARD were used.

A second set of modules explains the physiological models of diabetes and can be adapted to the patient data. The instruction is running like a movie with the possibility to be interrupted by the physician user. It is implemented on a PC with EGA colour card and runs for about 45 minutes without interruption and also contains steps to check the understanding.

In a third set of modules interactive blood glucose simulation is shown with instruction parts and graphical output. These modules are based on the physiological model. They are written in PASCAL and the instruction is developed also using STORYBOARD.

Conclusion

DIACONS is an approach to assist physicians, nurses and patients in the treatment of Diabetes mellitus. A second goal of this project is to get expertise and experience and to transfer this other ward oriented applications or models and standards to ensure the interpretation of information, to enhance the system and to build a platform for further development or integration of other components. For the standardization of the data structure there exists the MBDS (Minimal Basic Data Set for hospital statistics in Europe) which will serve as an example and will be extended to a reference for chronic care in the EURODIABETA project.

Looking at the DIACONS project other components may be identified. As hardware standard, PCs are used with a communication connection via PC network on the departmental layer. This enables the usage of a lot of interface cards and enhancements, e.g. to connect the PC to the blood-glucose meters which are used on the ward in an easy and reasonable way. Also connections will be installed via standard add-on cards to the IBM mainframe and SIEMENS mainframe in the hospital Bogenhausen. A connection to the computer of the clinical laboratory is installed on the basis of a standard interface. The decisions on the software were more difficult. On the PC level there are dramatic changes to be expected from the SAA concept, but software is not yet available. It has been decided to use dBase III file structures on the PCs to enable an easy access from different standard software packages, even to use dBase itself. The database model is the relational model of Codd and points to the SAA SQL approach.

On the mainframe the administrative hospital information system krw2 is available, developed by GSD (Gesellschaft für Systemforschung und Dienstleistungen im Gesundheitswesen), a company founded by the city of Berlin to develop a system which is adaptable to all needs of the hospitals of Berlin ranging from university hospitals to acute hospitals. This krw2 system is based on the database management system ADABAS, which can be seen as a relational one in connection with the programming system NATURAL and the SQL interface. From the PC network there is a user written interface to the mainframe which is SQL-oriented and is a system-conform link between applications on the PC and centrally stored and maintained data on the krw2 system.

A first evaluation of the DIAMON part is just in the final validation stage and will serve as a basis for the development of evaluation requirements in the EURODIABETA project. It will be based on a selected sample of 50 European cases.

Beside the medical aspects this project will serve as a testbed for using methods of knowledge based systems especially the knowledge acquisition process.

References

Engelbrecht, R., Kunze, I., Schneider, J.: Entwicklung eines Dokumentationssystems für Diabetespatienten. In: Informationsbedarfsermittlung und -analyse für den Entwurf von Informationssystemen, R.R. Wagner et al. (Eds.), Berlin Heidelberg: Springer, 244-257, (1987a)

Engelbrecht, R., Schaaf, R., Scholz, W.: Pharmaceutical consultation system for physicians and pharmacists - basis for an expert system ?, In: EFMI-MIE 87 proceedings, A. Serio et al. (Eds.), Rom, Edi.Press, 1106-115 (1987b)

Schneider, J., Piwernetz, K., Engelbrecht, R., Renner, R.: DIACONS - A consultation system to assist in the management of Diabetes. In: Expert Systems and Decision Support in Medicine, Rienhoff, O., Schneider, B., Piccolo, U., (Eds.), Lecture Notes in Medical Informatics 36, New York, Springer, 44-49, (1988)

Schneider, J., Renner, R., Engelbrecht, R., Piwernetz, K.: DIAMON - First Evaluation Results. MEDINFO 89, Singapore 10-14 December 1989, Barber, B., Cao, D., Qin, D., Wagner, G. (Eds.), North-Holland, 222-225, 1989.

CARTES - A Prototype Decision Support System in Oncology

Pentti Kolari[1], Jussi Yliaho[1], Kari Näriäinen[1], Simo Hyödynmaa[1], Antti Ojala[2], Jukka Rantanen[3], and Niilo Saranummi[1]

1 Medical Engineering Laboratory, Technical Research Centre of Finland, Tampere, Finland

2 Department of Radiotherapy, Tampere University Central Hospital Pikonlinna, Finland

3 Laboratory for Information Processing, Technical Research Centre of Finland, Helsinki, Finland

Introduction

Oncology, the study of neoplastic diseases, is generally referred to as the cancer problem (*Rubin, 1983*). It is the study of a large variety of tumors of malignant nature with lethal potential. In spite of its lethal character, it is nowadays far from synonymous with "an incurable disease". Much progress has been achieved to cope with all aspects of the cancer problem.

Characteristic to current cancer therapy is that there are more opinions than truths about the most suitable treatment. Since the etiology of cancer diseases is still partly unknown, the knowledge of these diseases is mostly empirical. In these circumstances, careful collection, recording and analysis of patient data is a necessity in monitoring the quality of care and in developing better treatment methods. Because of the chronic character of many cancer diseases, the treatment cycle of a cancer patient (diagnosis, therapy design and execution, follow-up) is often several years, even decades. Although there is an endeavor to uniform therapy in various cancer diseases, the response of patients to a given therapy varies necessitating in some cases a more individual therapy. This, in turn, makes it difficult to obtain statistical evidence for the most suitable treatment. The long treatment cycle and individual therapy jointly put special emphasis for patient management.

Information technology has been utilized in oncology for some decades to automate the complicated computations associated with radiotherapy dose planning (*Johns and Cunningham, 1980, Viitanen, 1989*). Computers have also been used to assist physicians and other health professionals treating cancer patients with their decision making tasks. The first systems used statistically oriented (*Feinstein et al, 1972*) and algorithmic approaches (*Wirtschafter et al, 1979, Lenhard et al, 1984*). Knowledge based techniques have also been experimented as a way to assist the oncologist. ONCOCIN (*Shortliffe et al, 1981, Langlotz and Shortliffe, 1983*) and its offsprings OPAL (*Musen et al, 1987*) and ONYX (*Langlotz et al, 1987*) are perhaps the best-known applications of this approach in oncology. Several other examples of activities in this domain can be found in the literature (e.g. *Rennels, 1987, Kalet and Jacky, 1987*).

The Nordic CART (Computer Aided RadioTherapy) program (1985 - 87) developed an integrated information system for radiotherapy (*Lamm, 1987*). The principal results of CART were functional prototypes of the modules in an integrated information system for radiotherapy, and parameter definitions and standards for information transfer between the modules. During CART it became evident that there are numerous situations in the cancer therapy process, where decision support is needed and applicable. A project named CARTES (CART Expert System) was launched as an associate to CART to address these decision support issues.

Cancer Therapy Process

The therapy process begins with diagnostic procedures and tests to verify the malignant character of the disease, the site, type and extension of the tumor. This is followed by planning of therapy. It starts with the definition of the intention of the treatment, whether it is to cure, to palliate, or just to support the patient. The next step, after the definition of the intention of therapy, is to consider, by which treatment modality (or combination of these) the goal is best achieved. Three different treatment modalities are used routinely in cancer therapy: surgery, radiotherapy and chemotherapy (including hormonal therapy). In some cancer diseases several treatment modalities are combined routinely - simultaneously or in succession. After choosing the treatment modality(-ies), a detailed treatment plan is worked out. This comprises the essential details of the planned treatment.

For the basis of therapy planning several additional tests may be needed to determine e.g. the stage of the disease, degree of microscopic differentiation and operability of the patient. The results of these tests as well as the patient's age, general condition, symptoms and his own wishes about therapy affect the decision. In most cases there are two or even more alternative treatment schemes to choose. The physician must choose between alternative treatment options, each of which may carry considerable risk. The risks and benefits of each strategy need to be carefully considered before undertaking treatment. The final decision in selecting treatment often requires some value judgement in balancing quality of life against quantity of life, or one state of ill health (e.g. painful disease) against another (e.g. side effects).

There are disease specific classifications for most cancer diseases that help to classify patients into homogeneous groups according to their prognostic factors. If a clinic has fixed certain treatment practices for prognostic groups, the physician's main tasks are to determine the relevant class for the patient and to assess, if there are any special factors that indicate deviation from the standard treatment scheme.

The treatment is executed according to the plan, if possible. During treatment the patient is monitored continuously. Modifications to the treatment plan are made if the patient is not responsive to the given therapy or if he experiences severe, unexpected complications. An essential part of the management of the patient during therapy are the various supportive measures such as treatment of infections, relief of pain, taking care of nutrition, and rehabilitation.

In cancer treatment permanent cure is not always achievable. Because of the chronic character of cancer, treatment outcome can be measured often only after a follow-up period of several years. This implies that a well-organized follow-up of the patient is necessary. At present, patient follow-up is often inadequate, which makes it difficult to draw conclusions of the suitability of therapy. Missing, too weak or erroneous feedback from therapy outcome to therapy decision making and design of therapy is considered one of the most serious problems in current cancer therapy.

Role of Information Technology and Knowledge Based Systems in Oncology

Some of the decisions that are made during the treatment process are simple, some are complex and require expertise from several medical specialities. General oncological knowledge derived from medical textbooks, reports of clinical trials etc. is involved in each decision making stage. This knowledge is applied at the institutional level according to the local circumstances (e.g. availability of radiotherapy units) and experience. Local experience is gathered by recording relevant clinical data in each phase of the therapy process and analyzing it afterwards.

The significance of careful data collection, recording and analysis has been recognized early in the monitoring and control of malignant diseases. It enables the evaluation of the current practice, i.e. quality assurance. On the basis of this, it is natural that the backbone of a computerized oncological information system is the clinical database system, which comprises all data that is generated during the diagnostic, therapeutic, and follow-up cycles of a cancer patient. In addition to data management, it includes facilities for entry and analysis of data.

In striving towards uniform therapies oncologists have set up local, national and international therapy programs, which define the best currently known therapy for a specific cancer disease. The concept "treatment protocol" usually is associated with the strictly specified protocols of the clinical trials, but it can also be used in context of the routine treatment schemes, which are often very diffusely specified. In routine treatment schemes also slight modifications to the basic protocol may be allowed, if considered acceptable for the purposes of the overall treatment. The protocols are often complicated and there are several of them in use simultaneously.

Knowledge based systems for decision support should be integrated with the overall oncological information system. They support by augmentation the physician during the therapy process of a cancer patient. Knowledge based techniques can also be applied in providing feedback from outcome analysis to decision making.

A prerequisite of the oncological information system is a data exchange standard, which facilitates the exchange of data between different components of the system. Integration of the oncological information system to other information systems of the hospital is essential in order to utilize existing, already recorded data and information.

System Model

Three stages in the cancer therapy process were identified where decision support with knowledge based techniques seems necessary and has an impact on the outcome of cancer therapy. The stages are:
- therapy decision making,
- design of new treatment protocols, and
- analysis of therapy results.

The chosen stages were taken as separate modules in the system. Figure 1 outlines the model of an integrated oncological decision support system.

Module 1 supports the primary therapeutic decision making at an oncological clinic after cancer diagnosis has been made. It checks the eligibility of the patients into existing treatment alternatives and classifies the patients into prognostic groups. On the basis of this information the module assists in the definition of the intention of therapy and in the selection of an applicable treatment protocol. If none of the existing protocols is relevant, the module assists in the design of individual therapy.

Module 2 supports the design of new and modification of existing treatment protocols. It includes knowledge of the existing treatment protocols and methods to change them and to design new ones based mainly on the results of clinical trials. The module includes oncological and statistical knowledge of the design and execution of clinical trials to test new and alternative treatment protocols.

Module 3 supports the analysis of treatment results. One purpose of the analysis is to derive relationships between treatment outcome (e.g. survival time) and other factors. This implies the need to use statistical methods. The module assists in the analysis and statistical processing of therapy results (problem formulation, execution of the analysis, interpretation of the results of the analysis). The module is also used to feed conclusions and hypotheses back to therapy decision making and therapy design. The objectives of the module are the evaluation of the correctness of current decision criteria, verification or falsification of heuristic hypotheses and automatic control of therapy results. The module is influenced by the principles used

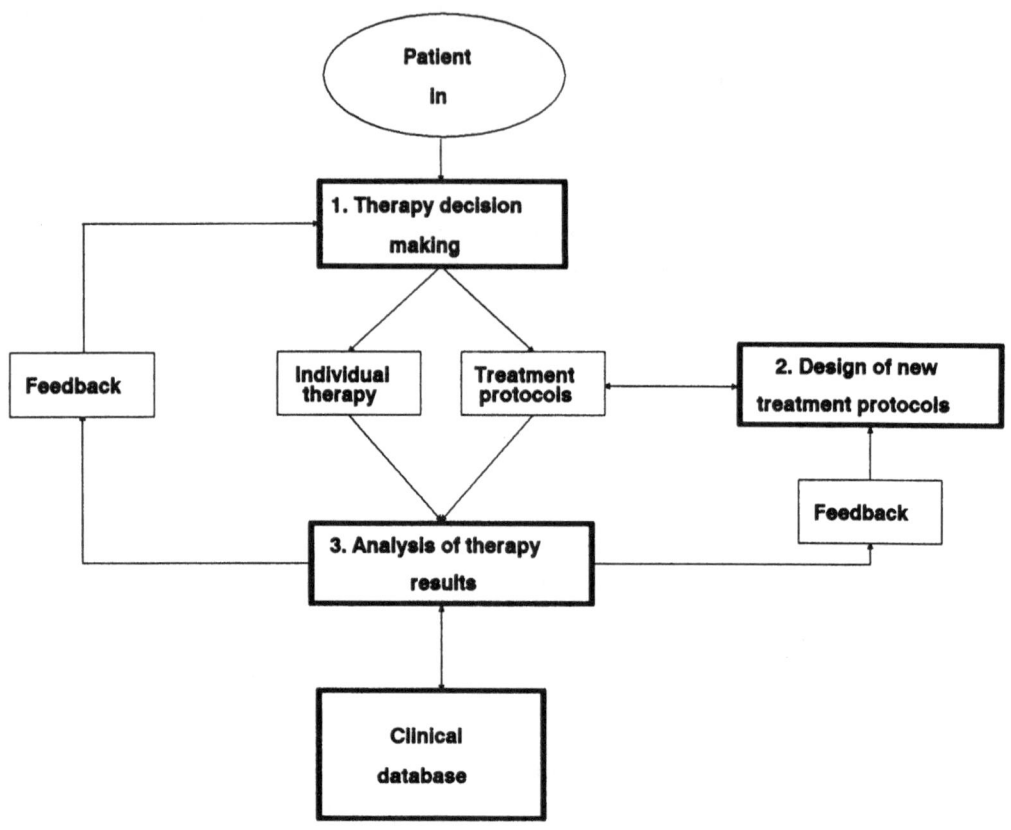

Figure 1: Proposed system model

in RADIX (*Blum, 1982*), which developed methods for automating the discovery and confirmation of scientific hypotheses from large databases.

Much of the functionality of the system is based on the intensive use of the *clinical database*. The use of the clinical database in the proposed system is twofold. It is used by Module 1 as a source of patient data to minimize the amount of data the user has to enter during consultation with the system. It is also a prerequisite in the analysis of treatment results. To be useful in the outcome analysis the data must be reliable and detailed enough.

The users of the system are physicians on the oncological department of a hospital, either in actual clinical work or in research activities. The main user of module 1 is a junior doctor without major experience in cancer therapy. The oncology expert himself is the main user of modules 2 and 3.

Specifications of all the modules have been worked out. Only module 1 has been implemented in the form of a prototype.

Prototype of Therapy Decision Support Module

Modality and functional specifications

To be acceptable in a clinical environment, the intended purpose of the system must be considered in the context of who will be its principal users before the system is created. A clear distinction between the roles of the system and users and the problem solving task must be made.

There are principally three ways an expert system might approach giving and justifying its advice (*Miller, 1984*):

- the system commits itself to a particular approach,
- the system produces a general discussion of viable alternatives and of their respective risks and benefits, and
- the system critiques user plans.

In the proposed system, the critiquing model is used where it seems applicable and relevant to the context. The system shall justify its recommendations in a medically sound way and with references to medical literature.

The user interface must be convenient for a busy clinician who is necessarily not familiar with computing and information systems. Intelligent forms and graphic presentations based on windows, icons, menus, and pointer device are used in the conversation between the system and the user.

A limited prototype has been constructed for module 1. The domain of the prototype is primary therapeutic decision making, i.e. specification of the intention of therapy, in inoperable non-small cell lung cancer. The treatment modalities supported by the system are restricted to radiotherapy.

Lung cancer was chosen as the domain of the prototype, because it is a common cancer disease and traditionally many patients are treated with radical radiotherapy, but only a few of them have a real advantage of radical treatment. Although groups of patients exist, who undoubtedly are candidates for radical treatment and others, who are not, there is a large group of patients, for whom the decision between radical, palliative and/or supportive treatment is not easily made.

Tasks of the system

The tasks of the prototype are:

- to check if the clinical picture of the patient matches with the diagnosis proposed by the physician,

- to find out if there are any such symptoms that indicate to start the treatment immediately (e.g. vena cava superior syndrome), and
- to check if the proposed intention of therapy (only local radical/locoregional radical/possibly radical/possibly palliative/palliative or supportive) is relevant in the case.

This last task is the main task of the system. Selection is affected principally by the age and performance status of the patient, and stage of the disease. For staging, several tests and examinations must be done, and the combination of these results yields the staging information. In addition, different symptoms and results of laboratory tests give hints about the clinical stage of the disease and may indicate more detailed staging examinations.

Development environment

The prototype is based on an object oriented design. It is implemented on a Xerox 1186 AI workstation using Interlisp and LOOPS (Lisp Object Oriented Programming System). LOOPS incorporates four distinct paradigms of programming (procedure, object, data and rule oriented programming) within the Interlisp programming environment to allow users to choose the style of programming which best suits their application (*Bobrow and Stefik, 1983*).

Knowledge representation

Domain knowledge is represented by a tree-shaped object taxonomy (Figure 2) describing the classification (based on microscopical type of the disease) of lung carcinoma and its subtypes. Each disease class contains several assertion sets, which capture different disease specific features like when to support or be doubtful about the diagnosis, when regional treatment is needed, or when radical treatment is possible.

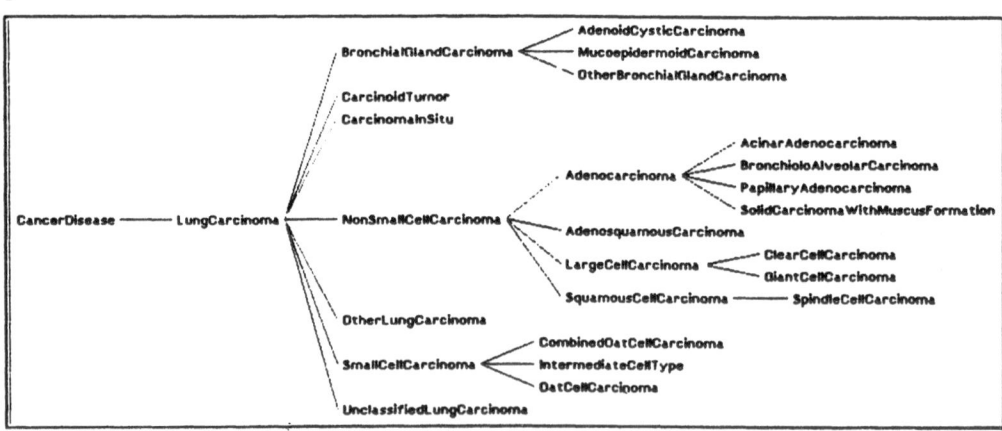

Figure 2: Classification of lung carcinoma and its subtypes

The system has an agenda-based control. When the reasoning is started all root tasks (tasks that are not activated by other tasks) that have to be executed (AssessDiagnosis, FixNeedOfImmediateTreatment, FixIntentionOfTherapy, CriticizeIntentionOfTherapy) are loaded to the agenda. Every task knows the name of the working memory (WM) variable whose value it can infer, its value class, and the names of the assertion sets that are used during the inference process. When the value of a WM variable which does not yet exist, is needed, the corresponding task is sought and invoked. This facilitates a kind of backward chaining in the system. Root tasks are executed one by one until all of them have been processed.

Each task infers the value of the corresponding WM variable as follows. All assertion sets that are needed are collected from all disease classes that are on a route which begins from the class that corresponds to the diagnosis (microscopical type of the disease) and ends to the root class of the disease taxonomy. The assertions in the set are evaluated one by one using the information about the current patient case and the contents of the WM. As the result, the system returns the truth value of each assertion set and as the justification for the conclusion the assertions that are either true or false.

When the system generates its critique prose, i.e. explains its reasoning, it transforms the assertions that are stored as justification of a conclusion into a prose form. Augmented Transition Network (ATN) formalism is used to connect the transformed prose segments to form stylized English prose. The ATN's are used in the way described by *Miller, 1986*.

The main LOOPS objects of the prototype are the following:

- Object *Desktop* consists of objects that are common resources for all cases in the system. These include windows, forms for data input, menus for controlling the system, global variables etc.
- Object *Agenda*, which controls the execution of tasks.
- Object *WorkingMemory*, which provides temporary storage for deduced values.
- Object *InferenceEngine*, which manipulates the assertion sets.
- Object class *Case* is instantiated whenever a new patient case is introduced in the system. Each instance contains attributes that describe the patient, symptoms, test results, diagnosis etc.

Agenda, WorkingMemory and InferenceEngine are instantiated as part of object Desktop. The tasks are implemented as LOOPS methods written in Interlisp.

Use of the system

For the basis of reasoning relevant data and information about the social and medical history of the patient, signs and symptoms, and results of various examinations and tests are needed. The system retrieves data from the clinical database automatically or data is entered by the user through input forms.

After the user has entered his proposal for the intention of therapy, the reasoning is started. During the reasoning phase the system deduces values for the key variables and, on the basis of these, forms its proposal for the intention of therapy. In addition, it compares the proposals of the user and its own, and shows the results of the comparison as critique text (sample output below).

> *I would not recommend radical treatment in this case. First, when the age of the patient is greater than 75 years, he probably won't tolerate radical treatment. Second, when Karnofsky performance is less than 70 or Zubrod more than 2, radical treatment seldom is useful. Third, since symptoms include weight loss, this may indicate more widespread disease than the actual stage III.*

Evaluation

A group of Scandinavian oncology experts has evaluated the principles of the system and the human computer interface. Clinical experiences have also been gathered from a group of physicians with varying backgrounds in oncology. In addition, the system is presently being tested retrospectively with a number of inoperable lung cancer patient cases.

On the basis of the experiences so far, it is evident that to be clinically acceptable, the system must have access to the clinical database. The present prototype is a stand alone system, and data entry has been seen as a bottleneck of the system. Response time is also an important factor that has to be addressed to make the system convenient to use. Flexibility of the system is significant, too. The system should e.g. be able to indicate the changes in the results of reasoning, if the user modifies some of the input parameters (what-if questions).

Evaluation has shown that the system is of greatest value for unexperienced physicians. It can assist in avoiding mistakes by reminding the user of missing information. In addition, it forces the user to justify his decisions by making the decision process and criteria explicit.

Conclusions

It seems evident that knowledge based decision support systems have many possible applications in oncology, if the right stages of application are identified. However, there are several difficulties, which may restrict the use of such systems in practice. In many common cancer diseases, the diagnostics and the treatment are often quite schematic. Uncommon diseases, although suitable in theory for expert systems, are seen so rare in a clinic that the efforts needed to build a decision support system are too high for occasional use of this system. In some cancer diseases, the diagnostic and/or therapeutic strategies may be changing so fast that major changes may occur already during the building of the decision support system.

Variations in diagnostic and therapeutic methods and in organization and resources between clinics diminish the usefulness and acceptance of the system. This is contrasted by the need for unified practices promoted by both collaborative national and international clinical trials and decision support systems like this. Information technology and knowledge based systems especially are a potential tool in making differences in practices and outcome measurable.

The final aim of the future work is to integrate knowledge based systems with the clinical database. The next step will be the specification and construction of an oncological clinical database for the system. Special regard will be given to the problem of coordination of the clinical database with other information systems of the department and hospital relevant to the delivery and evaluation of cancer therapy. The integration of the decision support subsystem and other subsystems as part of an oncological information system will also be addressed.

Acknowledgements

This work was a spinoff of the Nordic CART (Computer Aided RadioTherapy) R&D program. It was funded by the Board of Nordic Ministers, and by Technical Research Centre of Finland through its research program for AI Applications.

References

Blum, R. L.: Discovery and Representation of Causal Relationships from a Large Time-Oriented Clinical Database: The RX Project. Lecture Notes in Medical Informatics. Edited by Lindberg, D. A. B. and Reichertz, P. L. Berlin, Springer-Verlag, 1982, 242 pp.

Bobrow, D. G. and Stefik, M.: The LOOPS Manual. December, 1983. Xerox Corporation, 1983, 124 pp.

Johns, H. E. and Cunningham, J. R.: The Physics of Radiology. Third edition, sixth printing. Springfield, Illinois, USA, Charles G. Thomas Publisher, 1980, 800 pp.

Kalet, I. J. and Jacky J. P.: Knowledge-Based Computer Simulation for Radition Therapy Planning. Proc. of the 9th Int. Conf. on the Use of Computers in Radiation Therapy. The Hague, The Netherlands, 22 - 25 June 1987. North-Holland, Amsterdam, 1987, pp. 553 - 556.

Lamm, I. L. CART - Report on the Nordic Co-Operation Programme. Proc. of the 9th Int. Conf. on the Use of Computers in Radiation Therapy. The Hague, The Netherlands, 22 - 25 June 1987. North-Holland, Amsterdam, 1987, pp. 257 - 260.

Langlotz, C. P. and Shortliffe, E. H.: Adapting a consultation system to critique user plans. International Journal of Man-Machine Studies, 19, 1983, pp. 479 - 496.

Langlotz, C. P., Fagan, L. M., Tu, S. W., Sikic, B. I. and Shortliffe, E. H.: A therapy planning architecture that combines decision theory and artificial intelligence techniques. Computers and Biomedical Research 20, 1987, pp. 279 - 303.

Lenhard, R. E., Blum, B. I. and McColligan, E. E.: An Information System for Oncology. In: Blum, B. I. (ed.) Information Systems for Patient Care. New York, Springer-Verlag, 1984, pp. 385 - 403.

Miller, P. L.: Critiquing as a modality for explanation: Three systems. Proceedings of AAMSI Congress 84, 1984, pp. 105 - 109.

Miller, P. L.: Expert Critiquing Systems. Practice Based Medical Consultation by Computer. Computers and Medicine. Edited by Blum, B. I. New York, Springer Verlag, 1986.

Musen, M. A., Fagan, L. M., Combs, D. M. and Shortliffe, E. H.: Use of a domain model to drive an interactive knowledge-editing tool. Int. J. of Man-Machine Studies, 26, 1987, pp. 105 - 121.

Rennels, G. D.: A Computational Model of Reasoning from the Clinical Literature. Lecture Notes in Medical Informatics. Edited by P. L. Reichertz and D. A. B. Lindberg. Berlin, Springer-Verlag, 1987, 230 pp.

Rubin P. (ed.): Clinical Oncology for Medical Students and Physicians. A Multidisciplinary Approach. Sixth Edition. New York, American Cancer Society, 1983, 536 pp.

Shortliffe, E.H., Scott, A.C., Bischoff, M., Campbell, A.B., van Melle, W. and Jacobs, C.: ONCOCIN: An expert system for oncology protocol management. Proceedings of the 7th International Joint Conference on Artificial Intelligence. Vancouver, 1981, pp. 876 - 881.

Viitanen, J.: Development and evaluation of a dose planning system for radiation therapy. Technical Research Centre of Finland, Publications 52. Espoo, 1989, 148 pp.

Wirtschafter, D., Carpenter, J. T. and Mesel, E.: A Consultant-Extender System for Breast Cancer Adjuvant Chemotherapy. Annals of Internal Medicine 90, 3, 1979, pp. 396 - 401.

Questions from the discussion

V.d. Lei: Langlotz also produced a critiquing mode for ONCOCIN. What are the differences or similarities between his system and yours?

Saranummi: ONCOCIN offers as its treatment recommendation a comprehensive chemotherapy treatment plan. The treatment proposal provided by our system includes the intention of therapy. Main difference between the systems is that the treatment proposal of ONCOCIN is more complicated than that of our system.

APPLICATIONS
Management of the critically ill

Information Management and Decision Support for the Critically Ill

K. Autio[1], A. Mäkivirta[1], T. Sukuvaara[1], A. Kari[2], E. Koski[2], S. Kalli[1], J. Hunter[3], N. Saranummi[1]

1 Technical Research Centre of Finland, Medical Engineering Laboratory, Tampere, Finland

2 Kuopio University Central Hospital, Kuopio, Finland

3 University of Aberdeen, Department of Computing Science, Old Aberdeen, United Kingdom

Abstract

Some general features of future Patient Care Management Systems integrated with knowledge based systems are sketched. A general framework for this integration is presented. Within this framework the potential of knowledge based techniques has been investigated by building two experimental knowledge based systems integrated to a patient data management system. A description of these systems is given with some experiences gained during the development and evaluation of these systems. It seems that, although a lot of work remains to be done, knowledge based techniques together with other advanced informatics tools can improve the quality and cost-effectiveness of clinical care.

Introduction

The high dependency environment (HDE) comprises several medical activities sharing similar characteristics, e.g. intensive, coronary, neonatal, and burns care, operating theatre/anaesthesia etc. The common denominators are the disease process and its immediate consequences disturbing patient's physiological systems and leading into a de-stabilization spiral if the situation is not immediately corrected. The high dependency environment is specially set up to provide significant personnel and equipment resources for the care of critically ill patients, who have or who are at risk to get failures in vital functions.

Consequently, large amounts of data about the patient are generated and are available in HDE, and the medical personnel spends a notable part of their time collecting and/or assimilating that data. Furthermore, the unit must be staffed continuously, and decision makers often have to act in critical situations at times when they are not working most effectively, and when they are unable to consult colleagues.

Patient monitoring in the HDE has progressed from monitoring of vital signs to trending, and to computerized patient data management systems. The next step are systems for management and support of the care process. This could be done with advanced informatics methodologies, including, among others, knowledge based techniques. The application of advanced informatics tools should, however, improve the quality of patient care and the cost-effectiveness of the unit. It seems that the quality of care can be monitored and thereby improved, whereas the cost-effectiveness is difficult to prove (*Bradshaw et al, 1988*).

The use of computers in a high dependency environment is not yet widespread and is presently limited to patient data management systems (PDMS) for acquisition, storage, and display of data, as well as for reporting and calculation of derived parameters (*Gardner, 1986, Kari et al, 1988*). The use of knowledge based techniques for decision support is still experimental.

Architectural Considerations; Integration and Distribution

During treatment it is imperative that clinical data and decision support functions are accessible at all locations. At the bedside, the immediate patient data has to be interpreted and abstracted, artefacts detected and rejected, alarms recognized and analyzed, in the context of a known or a hypothesized clinical state of the patient. This information is then used in establishing or refining the hypothesized clinical state, in generating expectations for the future, in establishing therapeutic regimens to return the patient to an acceptable state, and in monitoring of the progress towards this desired state. Knowledge based techniques are considered as potential tools for providing decision support for these tasks (*Fagan et al, 1984, Rennels and Miller, 1988*).

The instruments are evolving into processor controlled modules. Standardization, will ultimately make it possible to interface and network modules from different manufactures (*Hawley et al, 1988*). In terms of hardware, functions closest to the raw data (e.g. filtering of data and alarming) are supported by the computing resources embedded in bedside instruments (monitors, ventilators, etc.). Longer time-scale functions are more likely to be carried out at workstations, where the user can access and display a large variety of data.

A considerable amount of work has been carried out to provide decision support in different critical care domains, e.g. management of ventilation (*Fagan et al, 1984, Miller, 1985*), fluid and electrolyte balance (*Kunz, 1984, Patil, 1981, Shamsomaali et al, 1988*), and regulation of cardiovascular system (*Long et al, 1987*). Likewise, various methodological approaches have been applied, e.g. mathematical modelling (*Flood et al, 1986, Hedlund et al, 1988*), causal modelling (*Patil, 1981*), knowledge based techniques (*Fagan et al, 1984, Miller, 1985*), mixed mathematical and knowledge based techniques (*Kunz, 1984, Shamsomaali et al, 1988*), and qualitative modelling (model based) techniques (*Bylander, 1988, Long et al, 1987*), etc.

However, little or no attention has been given to a comprehensive information system that provides in addition to the PDMS services also decision support. Similarly, little is available concerning the user requirements for such systems. A layered architecture is probably necessary in which the lower levels are concerned with autonomous reflex-like functions, monitoring and alarming and make use of detailed representations on short time scales (seconds to minutes). These levels are concerned with Intelligent Instruments. The higher levels can be referred to as Patient Management and they are involved with the support of strategic decisions, e.g. diagnosis, therapy planning, and setting of goals on a longer time scale (tens of minutes to hours).

Layered Architecture

The lower levels of the layered system architecture provide data abstractions for the higher levels, which, in addition, can assume that these data are free from artefacts. The higher levels establish the current clinical state of the patient, and generate expectations and goals to be used by the lower levels in monitoring and control.

Intelligent Instruments

The objective of the continuous patient monitoring is to detect immediately life threatening emergencies and deviations. A considerable amount of data is needed to achieve this, calling for different measurements and data processing techniques, including filtering for artefact rejection, and feature extraction. Intelligent data processing instruments must be able to handle noisy and missing data, even from various independent sources. This requires adaptiveness and standardization.

Furthermore, the alarm generation and processing must be exact and accurate. These levels should be able to give overall picture of the alarms, and to process in real time for the results of monitoring and alarming to be available in time for appropriate action to take place (perhaps at higher levels in the architecture). This calls for scheduling of resources and use of priorities. Intelligent instruments should provide a solid foundation for patient management.

Patient Management

Most patients enter the HDE with the initial diagnosis already made. The goal of patient management is to provide a summary of the status of a patient, prognosis of its expected development, and recommendations for actions.

Furthermore, different users may utilize a patient management system in various ways at different times. An experienced user, may wish to consult the system concerning a detailed aspect of, for example, fluid therapy or ventilator management. On the other hand, a less experienced clinician, possibly when expert advice is unavailable, may need an overview of the patient state, with general recommendations for action.

Two requirements for patient management seem to be of special concern here. Firstly, the system has to be able to reason over time. The patient history is an important guide to the current patient state, and for the prognosis. Secondly, uncertainty in the patient management should be handled, for example, with probabilistic techniques.

The architecture which seems relevant is that of consisting of a top level knowledge based system capable of identifying the patient state, formulating the relevant therapeutic courses of action, and generating the expectations. The top level will have access to a number of specialist modules competent in restricted subareas. This conceptual architecture of the patient management, in terms of generic tasks, can be seen as in Figure 1 comprising three modules: diagnosis, therapy, and monitoring. They communicate and are controlled by a manager providing planning and control of (i) communication and knowledge exchange between the modules, (ii) interface and integration to a patient database, (iii) user interface integration. The diagnosing module controls the entire diagnostic reasoning by abducting hypothesis and by requesting new information for conforming and rejecting them. The therapy module provides the user with advice for therapy planning and execution. The monitor module enables the user to measure the progress of therapy and in steering the therapy.

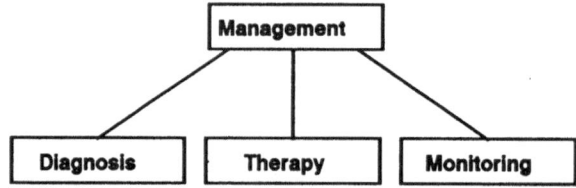

Figure 1:   High level generic tasks in patient management.

All data must be reliable and free from artefacts. Also, there should be no real time constraints i.e. sufficient computing resources must be provided to guarantee a conclusion within the required time. This has to be taken into account in designing the software/hardware architecture.

Prototyping of Decision Support Elements for HDE

Two experimental knowledge based systems were built and interfaced to an existing PDMS in Kuopio University Central Hospital to evaluate the potential of knowledge based techniques in information management and decision support in the HDE. The systems are separate modules of the framework presented above representing tasks at different levels of this framework. The first one identifies fluid and electrolyte disturbances. It can be seen as operating at the Patient Management level. The second is for intelligent alarms, operating at the Intelligent Instrument level. The essential part of these experimental systems is their integration to PDMS. The PDMS was manufactured by Kone Monitoring Systems, and handles all patient information, except natural language text of medical records, and maintains a duplicate copy of the patient data base for backup purposes. This system has been in routine clinical use for three years, and is well accepted. The general architecture of PDMS is depicted in Figure 2, comprising a network of five microcomputers, 14 patient monitors, and three workstations for physicians. The PDMS communicates with the clinical laboratory information system, and uses a MDBSIII database and a Xenix 286 operating system.

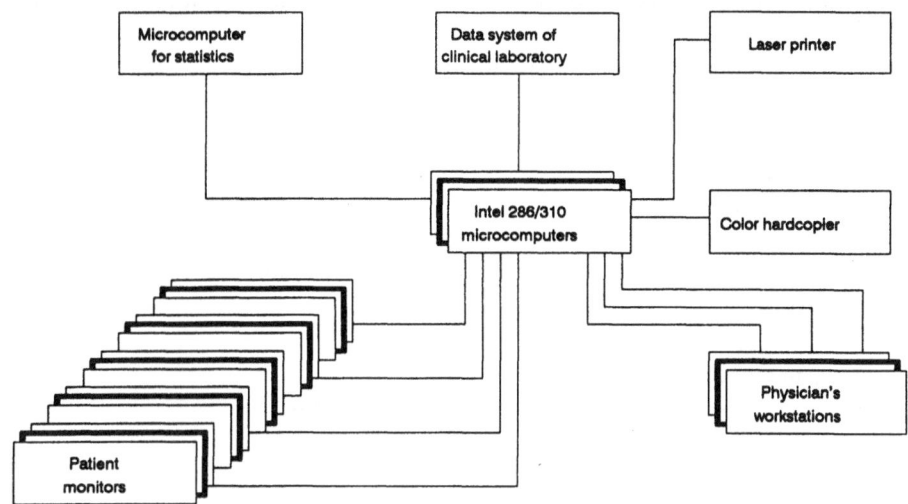

Figure 2:   The architecture op PDMS in Kuopio University Central Hospital.

Identification of disturbances in fluid and electrolyte balance

For most patients either at admission to the HDE or during their stay plasma electrolytes are measured. Frequently abnormal values and disturbances are encountered. The corrective fluid and electrolyte therapy involves usually intravenous administration of, for example, water, sodium and potassium, and is a vital treatment for many critical care patients.

The current practice of fluid therapy is broadly as follows. The physician generates an infusion plan to satisfy the patient's estimated fluid and electrolyte needs and to replace losses estimated to occur over the following 24 hours. A nurse administers this plan and records all inputs and outputs (e.g. urine, vomit) during the period. At the end of each period the current balance is calculated using the inputs and outputs, and the infusion plan for the next 24 hours is generated, taking into account the calculated balances, and clinical and laboratory data. If essential changes in the state of the patient are identified during the current infusion period, the state of the patient has to be re-evaluated and corresponding changes made to the infusion plan. Because all critical situations should be identified in time, the monitoring of the patient state has to be continuous. Our system was designed for the continuous monitoring and identification of the disorders.

Disorder identification system

The prototype knowledge system retrieves all data needed in problem solving from the database of PDMS enabling operation in the background, invisible to the user. The PDMS database includes physiologic monitoring data, laboratory data, patient specific data, and diverse clinical observations up to two weeks per patient.

The knowledge system interprets the data looking for disorders (e.g. isotonic dehy-dration). These disorders may be explained by external influences (e.g. caused by renal loss), in which case the program attempts to provide possible etiology of the identified disorder. The domain of the system covers four categories of disorders:

- organ system function, including general knowledge about vital disturbances e.g. the circulating blood volume,
- water and sodium metabolism,
- potassium metabolism,
- acid-base balance.

The system covers disorders that are common in intensive care, and potentially dangerous, and which can be cured or stopped. The system is able to identify 19 different disorder states (Table 1).

Circulating blood volume	Hypovolemia
	Hypertonic hypervolemia
	Isotonic hypervolemia
Water and sodium metabolism	Hypertonic dehydration
	Isotonic dehydration
	Hypotonic dehydration
	ECF expansion
Acid-base metabolism	Compensated respiratory alkalosis
	Uncompensated respiratory alkalosis
	Compensated metabolic alkalosis
	Uncompensated metabolic alkalosis
	Combined respiratory and metabolic alkalosis
	Compensated respiratory acidosis
	Uncompensated respiratory acidosis
	Compensated metabolic acidosis
	Uncompensated metabolic acidosis
	Combined respiratory and metabolic acidosis
Potassium metabolism	Hyperpotassemia

Table 1:   List of the individual disorders that the knowledge system is designed to identify.

It uses 31 PDMS parameters ranging from laboratory results to hemodynamic and respiratory measurements (Table 2). Because simultaneously occurring disorders, that alter the presentation of each other, are not covered, the rule-based approach is sufficient.

Each disorder class comprises a rule base. The rule bases are executed in a fixed order. The knowledge based system is invoked once per hour to check each patient in the intensive care unit (up to 16 patients). First, the system opens a connection to the PDMS database requesting the parameter values of the selected patient. The

Weight	Oxygen arterial pressure
Height	OC2 arterial pressure
Sex	Arterial blood acidity
Age	Base access
Body surface area	Blood hematocrit
Systemic arterial pressure (mean)	Blood leucocytes
Cardiac output	Blood platelet content
Level of consiousness	Serum albumin
Pulmonary arterial pressure (diastolic)	Serum urea
Pulmonary capillary wedge pressure	Serum creatinen
(mean)	Urine osmolality
Mean central venous pressure	Bilirubine total
Peripheral temperature	Gammaglutamylic transpeptidase
Urine output rate	Blood glucose
Fraction of inspiratory oxygen	Plasma sodium

Table 2:   The list of the PDMS parameters used in the knowledge system.

parameter values are valid only for a certain period, ranging from 1 to 48 hours depending on the parameter. The reasoning begins by comparing a patient's parameter values to fixed reference values. The reasoning method is mostly data driven forward chaining, and the length of the inference chain is typically only a few rules. Probabilistic or fuzzy reasoning methods are not used. As an output, the system produces a list of identified fluid and electrolyte disturbances for each patient. Then it generates explanations about its reasoning. The explanation mechanism is based on tracing the fired rules and a piece of explanatory text associated with each rule. This was found to be sufficient.

It is important that a system's intended purpose is considered in the context of its principal users. This should be reflected in the architecture and explanation facility of the system. The knowledge system was built for automatic identification of disturbances in fluid and electrolyte balance and it can potentially guide an unexperienced physician or nurse to pay attention to significant disturbances considering the fluid therapy, ensuring that relevant disturbances are not ignored. The user interface design has been a secondary task so far.

Many knowledge systems have demonstrated competence, but they require large amount of user's time simply for data input, which has a negative effect on user-acceptance. Our system differs from these conventional knowledge systems, because there is no dialogue with the user. Instead, all input data is automatically retrieved from PDMS. Perhaps the best known example of a knowledge system designed in similar fashion is PUFF (*Aikins et al, 1984*). Our disorder identification system was designed to be data driven (initiated automatically when certain set of new parameter values are stored in the PDMS). However, the user should still have control over the execution, and a possibility to start it whenever needed. To this extent, the user initiates the system and after the results of the identification process have been listed on the computer screen there is the possibility to investigate explanations for these conclusions. The primary function of the explanation is to prove that the conclusions are reliable.

Methods and tools
Our knowledge based system is a loosely coupled one (Figure 3), consisting of a front-end knowledge based system and a backend database. The knowledge based system serves as the repository for the domain-specific and problem solving knowledge as well as the implementation of the reasoning mechanism required for the identification task. The database of PDMS contains the facts required for knowledge based reasoning. The knowledge based system and PDMS communicate with messages. Physically, integration is accomplished with a standard serial interface, and special interface software. The knowledge based system is developed using the Guru expert system shell, and the interface software is programmed with C and Pascal. Guru was chosen, because it supports the MDBSIII database used in PDMS.

The system was realized using shallow rule based knowledge representation, because the objective was rather to build a running prototype to be used in clinical practice than to concentrate on causal or qualitative modelling of physiological systems. We wanted to extract high abstraction level heuristics only to model clinical decision making in our particular application domain.

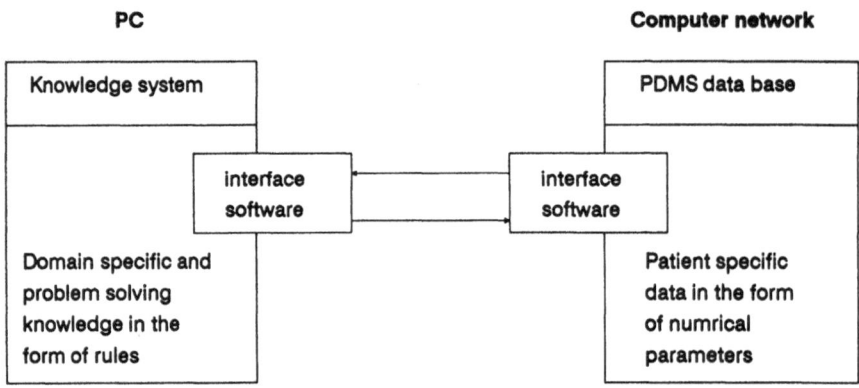

Figure 3:   The architecture of the knowledge system for fluid and
electrolyte balance.

Evaluation and experiences
The knowledge system was tested against two junior clinicians experienced in anaesthesia and at least one month working experience in the intensive care unit. They were asked to identify the 19 diagnosis covered by the knowledge system. The knowledge based system also evaluated the patients. An experienced anaesthesiologist working full time in the intensive care unit evaluated the results as the "gold standard" to which the performance of the junior clinician and the knowledge system were compared. These clinicians were not involved in the development of the knowledge system.

During this primary study 62 cases were analyzed. The expert identified 96 disturb-ances in the blood volume status, fluid, electrolyte or acid-base metabolism. The overall performance of the knowledge system compared to the junior clinicians is shown in Figure 4. The junior clinicians' diagnosis were more sensitive and more specific than those made by the knowledge system.

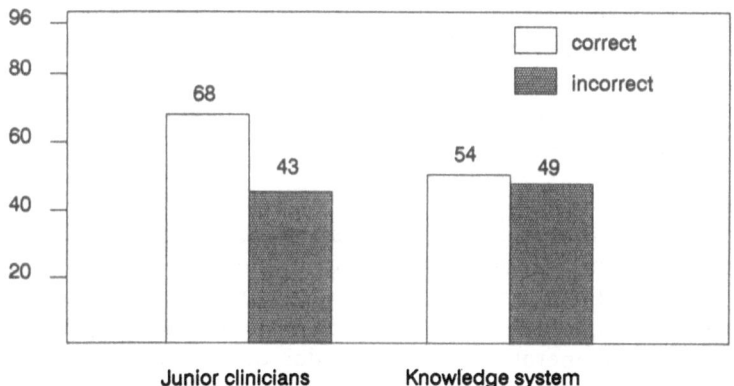

Figure 4: Frequencies of the correct and incorrect diagnoses made by junior clinicians and a knowledge system for 96 disorders of the fluid, electrolyte and acid-base metabolism identified by an experienced clinician. The junior clinicians worked alternately during the evaluation and their individual contributions are added.

Taking into account the limitations of the integrated knowledge system (e.g. it bases its reasoning on only the 31 PDMS parameters whereas the clinicians made their diagnosis using full PDMS data and personal clinical observations) the prototype system evaluated in this study performed considerably well, although it did not reach the level of the junior clinicians. There was, however, a distinct trend of learning in the performance of the young clinicians. During the first half of the study the clinicians and the knowledge system made 26 and 24 correct diagnoses, respectively, of 33 disorders identified by the experienced clinician. The knowledge system was then distinctly more specific (7 incorrect diagnoses whereas the clinician made 11 incorrect diagnoses). The test revealed to the junior clinicians the defects in their knowledge, inspiring them to further studies. The knowledge based system per-formed worst when the diagnosis was more based on clinical observations and prior knowledge of the patient than on data stored in PDMS database.

The results show that integrated knowledge systems might become useful compo-nents of information management systems for critical care. Careful selection of application domains and tasks and further development in methods for preprocess-ing the data may enhance their performance significantly. The knowledge base of the tested system should be refined and built at a more detailed level. At present, the knowledge system and the PDMS are located on separate machines for conveni-ence. In the future, the knowledge system should be embedded within PDMS.

Intelligent alarms in intensive care monitoring

An intelligent alarming system

The reliability of the current limit alarms of patient monitoring systems in critical care is poor. A small study conducted by us with patients recovering from cardiac surgery revealed that the majority of alarms (89%) were insignificant and did not result in any new therapeutic actions. Furthermore, a large portion of these alarms (30%) were caused by short transients and technical artifacts. Specificity of alarms should therefore be improved.

The approach we are proposing is based on two stages. First the signal is preprocessed using digital (median) filters to remove technical artifacts and noise and to detect slopes. Then the signal values and slopes are quantified and used as input data to a knowledge based alarm.

Preprocessing

The median filter is a non-linear signal processing method able to remove noise and transients from the signal without distortion of its base line. A causal median filter is defined by Eq. (1), MED denoting calculation of the median. The delay introduced by the filter is k samples, for the length of the data window of $2k + 1$ samples. Median filtering is a nonlinear operation, and the order of consecutive median filters is critical and can not be interchanged.

$$y(n) = MED\{ x(n-2k),..., x(n) \} \tag{1}$$

When a signal is repeatedly filtered with a median filter, a remainder of the signal not changed by further filtering is called the *root signal*. Being signals unchanged by filtering, the root signals determine the "passband" of a median filter.

This filter can reduce drastically the incidence of false alarms. However, when the delay of the filter is increased some true positives are also lost (Table 3). This example did not seek to optimize the delay of the filter. The optimum delay is different for various physiological signals and possibly even individual. It is improbable that a perfect rejection of false alarms could be achieved with this method without missing some true alarms simultaneously.

The ability of the median filter to remove activity lasting less than the delay of the filter can be employed to extract the variability in a desired time band. The extrac-

	565	M1	M2.5	M10
false total	8.063 (100%)	1.609 (20%)	0.463 (6%)	0.078 (1%)
true total	2.517 (100%)	2.049 (81%)	1.191 (47%)	0.210 (8%)

Table 3: The mean of the total number of alarms from HR, SAP, PAP and CVP mean, standardized to one patient hour. Legend: "True"alarms classified as true and requiring some therapeutic activity. "False"alarms not requiring such activity. "565"alarms produced by the patient monitor with conventional limit alarms."M1", "M2.5", "M10"alarms after median filtering of the monitor data with the delay of the median filter, 1, 2.5 and 10 minutes, respectively.

tion of a variability band B can be done simply by subtracting the (time synchronized) outputs of two median filters, i.e.

$$B(n) = MED1(x(n)) - MED2(x(n)) \qquad (2)$$

The trend quantifier of Figure 5 uses a 10 minute median filter. A least squares estimate of the trend content is calculated from the output signal. A provision for step-like changes is made by a mechanism that resets the least squares estimate in such cases. This speeds the estimation e.g. when fast acting medication is being used.

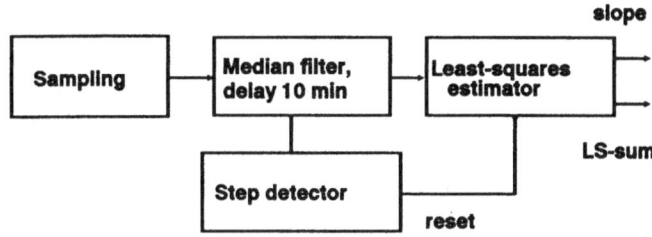

Figure 5:   Schematic presentation of the trend detector for patient monitor signals.

Knowledge based alarm

The knowledge based alarm comprises a preprocessor and a rule based system, and uses two IBM-PC/AT computers. The preprocessor was written with C-language, and the knowledge based system with Guru.

The data used by the knowledge based system originates from two sources: the patient monitor and the PDMS. Patient monitor signals (heart rate, blood pressures, temperatures) are fed through the preprocessor. The PDMS provides all other data (patient related data, lab results, clinical observations). No manual input is necessary. All trend contents are expressed as a qualitative measure (increasing, stable, decreasing). Trends of the PDMS data are determined in the knowledge based alarm. The knowledge based alarm displays values and trends of the monitored data, and the alarm messages. Multiple alarms can be active simultaneously. The values associated the alarms are highlighted with a different color.

The knowledge based alarm looks for serious data combinations, i.e. findings, in monitored data. A finding can be a value and/or a trend of parameter(s). Each finding contains either an indication of being an absolutely supporting or rejecting evidence for any of the possible alarms or it contains a number indicating the scoring of this finding associated with any alarm. The score number can be positive (supporting finding) or negative (opposing finding). The calculated score is also used in determining the importance of an alarm. An alarm is given on the basis of absolutely supporting or rejecting evidence, or on basis of a score calculated using the partially supporting and opposing findings. The knowledge based alarm currently covers four clinical alarms: (1) hypovolemia, (2) hyperdynamic state, (3) hypoventilation and (4) left heart failure. The alarms are given on two levels of importance, as the less critical "notices" and as "alarms". A short explanatory text accompanies the alarm message.

Preliminary evaluation was conducted with ten patients recovering from an open heart surgery at the ICU. 26 alarms occurred, of these eight were false, in seven cases the alarm was considered right but premature (too sensitive), and in eleven cases the alarm was correct. In five out of the eleven correct alarms the knowledge based alarm was the first one to notice the medical failure.

Conclusions

Patient monitoring in the HDE has evolved from simple monitoring of vital signs to a complex task of assimilating large quantities of data from several sources. Systems providing the management of the large amount of data have been built. These systems merely store and display the intensive monitoring data in a clinically meaningful manner. Users require rationalization of the manual tasks and embedding of intelligence to improve the quality and usability of the stored data.

The trend is towards patient management instead of managing only the patient data. The special issue of concern in future patient care management systems (PCMS) is the integration of knowledge based systems into the patient management systems.

Monitoring systems develop into platforms with a patient database, into which decision support applications can be integrated. A number of prototype knowledge based systems have been built in critical care, including the ones described above. However, a unifying framework for integrating these modules is missing. A dynamic model of the patient states may enable a system to abstract the physiological status of the patient based on data and observations stored into a database and to create strategies and expectations on how the status can be treated (*Kalli and Sztipanovits, 1988*).

Several information systems are in clinical use. Existing systems use different and incompatible types of hardware. Even when the hardware is compatible, the software is not. Frequently the user must leave one system before he can use another, and user interfaces of the systems are different. Every system has to be learned and operated separately, and there is little cumulative learning from one system to the next. The architecture of the future PCMS (not only in the HDE, but in health care generally) must allow applications to be integrated in a unified framework. The architecture is one of cooperating experts coordinated by a manager communicating with the user. This architecture should provide a unified user interface. Applications should be encapsulated behind and should communicate with the user only through the common user interface. The user should be unaware of a transition between applications.

Acknowledgements

This research was a part of the FINPRIT research programme. It was funded by Technology Development Centre, National Board of Health, Nordic Industrial Fund, Kone Corporation, Leiras Pharmaceuticals, Nokia Data, Datex Instrumentarium Corporation, Wallac, and COST 13 programme. Some of the ideas presented in this paper originate from discussions between the writers in writing a proposal for EC's research and development programme Advanced Informatics in Medicine.

References

Aikins J.S., Kunz J.C., Shortliffe E.H., Fallat R.J.: PUFF: An expert system for interpretation of pulmonary function data. In Clancey W.J., Shortliffe E.H. (eds.) Readings in medical artificial intelligence, Reading MA, Addison-Wesley, 1984, pp. 444-455.

Bradshaw K.E., Sittig D.F., Gardner R.M., Pryor T.A., Budd M.: Improving efficiency and quality in a computerized ICU. Proc. of SCAMC, IEEE New York, 1988, pp. 763-767.

Bylander T.: Qualitative representation of behavior in the medical domain. Computers and Biomedical Research, 21(1988), pp. 367-380.

Fagan L.M., Shortliffe E.H., Buchanan B.G.: Computer-based medical decision making: from Mycin to VM. In Clancey W.J., Shortliffe E.H. (eds.) Readings in medical artificial intelligence, Reading MA, Addison-Wesley, 1984, pp. 241-255.

Flood R.L., Cramp D.G., Leaning M.S., Carson E.R.: Mathematical modelling of fluid-electrolyte, acid-base balance for clinical application, MEDINFO 86, Elsevier North-Holland, 1986, pp. 133-137.

Gardner R.M.: Computerized management of intensive care patients, MD Computing, 1986, 3, pp. 36-51.

Hawley W.L., Tarig H., Gardner R.M.: Clinical implementation of an automated medical information bus in an intensive care unit. Proc. of SCAMC, IEEE New York, 1988, pp. 621-624.

Hedlund A., Zaar B., Groth T., Arturson G.: Computer simulation of fluid resuscitation in trauma. I. Description of an extensive pathophysiological model and its first validation. Computer Methods and Programs in Biomedicine, 27(1988), pp. 422-438.

Kalli S., Sztipanovits J.: Model based approach in intelligent patient monitoring, Proc. of IEEE Engineering in Medicine and Biology Society, IEEE New York, 1988, pp. 1262-1263.

Kari A., Saijonmaa J., Ruokonen E., Takala J.: The assessment of a data management system for critical care, Proc. of IEEE Engineering in Medicine and Biology Society, IEEE, New York, 1988, pp. 1783-1784.

Kunz J.: Use of artificial intelligence and simple mathematics to analyze a physiological model, Stanford University, PhD dissertation STAN-CS-84-1021, 1984, 169 p.

Long W.J., Naimi S., Criscitiello M.G., Jayes R.: The development and use of a causal model for reasoning about heart failure, Proc. of SCAMC, IEEE New York, 1987, pp. 30-36.

Miller P.L.: Goal-directed critiquing by computer: ventilator management, Computers and Biomedical Research, 18(1985), pp. 422-438.

Patil R.: Causal representation of patient illness for electrolyte and acid-base diagnosis, Massachusetts institute of technology, PhD dissertation MIT/LCS/TR-267, 1981, 137 p.

Rennels G.D., Miller P.L.: Artificial intelligence research in anesthesia and intensive care. Journal of Clinical Monitoring, 4(1988)4, pp. 274-289.

Shamsomaali A., Carson E.R., Collinson P.O., Cramp D.G.: A knowledge-based system coupled to a mathematical model for interpretation of laboratory data. IEEE Engineering in Medicine and Biology Magazine, 7(1988)2, pp. 40-46.

On Knowledge Based Systems in CCU's: Monitoring and Patients Follow-up

J. Mira[1], R.P. Otero[2], S. Barro[2], A. Barreiro[2], R. Ruiz[2], R. Marín[2], A.E. Delgado[2], A. Amaro[3], M. Jacket[3]

1 Departamento de Informática y Automática, Facultad de Ciencias de la UNED, Madrid, Spain

2 Departamento de Electrónica, Facultad de Física, Universidad de Santiago de Compostela, Spain

3 Unidad de Cuidados Coronarios, Facultad de Medicina, Hospital General de Galicia, Santiago de Compostela, Spain

Abstract

*This paper sketches the design methodology, knowledge representation and inferencing techniques and development tools used in our group by the abridged description of two systems, SUTIL, and AMIS, and a tool, MEDTOOL. SUTIL is a monitoring system for the main biosignals of interest in the CCU context, which are the **electrocardiogram (ECG)**, and the **cardiovascular pressures**. AMIS is a therapy adviser for patients follow-up oriented towards Acute Myocardial Infarction. AMIS and MEDTOOL can run on any **PC-AT** compatible under MS-DOS and SUN Workstation under UNIX. The hardware architecture of SUTIL consists of two main blocks: an IBM PC compatible computer and a real time parallel processor based the VME bus and the MC 68000 microprocessor. We are currently evaluating AMIS and SUTIL at the Hospital General de Galicia (CCU), Santiago (Spain).*

Statement of the Medical Problem

It is a differentiating fact that systems based on knowledge and in particular expert systems have emerged from the laboratory to become products in medicine. Medical experts systems are on principle static systems for consultation, but the present trend is to endow them with more flexibility seeking: (1) Structures for critique and dialogue, (2) "Explanation" modules, (3) Possibility for learning, (4) Dynamic systems for follow up, (5) Handling of temporal reasoning, (6) Real time processing.

The case of **coronary care units (CCU)** is peculiar and particularly important. Here the theoretical and conceptual aspects are usually not questioned but a narrow domain of knowledge is selected. Its computational part elicited, the appropriate tools for its representation, management and control used and a configuration of the target machine on which the program is finally going to run is studied. As an important additional question, we have the acceptability and evaluation of the system in a real environment.

The medical problem in high risk units, where CCU's are paradigmatic cases, is not to cure the patient but merely to counter the immediate threat of death and lead him to a stable non-critical condition in which he can safely be transferred to less care-intensive departments for treatment of the underlying pathology responsible for his crisis. Accordingly, the therapies applied in high risk units generally act quite directly upon the main vital parameters, and the model of the critical patient is relatively well defined in terms of correspondingly low-level "microstates" determined by just one or two parameters. For instance, the fact that
Pulmonary Capillary Wedge Pressure > 18 mm Hg
determines the microstate
Pulmonary Congestion,
which calls for the patient's progress to be re-routed along the path
Decongestion
by means of the treatment
Administration of a dose x of drug D.
The fact that microstates are often separated by relatively small differences in parameter values makes exact measurement of the latter of vital importance. Since an unattended high risk patient is likely to pass rapidly through a series of worsening microstates, or to jump suddenly to a highly critical state, measurements must also be practically continuous and the treatments applied must take effect rapidly. These conditions justify the use of invasive monitoring of haemodynamics, for example, and of drastic therapies such as defibrillation.

At present, the bed of a patient in a high risk unit is surrounded by a swarm of diverse apparatuses that monitor the patient's condition or apply therapy. In coronary care units, for example, all patients are wired to electrocardiographs, and the most critical may have one or more catheters installed for continuous monitoring of haemodynamic parameters, for withdrawal of blood samples (for determination of levels of oxygen, CO_2, etc.) or for pacemaking, as well as being connected to drips for intravenous medication, etc.

The effectiveness of a CCU depends basically on the skill of its medical staff in taking rapid decisions based on detection of foreground symptoms associated with clinical situations endangering the life of the patient. Examples of such symptoms are ventricular fibrillation and flutter, which produce serious haemodynamic abnormality and inevitable lead to the patient's death if suitable treatment is not rapidly received. In this context, more thorough conventional examination, diagnosis and treatment are of secondary importance compared with the taking of immediate action to restore normal values of the patient's physiological variables.

In this context a doctor may be regarded as a real time **control system** regulating the health of his patients in accordance with certain informal models (**state variable representation**) in which the following entities can be distinguished (*Otero et al, 1988*):

1. A set of **patient states**, i.e. pathologies and similar entities.

2. A set of **state-variables** determining the patient states. These state variables includes symptoms, signs, analytical data and physiological signals of clinical value in a CCU environment (ECG and cardiovascular pressures) taking charge of detecting dangerous situations.

3. A set of **control procedures** corresponding to medically possible paths between states which represent a serious threat to the life of a patient (i.e. recuperating from Myocardial Acute Infarction, MAI), and normal states. **Real time monitoring** closes the control loop.

4. A set of **treatments** (drug administration and other therapies) capable of favouring certain paths.

So, limiting ourselves to CCU environments, two basic functionalities we need in a knowledge based information system are:

1. Real time "intelligent" monitoring of ECG (SUTIL).

2. Patients integral state follow-up (AMIS)

The monitoring of the patient is done, to a great extent, through physiological parameters directly related to cardiac mechanical or electrical activity: electrocardiographic signal (ECG) and haemodynamic variables (pressures in heart cavities and great vessels, etc.). The continuous monitoring of physiological signals implies a degree of attention, analysis and storage of large numbers of situations, which is beyond the capabilities of the clinical staff. Therefore, the automatic monitoring of these signals increases the reliability of this process, and allows the clinical staff a greater dedication to assistential tasks, for which they cannot be substituted.

SUTIL

SUTIL is a real time monitoring system for the main biosignals of interest in the CCU context, which are the electrocardiogram (ECG), which faithfully reflects arrhythmias menacing the life of the patient, and cardiovascular pressures, of great importance in certain complications of acute myocardial infarction (AMI), such as grave left ventricular insufficiency, unstable angina, etc. Apart from the information derived from these signals in an autonomous way, the system takes into account other parameters (such as temperature and cardiac output) that are introduced by the user via the keyboard. This system has two fundamental objectives: (1)**To detect situations** and events that can mean risk, and (2) **to acquire and adequately present information** of clinical value so that the state and evolutive trend of the monitored patient can always be followed.

The hardware architecture of the SUTIL consists of two main blocks: an IBM PC compatible computer (with a colour monitor, 20 Mbyte hard disk and 512 Kbytes of

RAM memory) which is used as a system-user interface element and as a massive storage device for the information extracted from the signal in the monitoring process. The other block, based on the VME bus (*Barro et al., 1988a*), is responsible for the real-time processing of the ECG signal corresponding to a peripheral lead and of the two cardiovascular pressure signals, including the following modules: two microprocessor boards, based on the MC68000 16 bit microprocessor, an analog/digital conversion board, with 12 bit resolution, and a memory board with 128 Kbyte static RAM memory.

The functionalities of SUTIL are: **Cardiovascular pressures** monitoring and **ECG monitoring**, with beat characterization and classification and arrhythmia detection with the emission of diagnosis and therapeutic advices.

Cardiovascular pressures monitoring.

It's invasive character means that it is only used on patients that present certain infarct complications. In these cases it computes the magnitude and trend of the changes in certain parameters which are derived from the two pressure waves that the system can monitor simultaneously. The incoming signals are from a Swan-Ganz catheter (pressures). Each pressure signal is sampled at a rate of 100 samples/second.

ECG monitoring.

ECG monitoring comprises two main blocks, one for primary processing and a second block that executes in parallel under certain conditions on the input signal. The "primary" block is responsible for processing the ECG signal in the time domain on a beat to beat basis. It includes the following main tasks:

- **Extraction of QRS characteristics.** Extractions of the timing and morphological characteristics of each QRS complex allows the complexes to be grouped in families that facilitate subsequent more rigorous classification.
- **Basal beat analysis.** Averages the beat signals recorded during one minute, and characterizes the "typical" complex so obtained by calculating parameters such as the ST rise.
- **Fuzzy beat classification.** The information obtained in previous stages is used for fuzzy classification of each beat in the following set of classes: normal beats, supraventricular ectopic beats and ventricular ectopic beats.
- **Diagnosis of rhythm.** Contextual processing of beat sequences that takes into account both the classification of individual beats and global rhythm parameters allows continuous detailed diagnosis of cardiac rhythm. The fuzzy classification of individual beats induces a corresponding fuzzy diagnosis of rhythm. It is at this stage that a series of warnings and alarms of different priorities may be activated on the basis of the diagnosis arrived at. The parallel processing block is activated by "suspicious" conditions detected by the "primary" processing block, associated to ventricular arrhythmias.
- **Periodic report generation.** The most significant information acquired during monitoring is periodically reported in compact, easily interpretable form. For example, fig. 1 shows the IdN-RR graph, which contains, at all times, the last

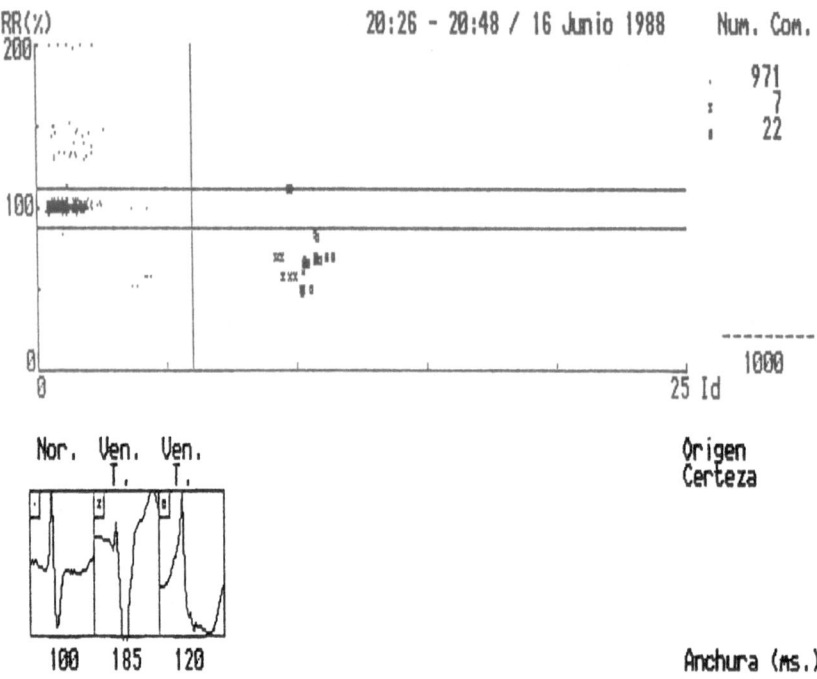

Figure 1: I – RR graph and templates associated to different morphological famlies of complexes detected in a monitored patient.

1000 QRS complexes detected by the system. This graph's abscissas axis represents the value of a dissimilarity index ($I \overset{N}{d}$) (*Ruiz et al., 1984*), and the ordinates axis the % of the distance to the previous complex (RR interval) with respect to an average value representative of normality in each instant. The templates or patterns associated with the different morphological families of QRS complexes detected by the system from the beginning of monitoring are also shown, indicating the situation of their originating focal point and their width. This graph presents, in a compressed and easily interpretable way, rhythm information referring to the preceding minutes of monitoring. To consider 6 areas on the graph, according to the morphological normality or aberrance of the complexes and their temporal normality, prematurity or lateness, permits the identification in a very approximate way of the type of beats present in the monitored patient. Another example of a report with a great clinical value is the tendency diagram in which the value of the heart rate (maximum, average, minimum values) and the number of ventricular (VEBs) and supraventricular (SEBs) beats in each minute of monitoring is shown (fig. 2). It is interesting to emphasize the possibility of introducing notes of relevant situations for the later interpretation of the information acquired by the system (drugs and doses administered, etc.). These notes are stored and presented on trend graphs in the corresponding positions.

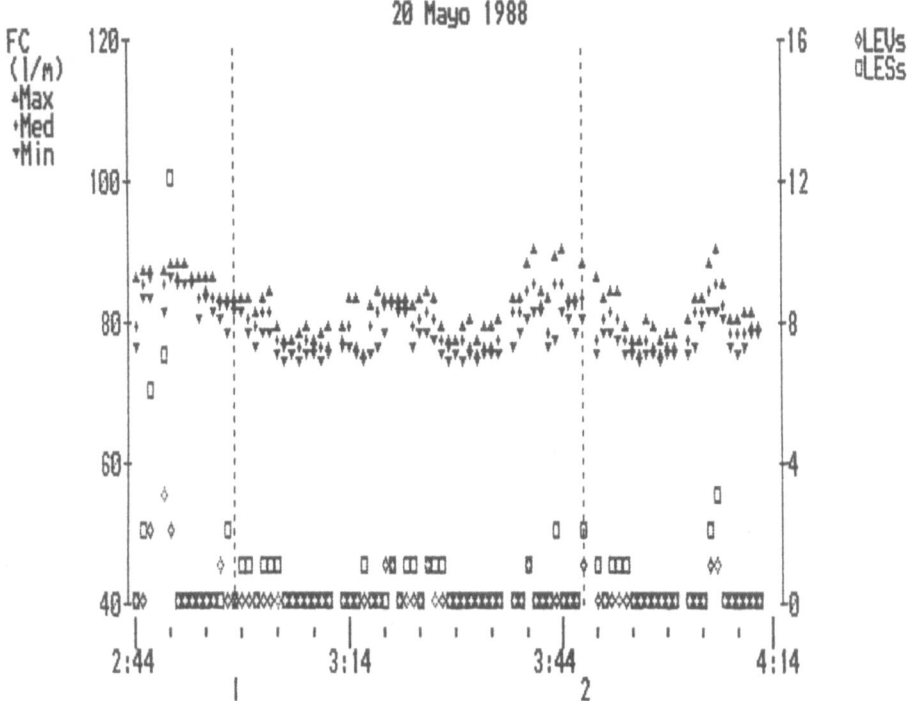

Figure 2: Cardiac frequency trends diagram (representing maximum (Max), mean (Med) and minimum (Min) values in each minute of monitoring) (FC [1/m] → heart rate [beats/minute])

The "Parallel" Processing Block: This block, which comes into operation when the primary block detects the presence of certain features in the ECG signal, analyzes the ECG in the frequency domain (*Barro et al., 1989*) to classify it in one of three categories (ventricular fibrillation or flutter; ventricular rhythms with morphologically aberrant complexes; and signals with artifacts) on the basis of a set of descriptors quantifying the regularity of its amplitude spectrum.

Knowledge Representation in SUTIL

In SUTIL, we consider a process for fuzzy classification of beats that uses heuristic criteria in order to mimic as much as possible the cardiologist's criteria in the realization of this task. We have considered a classification of beats founded on their etiology or focus of origin, leaving the temporal considerations that permit the discrimination, for instance, between a premature ventricular ectopic beat and an escape beat, for the later stage of rhythm diagnosis. We differentiate among the following three types or classes of beats: **normal** (associated with beats that originate in the sinus node, normal physiological focal point), **supraventricular** (associated with beats that have an origin in a supraventricular ectopic focal point, auricles or auricle-ventricular union) and **ventricular**. The "labeling" or beat classification process, is analogous to that developed by the medical expert. Thus, the semantically ascendant definition process of a set of objects (QRS complex, T and P waves), with a series of attributes (QRS width and morphology, RR interval length, etc.) and on these, a process of delimitation of values of interest (aberrant morphology, wide QRS complex, etc.), to consider them finally in a diagnosis or classification process, allows a structure for computable processes and representations that conforms, from a functional point of view, a computational space homomorphic to the clinical environment.

The type of quantifiers used in a "natural" way in the systematization of knowledge are particularized into "linguistic variables" (*Zadeh, 1973; Adlassnig et al., 1985*) more related to the synthetic capacity of the information inherent to the processes of human reasoning.

With all the premises mentioned, the previous step in the construction process of the classifier can be summarized as the need to establish a big enough set of "descriptors" for the attributes considered by the human expert that allow a "literal translation" from the medical language to knowledge usable by the computer. On table I the set of descriptors that are extracted automatically from the electrocardiographic waves each cardiac cycle are indicated together with the fuzzy sets that define a series of values of attributes useful for the classification process.

After this, the classifier designed applies a fuzzy conditional statement structure which represent the knowledge of the cardiologist expert. The fuzzy sets defined from the numerical descriptors (shown on table I) are used almost exclusively, introducing degrees of fuzziness in the inference structure itself. Even in the case in which the membership functions to the fuzzy sets defined had only the extreme values of their variation interval, the criteria used in the classification process have in some cases a component of uncertainty which has to be added to the procedure itself. Let us consider an example of fuzzy conditional statement as implemented in **SUTIL**:

> **IF**
>> 1.very_aberrant_QRS_morphology **AND**
>> 2.wide_QRS **AND**
>> 3.premature_beat
>
> **THEN**
>> ventricular_beat(μ^c = absolute; μ^e = low)

where μ^c (confirmation degree) and μ^e (exclusion degree) are associated with the confirmation and exclusion between antecedents and consequents in the fuzzy conditional statement.

The process of classification is completed with information derived from the consideration of "families", which group beats that have QRSs of similar morphology, and with information brought in by the user himself in the monitoring process.

Finally, the information given by the beat-label assigning degree "generator" designed, constitutes the entrance of a block for the identification of cardiac rhythm which considers the sequences of fuzzy classification labels as a basis for constructing the rhythm diagnosis (*Barro, 1988b*) by a finite state automaton. The input to this

SYMBOL AND DEFINITION	TYPE	FUZZY SETS
P_Wave_exists	Boolean	--
$I_{PR} = X_{PR} / \overline{X}_{PR}$	Real	Long_PR_Interval $\equiv$ S(I_{PR}; 1.06, 1.13, 1.20)
D_P = Dissimilarity index normalized with respect to normal P wave template	Real	Normal_P_Wave_Morphology $\equiv$ $1-S(D_P; 0.1, 0.12, 0.14)$
$L = X_{RR} / \overline{X}_{RR}$	Real	Premature_Beat $\equiv$ 1-S(L; 0.75, 0.85, 0.95) Late_Beat $\equiv$ S(L; 1.06, 1.15, 1.24)
W	Real	Wide_QRS $\equiv$ S(W; 0.1, 0.115, 0.;13)
WT	Real	Wide_QRS_Template $\equiv$ S(WT; 0.1, 0.115, 0.13)
$C_N = (X_{RR} + X_{RR+})/2*\overline{X}_{RR}$	Real	Compensatory_pause_following_the_beat $\equiv$ Premature_beat $\wedge$ S(C_N; 0.85, 0.9, 0.95) $\wedge$ [1 - S(C_N; 1.05, 1.1, 1.15)] Interpolated_Beat $\equiv$ S(C_N; 0.4, 0.42, 0.44) $\wedge$ [1 - S(C_N; 0.55, 0.57, 0.59)]
$C_P = (X_{RR-} + X_{RR})/2*\overline{X}_{RR}$	Real	Compensatory_pause_previous_to_the_beat $\equiv$ Late_beat $\wedge$ S(C_P; 0.85, 0.9, 0.95) $\wedge$ [1 - S(C_P; 1.05, 1.1, 1.15)]
$\int = \int_{QRS} / \int_T$	Real	Inverted_ventricular_repolarization $\equiv$ [1-S($\int$; -0.9, -0.5, -0.1)] $\wedge$ S($\int$; -3, -2, -1)
D_{QRS} = Dissimilarity index normalized with respect to normal QRS template	Real	Normal_QRS_Morphology $\equiv$ 1 - S(D_{QRS}; 0.1, 0.12, 0.14) Aberrant_QRS_Morphology $\equiv$ S(D_{QRS}; 0.1, 0.2, 0.3)

$X_{PR} \rightarrow$ PR interval value of the beat (sec); $\overline{X}_{PR} \rightarrow$ Normality average of the previous X_{PR} (sec);
$X_{RR} \rightarrow$ RR interval of the beat (sec); $\overline{X}_{RR} \rightarrow$ Normality average of the previous X_{RR} (sec);
$X_{RR+} \rightarrow$ RR interval between the beat and the following one;
$X_{RR-} \rightarrow$ RR interval between the two beats preceeding the beat under study (sec);
$W \rightarrow$ Width of the QRS complex (sec); $W_T \rightarrow$ Width of the standard complex of normality (sec);
$\int_{QRS} \rightarrow$ Area under the QRS complex (v*sec); $\int_T \rightarrow$ Area under the T wave (v*sec)

Table 1: Description of attributes and values of attributes (defined through the fuzzy subsets), considered in the process of beat classification. The fuzzy sets are defined by means of standardized "membership functions" of adjustable parameters, functions 'S' of **Zadeh** (1979), S(u; α, β, Γ).

automaton are the labels associated to each classified beat. The presence of a specific sequence implies the analysis of a series of additional conditions, the objective of which is to confirm or discard possible situations associated with the recognized sequence, for example:

> Detected sequence: ...**NVNNV** =
> (N sinusal beat; V ventricular beat)
> Additional analysis:
> **if** last QRS on preceeding T wave **then R-on-T**
> **if** late ventricular beats **then Ventricular Escape Rhythm**
> **else Ventricular Trigeminy**

The detection of those arrhythmias not linked to specific beat sequences (asystolia, etc.) or the detection of which is not viable from a beat by beat analysis (ventricular flutter fibrillation and certain ventricular tachycardias) is done by a specific analysis of the ECG signal.

AMIS

A MIS is a patient follow-up system for Coronary Care Units (CCU) oriented towards Acute Myocardial Infarction and has been developed using the **MED-TOOL** system, a teachable medical expert system development tool. It can run on any computer under MS-DOS. A new version can also run on SUN under UNIX.

The outputs of **SUTIL** are the inputs of **AMIS** complemented with additional information (via keyboard) on other clinical variables.

Although **SUTIL** process its inputs to provide detection and classification of arrhythmias and other information, it only deals with just a few of the relevant parameters. Attempts to construct complete diagnostic and follow-up systems based exclusively on the ECG and pressure signals have been usually unsatisfactory. **AMIS** integrates monitoring and processing of all accessible parameters: diuresis, laboratory data, diet, medication, "micropathologies" (arrhythmias, etc.) and other events (pain, surgery, etc.) to be continually recorded from the patient's entry in the high risk unit.

AMIS has the following parts:
- A medical database with utilities.
- A frames-based data-driven expert system for continuous diagnosis and patient monitoring.
- Symbolic keyboard interaction with the user.
- Graphics facilities.
- Multi-patient concurrent management (different instantiations of the same patient-model).

Specifically, **AMIS** accommodates all kinds of data (parameters, pathologies, treatments, etc.); stores all data chronologically to allow trend analysis; allows rapid display of any data stored; produces trend charts of any parameter, with optional comparison with other parameters; stores mathematical formulae for calculation of inferred parameters; and sums and integrates specified parameters for inflow/outflow analysis, etc. Further, it is highly teachable. The first step in the AMIS development is the Knowledge injection in the DICTIONARY, namely parameter's definition according to the form: < symbolic keyboard position, in/out name, reference name, set of coherent values > as well as the inference means for the parameters to be inferred. The user can at any time include new parameters in the system, change the way in which data are displayed, program new calculations, and control automatic data acquisition and report generation by setting up an agenda.

To obtain sufficient speed, most low-level input to the system by the "normal" user takes place using the function keys of the PC keyboard to specify the code numbers of parameters and commands.

The commands may be classified in five categories:

1) basic commands handling the values of parameters describing the subjects being monitored (STATE, TRENDS, ENTRY, TREND CHART and RELATIONAL CHART);

2) more sophisticated commands that likewise act mainly on subject parameter values (CALCULATION OF IST PARAMETERS, AUTOMATIC DATA ACQUISITION and REPORT);

3) subject-group management commands (SELECT SUBJECT, LIST SUBJECTS, DELETE SUBJECT, SEARCH SUBJECT);

4) the AGENDA MANAGEMENT command for programming repeated execution of other commands at regular intervals;

5) high-level dictionary management commands enabling the teacher to configure the system.

A relevant utility of the system **AMIS** is the facility to display the **state** and **evolution** of the patient in the follow-up functional mode with items such as: tendency, relationships between parameters, search with logical zoom and time remarks.

The STATE command displays part of the monitored subject's current state, specifically, the set of all the latest values of the descriptive parameters belonging to the specified type and subtype.

Knowledge Representation in AMIS and MEDTOOL

In **MEDTOOL** (*Otero and Mira, 1988*) and hence in **AMIS** (*Otero et al., 1988*) there are **numerical** and **alphanumerical** parameters. All of these are defined as **frames** from the operational point of view. For teachability reasons, these frames are not included as fixed elements of the system but as elements in a structure called the DICTIONARY (fig. 3). With this facility MEDTOOL becomes a **true expert system development tool**.

The DICTIONARY is a tree-level tree of frames where the application dependent features (knowledge, end-user interactions) are inserted in the development stage. Given that there is not a standard for **modelling non mathematical parameters** we have designed a lexicon and the corresponding syntax for frame elements inference representation:

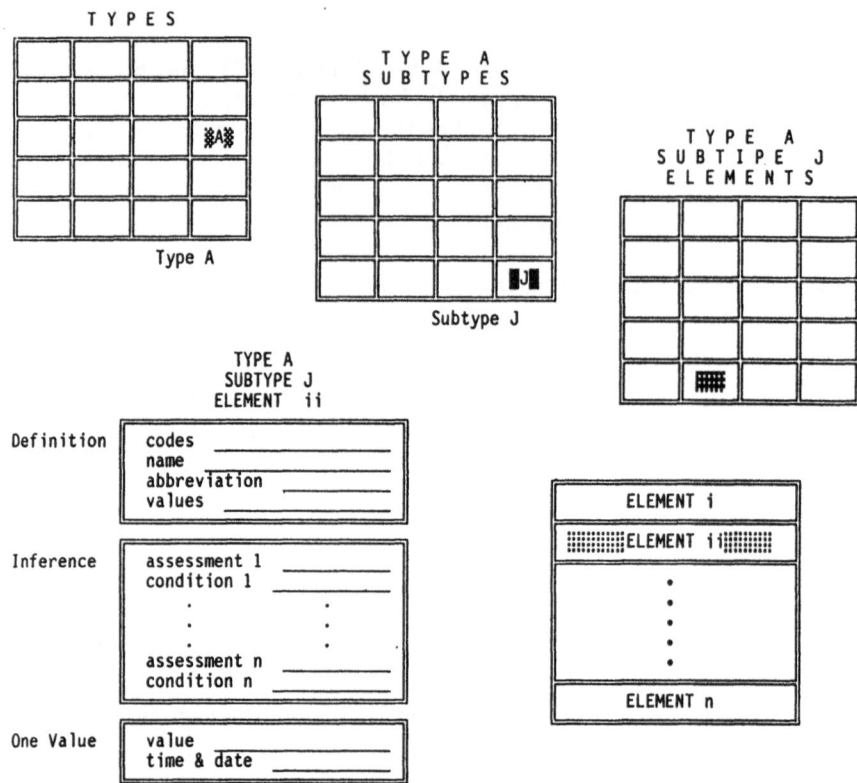

Figure 3: The structure of the DICTIONARY in MEDTOOL.

<assessment 1> **if** <condition 1>

<assessment 2> **if** <condition 2>

••••

<assessment N> **if** <condition N>

Where each slot **<assessment i>** is in general a concrete value or an "extended formula" and the slot **<condition i>** is a logic-relational "formula".

To relate this structure with the conventional one in frames-based expert systems let us consider the **frame** corresponding to a parameter modelled using type frame element as specified by definition plus inferent. As an example we consider the operational way of knowledge injection in the DICTIONARY corresponding to 'HYPERTENSION' parameter(see next page).

With the previously proposed frame-structure the modules of **knowledge are distributed** through the DICTIONARY (a knowledge-base from the operational viewpoint). The system has a minimum syntax for logic-relational basic conditions but can include approximate fuzzy reasoning as well as macro-functions to make the knowledge entry more user-friendly.

Once the DICTIONARY has been created for AMIS, the execution of the knowledge injected in the DICTIONARY is as follows. The teached system proceeds obtaining

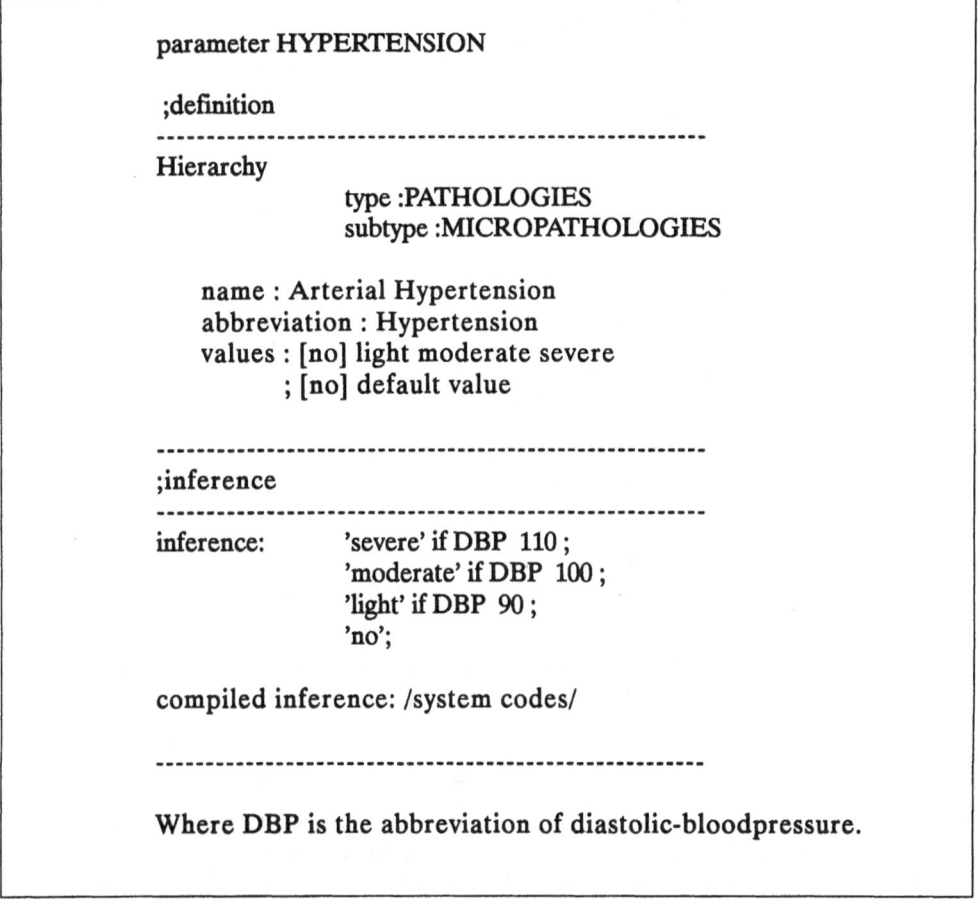

```
      parameter HYPERTENSION

      ;definition
      --------------------------------------------------
      Hierarchy
                     type :PATHOLOGIES
                     subtype :MICROPATHOLOGIES

          name : Arterial Hypertension
          abbreviation : Hypertension
          values : [no] light moderate severe
                 ; [no] default value


          --------------------------------------------------
      ;inference
          --------------------------------------------------
      inference:       'severe' if DBP  110 ;
                       'moderate' if DBP  100 ;
                       'light' if DBP  90 ;
                       'no';

      compiled inference: /system codes/


          --------------------------------------------------

      Where DBP is the abbreviation of diastolic-bloodpressure.
```

the values of the parameters defined as inferred (determined by an associated inference slot into the frame), using the input parameters (without inferred knowledge attached). Knowledge is used in a recursive manner, when needed, to determine all the inferred parameters. The system display to the user all the contingencies rised when applies domain-dependent knowledge (inference engine): presence of loops, not valuated input parameters, ... The classic conclusions of expert systems about the applied knowledge are obtained as values for some inferred parameters, previously defined as possible conclusions.

As an example of other utilities of **MEDTOOL** in the **AMIS** application, we show in figure 4 a case study corresponding to the temporal evolution of the patient's state into the Forrester's square: values of patient's cardiac index (CI) temporally related to patient's Pulmon-capilar pressure values (PCP). The current position and path of the patient in the Forrester's square is of extremely importance in Coronary Care Units because of his relation with patient's good evolution.

186   *J. Mira et al*

Relational graph of values   medtool&amiss   17:56:2   8-9-1988
Patient's Data. Numerical. Monitoring Cardiac Index
Number:1 Christian name:E. Surname:L.P. Sex:f
Hospital number:----- Unit number:-----

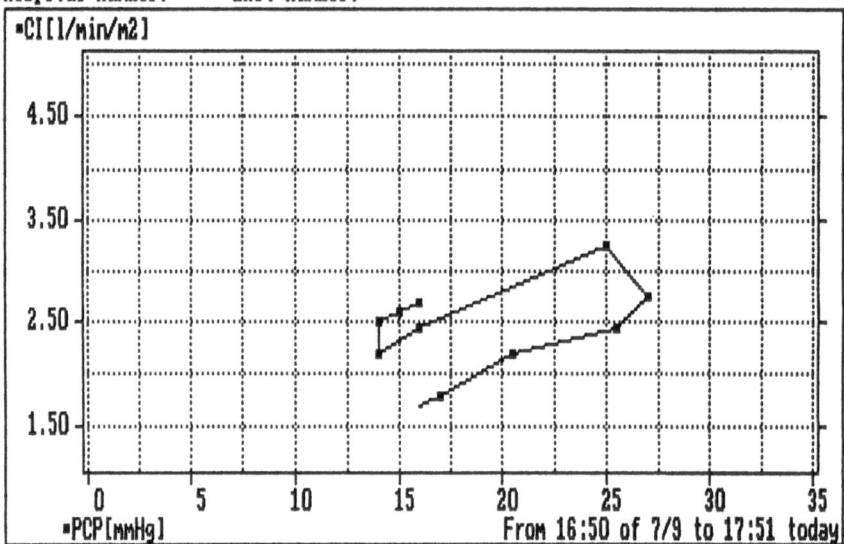

Figure 4:   Temporal evolution of the Patient's state in the Forrester's square. CI is cardiac index, PCP is Pulmocapilar Pressure.

Temporal Considerations in AMIS Using MEDTOOL

The problem of temporal knowledge representation and its manipulation in inference processes, has a growing interest in the field of artificial intelligence and expert systems. From the point of view of theoretical approximations, various solutions which attempt to formulate general theories of time have been proposed. *McCarthy and Hayes, 1981* proposed a theory that implies a formalization of the concept of state space, situational calculus. *Allen, 1984, McDermott, 1982,* and *Shoham, 1988*, propose several theories in the frame of temporal logic.

As an example of an actual application of the concept of sequence of states, we mention VM (Ventilation Manager), a system designed for the on-line interpretation of physiological data in an intensive care unit. VM assists in the treatment of postoperative patients that receive assisted mechanical respiration. The use of this approximation is due, to a great extent, to the existence of a model that can identify the state towards which the patient is moving.

In ONCOCIN (*Kahn et al., 1985*), an expert system in the domain of chemotherapy of cancer, each patient is associated with a temporal graph whose nodes represent important clinical events (chemotherapy, cycle, visit, etc) and can be open or closed depending on whether the event that they represent has ended or is currently happening; however, this elegant solution has the drawback that the patient's graph has to be stored in the data base and reloaded for the next consultation, which means that knowledge (relationships within the graph) is strangely mixed with the data base.

Time as a reference: representation and reasoning

An expert system in a medical monitoring context must handle time in a real way. This implies the assumption that "things happen in time" and, therefore, time is a reference. This is the main difference between those first diagnosis systems that only handled the static aspect of things and the actual monitoring systems that can handle the dynamic aspect. In particular, let's see the tasks that MEDTOOL manages automatically in **AMIS**:

Assignment of the time associated with each primitive event:

A primitive event is one in which the value associated with an input parameter is indicated by the user. The time associated with this event can also be introduced by the user or, by default, **MEDTOOL** uses the time in which the value was introduced in the system.

Causality:

The causality is associated with the fact that one or more events produce another event, associated with an inferred parameter of the knowledge base. In this case, an inference must produce not only a value, but also an associated time. MEDTOOL obtains, as time associated with an event, the largest of the times associated to the causing agents, taking as causing agents not only the causing events (parameter-value pairs and their associated times), but also any other temporal condition expressed in the description of the inference. For example, let's suppose two inferred parameters, B1 and B2, from the knowledge base. In **MEDTOOL** we could express the following inferences:

> For B1: "B1 = 0 if A5"
> For B2: "B2 = 0 if A5 and C = 3 more than two days ago"

The time associated with the value of B1 will always be the same as that associated with the value of A expressing that event "B1 = 0" is caused instantaneously when event "A5" occurs. Both events start being true at the same time. This does not have to be true in the case of B2. The event "B2 = 0" will be true if "A5" occurs, and two days must have elapsed since "C = 3" started being true.

With this methodology, the system defines a current state of the patient from all the events that are true now. This is a multitemporal current state. Therefore it is not a description by states as found in situational calculus.

Time as explicit knowledge: representation and reasoning

When working with MEDTOOL, the designer of the application can endow the inferred parameters he defines with temporal meaning, at a different interpretation level from that of the reference, automatically managed by **MEDTOOL**. The time functions provided by the tool are used for this purpose.

Access to an event in time

MEDTOOL is a tool aimed at the construction of expert systems in medicine (**AMIS**) and we believe that most of the reasoning in this domain is established based on the current and/or recent state of the patient, and that events which occurred a long time before are only occasionally referenced. Due to this, the basic modes of access to an event in MEDTOOL are:

- **Access** to an event that is true now (to the current value of a parameter). The name of the parameter is referenced.
- **Access** to an event that was true before (to the previous value of a parameter). The previous operator is used.

Access to the time of an event

MEDTOOL assumes that the events are true over temporal intervals, but permits the access to points in time, which facilitates the injection of temporal aspects into the knowledge base. Let's take a look at the facilities for access to points in time:

- **timeof (PARAMETER)**. Returns as a true result the hours elapsed from the time origin (date 1/1/1980) to the time associated with the last value of PARAMETER.

  timeof can be used with the ant operator: timeof (ant(PARAMETER)). This way the hours elapsed from the origin of times to the time in which the previous event for a parameter started to be true are obtained.
- **now**. Is a reference to the current moment (i.e., the time in which the inference motor finds it in the execution of knowledge).
- **inclusion**. Is a reference to the time associated with the inclusion of a patient in the system.

To accede to now and inclusion, the function timeof must be used: timeof(now), timeof(inclusion). Figure 5 shows an example of use of temporal functions in CCU's. With the use of previous (---) and timeof (---) operators, a temporal integration over user defined time intervals, can be made.

Proposal for the Evaluation of Knowledge Based Systems for CCU's

The evaluation of expert systems in the past has been generally done after the system's development stage, and has been focused on the validation of the knowledge (evaluation of the knowledge base). The final objectives of the evaluation process are to give a measure of the acceptance of the system by different users and its utility, and consequently, suggest modifications to the system to increase the value of these parameters. Thus, the evaluation of a system must be performed in a dynamic manner, increasing the communication between the technicians and users during all stages of development and increasing the responsibility of the latter in the design of the system, evaluating all its modules.

Next, we propose the stages to follow in the evaluation of **AMIS/ MEDTOOL** (*Grant et al, 1989*).

```
parameter ORAL_INPUT;
[...]
        values: ml 0 0 2000
                ; no inference
```
_____

```
parameter PARTIAL_ORAL_INPUT
[...]
        values: ml [0] 0 2000
                ;[0] default (initial) value
        inference: previous (partial_oral_input) + oral_input if
            time_of (oral_input) - time_of (previous(total_one_hour_input))) < 1;
                        oral_input;
```
_____

```
parameter TOTAL_ONE_HOUR_INPUT;
[...]
        values: ml [0] 0 2000
                ;[0] default (initial) value
        inference: previous (partial_oral_input) if
            time_of (oral_input) - time_of (previous (total_one_hour_input))) > 1;
```

Figure 5:   Temporal integration of parameters of clinical interest using temporal integration.

Validation of the knowledge base

The first aim in the evaluation of any expert system related to medicine is the agreement between the experts and the results of the system for the acceptance of its efficiency. In the past, this evaluation has not been done in a dynamic way due to an important reason related to one of the weak points of the technology: the maintenance of expert systems, specially the updating of the knowledge bases. A relevant utility in MEDTOOL, and hence in AMIS, is the editor of the DICTION-ARY, which is being used by the physicians of the Coronary Care Unit at the Hospital General de Galicia. This facility allows a continuous refinement of the knowledge base while the system is working in the CCU.

The comparison of results between the experts and the system must be done accordingly with the following tasks that AMIS performs:
- diagnosis of acute myocardial infarction
- considerations about the patient's stability: analytic and haemodynamic
- diagnosis of micropathologies
- continuous intravenous treatment.

We propose the following steps for the validation of the knowledge:
- previous discussion between the experts and the technicians about the contents of the dictionary, focusing on the working inferences. Our feeling is that before

the system begins to run in the hospital, the physicians want to be sure of the correctness of the implemented knowledge.

- real evaluation with cases of patients, simulated and real. Finally, the physicians must choose significant cases where the tasks to be performed (see above) involve a high level of complexity.

Acceptance

All the possible users of the system must evaluate it including experienced doctors who have taken part in the development of the system, experienced doctors who have not taken part in the development of the system, doctors in training, students, in the last year of their studies and nurses. The appropriate methodology is to use detailed questionnaires about the following general criteria: (1) Presentation of the information: contents and clearness. (2) Adequacy of the explanations to the user's expectations. (3) Learning of the system: measurement of the difficulty and time required. (4) Assessment of the time required by the system for the different tasks.

Clinical usefulness

Clinical usefulness includes assistential usefulness with the reduction of routine work and the work required by the different users for the introduction of the system, impact on the organization of the clinical environment and benefits for the patient

Two additional points to be considered are usefulness in investigation and usefulness in education. These aspects are related to the usefulness of the system to store clinical histories, to perform studies on these histories and to teach students on the knowledge representation, use and control strategies.

Conclusions

Knowledge Based Systems (KBS) are now a well established field of research, development and evaluation in medical domains. In fact, the existence of specific programs such as AIM (Advanced Informatics in Medicine) is the confirmation on a European scale of the social interest of this action line. Some strategic reasons has been agreed: 1) An increasingly elderly population, 2) Use of KBS as teachers and/or tutors of paramedical people, 3) Possibility of self-help and home care in connection with telemedicine and 4) Usefulness for rehabilitation and monitoring.

Coronary Care Units (CCU's) are possibly one of the best domains for the evaluation of the KBS's appropriateness in medicine for two reasons: 1) The comparative absence of ambiguous knowledge and 2) The urgency of decision. At the same time evaluation is easier than in other medical fields because the low "time-constant" of pathological patients state evolution.

The main point that characterizes the present state of knowledge based systems in critical care contexts is the search for dynamic systems for "intelligent" monitoring and follow-up. These two topics are connected in the specific case of diagnostic and/or therapeutic advice systems for hospital patients, and specifically for critically ill patients, because the need of integration of intelligent systems and units for automatic monitoring of the physiological variables relevant to the patient's condition.

This is our approach to the specific case of acute myocardial infarction patients in CCU's where the main biosignals of interest are the ECG and cardiovascular pressures. The need of real time processing demands multiprocessing architectures like SUTIL's one. The patient's follow-up demands a highly teachable system with real time management (like AMIS/MEDTOOL) capable of dealing with relevant information from different sources (diuresis, laboratory data, diet, medication, "micropathologies", etc.). These systems should produce a wide range of aids to the physician (reports about the patient's data and the system's conclusions, trend analysis, relationships between parameter, etc.).

Acknowledgements

We acknowledge the support of the Spanish CICYT under project 0615/84, the European Community support under ESPRIT project 1592/86 and the CICYT counterpart of this project.

REFERENCES

Adlassnig K. P., Kolartz G., Scheithauer W.: Present state of the medical expert system CADIAG-2. Methods of Information in Medicine, No. 24, 13-20, 1985.

Allen J.F.: Towards a general theory of action and time. Artificial Intelligence, 23 (2), 123-154, 1984.

Barro S., Ruiz R., Mira J.: Physiological monitoring in a CCU: a VME-based prototype. In "VMEbus in Research". Ed. C. Eck and C. Parkman. North-Holland, 167-175, 1988a.

Barro S.: SUTIL: sistema cuasi-integral de monitorización inteligente en UCC. Ph.D. Thesis, Universidad de Santiago de Compostela. In Spanish, 1988b.

Barro S., Ruiz R., Cabello D., Mira J.: Algorithmic sequential decision-making in the frequency domain for life threatening ventricular arrhythmias and imitative artifacts: a diagnostic system. J. Biomed. Eng., Vol. 11, 320-328, 1989.

Fagan L.M., Kunz J.C., Feigenbaum E.A., Osborn J.J.: Extensions to the rule-based formalism for a monitoring task. In B. Buchanan and E. Shortliffe (eds.): Rules-Based Expert Systems. Reading, Mass: Addison-Wesley, 397-423, 1984.

Kahn M.G., Fergusson J.C., Shortliffe E.H., Fagan L.M.: Representation and use of temporal information in ONCOCIN. Proceedings of the Ninth Annual Symp. on Computer Applications in Medical Care, Ackerman M.J., ed., IEEE Comput. Soc., Baltimore, MD, 172-176, 1985.

McCarthy J.M. and Hayes P.J.: Some philosophical problems from the standpoint of artificial intelligence. Readings in Artificial Intelligence, Tioga Pub. Co., Palo Alto, CA. 431-450, 1981.

McDermott D.V.: A temporal logic for reasoning about processes and plans. Cognitive Science, 6. 101-105, 1982.

Otero, R. P., Amaro, A., Yañez, A., Mira, J.: AMIS: A System for Intelligent Monitoring of Coronary Care Patients. Procc. of MIMI'88. Sant Feliu, Spain, 557-560, 1988.

Otero, R. P., Mira, J.: MEDTOOL: A Teachable Medical Expert System Development Tool. Proc. of the Third International Symposium on Knowledge Engineering, Madrid, 191-200, 1988.

Ruiz R., Hernandez C., Mira J.: Method for mapping cardiac arrhythmias in real-time using microprocessor-based systems. Med. & Biol. Eng. & Comput., No. 22, 160-167, 1984.

Shoham Y.: Reasoning about change: time and causation from the stadpoint of artificial intelligence. The MIT Press, Cambridge, Mass, 1988.

Zadeh L.A.: Outline of a new approach to the analysis of complex systems and decision processes. IEEE Trans. on Systems, Man and Cybernetics, Vol. 3, No. 1, 28-44, 1973.

Zadeh L.A.: A theory of approximate reasoning. In: "Machine Intelligence", Hayes J.E., Michie D. and Kulich L.I. Eds., Wiley, New York, 149-194, 1979.

ARCA - An Integrated System for Cardiac Pathologies Diagnosis and Treatment

Joäo Rocha and Eugénio Oliveira

D. E. E. C., Faculdade de Engenharia da Universidade do Porto, Porto, Portugal

Abstract

ARCA, which is being developed at Oporto University in cooperation with S. Joäo Hospital, is an Integrated System for Cardiac Pathologies Diagnosis (Oliveira et al 1987, Abreu-Lima and Marques de Sá, 1988). ARCA aims towards the development of an autonomous aid system for the treatment of cardiac patients, from the automatic extraction of the ECG signals to the final diagnosis, followed by a therapeutic prescription plan.

Introduction

In the real world it is necessary that doctors not only understand the statistical relations of signs and symptoms to the various possible diseases, but also have the wisdom and common sense that derive from the understanding and experience of everyday human existence. It is this last requirement that represents the greatest weakness (and perhaps the ultimate limitation) of computer technology in dealing in any comprehensive fashion with the problem of clinical diagnosis (*Barnett, 1982*). The diagnosis of a cardiac arrhythmia, based on the observation of an ECG, is difficult for non-experts.

This difficulty is not only due to alterations in the diagnosis caused by apparently insignificant variations in the signal, but also to the high number of existing malfunctions.

The objectives of our system are:

- to provide the non-experts with an easy manner of detecting the existence of cardiac arrhythmias (and their type);
- to provide the experts with an auxiliary aid that helps in diagnosing arrhythmias and that presents, whenever required, the explanation of the inference steps used to reach a certain conclusion;
- to allow its consultation as a "tutor", thus permitting novices to acquire greater specialization in the field;
- to produce an adequate therapeutic prescription, considering not only ECG observations, but also other kinds of complementary information.

It was considered that the most viable and practical way of achieving these objectives was to build a completely automated system. This system should include the ECG signal acquisition, the interpretation of these systems as well as the prescription of therapies.

The ARCA system is made up of several different modules, such as an electrocardiogram acquisition and processing module, an Expert System which is responsible for the diagnosis and a planning module for the therapeutic prescription.

Another approach to this domain is found in (*Shibahara, 1985*).

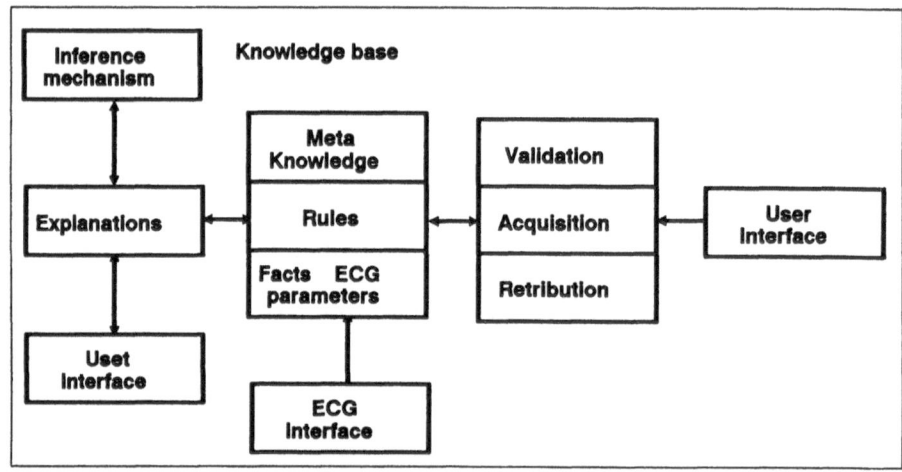

Figure 1:   ARCAs block diagram.

ARCA Knowledge Based Subsystem contains a Selfknowledge module that helps to decide which chaining inference mechanism is best suited. It also provides detailed knowledge about the domain.

The inclusion of this non-procedural knowledge allows the expert to develop a deep model of useful knowledge. This eases user interaction and improves the efficiency of the inferences.

Special attention was paid to the user's interaction through the presentation of various windows which also allow, using simplified techniques of natural menus, to volunteer information according to the user's needs.

In order to be completely automated, the system includes a hard- and software interface which achieves the automatic acquisition of the ECG and supplies a PROLOG file with the necessary quantitative data for posterior inference and diagnosis. Once this diagnosis is reached, another process starts, trying to give advice about possible therapies.

We think that ARCA is particularly well suited both for routine tests on cardiac arrhythmias and related diseases and as a tutor in this specific domain.

It is possible to use the system in a more relevant way, but this depends on the knowledge reliability and on special rules that can be introduced into the Knowledge Base. This is a very hard work, since two different physicians will not always agree on the same diagnosis and even if they would, their reasoning procedures would, probably not be the same.

The credibility and confidence degree of the provided explanations are also important factors to influence the acceptance of this system.

Soon we foresee a crucial enhancement on ARCA when learning capabilities through experience will be included.

ECG Acquisition and Processing

The ECG acquisition and processing subsystem allows ECG signal extraction from an ordinary electrocardiograph. It supplies a data file that is read and interpreted by the expert system.

In a first stage, the most important characteristics of the acquired waves (those who have been considered of interest for arrhythmia diagnosis) are processed (*Wartak, 1978*).

Frank's ECG model of three leads is used and is transformed into the derived ECG (leads AVR and D2) by mathematical manipulations. Specialists find these transformations adequate for pathological cardiac diagnosis, at least in the case of adults.

From the AVR and D2 leads, 11 and 5 parameters are extracted respectively for each of the considered cardiac cycles.

They mainly concern temporal positions and durations as well as amplitudes of P and T waves and QRS complexes. Other important information is also gathered, like the possible existence of a baseline and cardiac and P wave frequencies.

The automatic ECG acquisition and processing module ("Sistema de Electrocardiografia Computorizada do Porto" - Oporto Computerized Electrocardiograph System) (*Abreu-Lima and Marques de Sá, 1988*) is installed in Oporto S. João Hospital. Some programs have been implemented to establish an interface between this subsystem and the PROLOG fact base.

Knowledge

The domain

The ECG is a graphic representation which registers electric potentials produced in association with the cardiac pulses.

The cardiac muscle is the human muscle that has automatic and rhythmic contraction quality. The formation of pulses and their conduction produces electrical currents which diffuse through the body. The ECG is obtained by connecting electrodes to different parts of the body and to the electrocardiograph.

The arrhythmia constitute a group of physiological cardiac states characterized by alterations in the depolarization and repolarization processes of the heart. They need not always indicate a heart disease. The relevant parameters for the detection of cardiac arrhythmias (*Wartak, 1978*) are represented in figure 2.

Morphology and timing of the QRS complexes are the most reliable data in diagnosing arrhythmias. They are employed early in our evaluation of the electrocardiogram.

It is also possible to discuss how long (1 hour, 1 day,...) and in which situations (stress, rest,...) the ECG's should be recorded that will provide the initial data for further analysis.

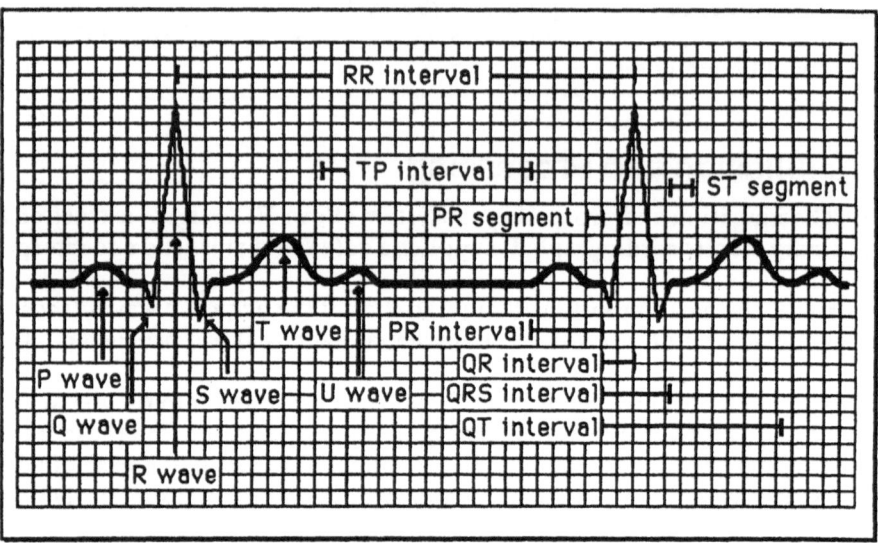

Figure 2:   ECG parameters.

Knowledge Base and Reasoning Process

The domain knowledge is basically represented in three different forms:

- production rules also incorporating inexact reasoning capabilities;
- semantic networks including specific domain concepts, all the relationships among them and other useful attached information (concept meanings, domain values, etc);
- ECG measurements asserted as facts with an associated certainty factor in PROLOG clauses.

To assembly small pieces of expert reasoning into rules and to explicit the existing knowledge in the domain, is somewhat difficult, due to the large number of patterns necessary for a realistic approach in any area of medicine.

An aspect also considered of vital importance, is the attempt to establish rules at the lowest possible level. These fine grained rules explicit all inference steps from the ECG data to the more elaborated and higher level diagnostic rules.

These lower level rules together with more sophisticated knowledge also embedded in the same form (rules), make the Knowledge Base completely modular and easy to increment. They avoid the use of implicit knowledge in procedures that are not completely visible neither easily modified.

The established model divides the arrhythmias into the classes defined in *Wartak, 1978* (Table 1).

- regular rhythms
  - tachycardias
  - normal or shifted pacemaker
  - blocks and AV dissociation
- periodically irregular rhythms
- completely irregular rhythms
- beats outside the dominant run
  - extrasystoles
  - blocked beats

Table 1: Classes of arrhythmias considered in ARCA.

Each of these classes is considered independently, thus constituting the superior level of chaining of the diagnosis. So, ARCA initially attempts to choose a Knowledge Source (subset of rules) according to the selected arrhythmia class.

Therefore, the initial characteristics taken from the ECG, trigger knowledge sources that are activated in backward chaining (during the diagnosis) in a more efficient way.

The system, although oriented towards efficiency in the presentation of the diagnosis, can present alternative answers even belonging to classes initially excluded. The idea behind this behaviour, even though the degree of certainty is reduced, is to call expert's attention towards malfunctions which could, otherwise, have been missed.

The system, after choosing one of the possible classes, will try to satisfy rules that become more specific and dependent on the values read directly from the ECG, and which are also associated with the arrhythmia model being analyzed.

Knowledge inherent to the rules is enhanced by types of frames with associated declarative knowledge enabling more interesting and friendly explanations.

On the other hand, selfknowledge relating qualitatively all the concepts involved, provides also an aid in focussing the inference as well as a semantic validation of new acquired knowledge.

Example 1 - meta rule:
IF diagnosis in known
AND prescription is not known
THEN select forward chaining

Metaknowledgeis also important. Rules can act upon object rules during execution. An example is the application of metarules which, according to the situation, choose between proceeding the inferences in backward chaining, forward chaining or event driven mode.

Knowledge Representation

Concepts are represented using object-attribute-value triplets.This representation allows an easier acquisition of new concepts and detailed explanations about all know concepts.

Example 2 - concepts representation

concept(name, attributes list, attributes values list)

concept('dominant run', [existence, type], [[exists, 'not exists'], ['A', 'C']]).

concept('QRS type', [type], [['A', 'BL', 'BR', 'C']].

Selfknowledge plays an important role in ARCA's knowledge representation containing not only information concerning known concepts and rules, but also relations between them.

Selfknowledge is represented using the above notation:
  sk(concept, predicate, dependencies, contributions, meaning)

The slots have the following meaning:
concept — represents the name of the concept as ARCA will know it;
predicate — is the name of the Prolog predicate that corresponds to the concept;
dependencies — contains the names of concepts - if any - on which this concept depends;
contributions — contains the names of the concepts - if any - that depend on this one;
meaning — used to give explanations about the meaning of the concept.

This representation permits a 'frame based representation'. The slots 'dependencies' and 'contributions' allow a semantic network to be used that links all concepts and helps the representation of the reasoning process.

Figure 3 summarizes the three level knowledge representation that is used in ARCA.

Volunteer Information

The user can, at every moment during the diagnosis, provide the system with information that he considers to be of interest. The evaluation of the relevance of the information is however, made by the system.
This possibility permits that, whenever the information is considered of significant importance, certain actions will immediately be triggered. Therefore, some intermediate steps may be eliminated, simplifying the path to the conclusion. All the information is introduced using simplified techniques of natural menus.
It was decided to use this technique for two fundamental reasons:

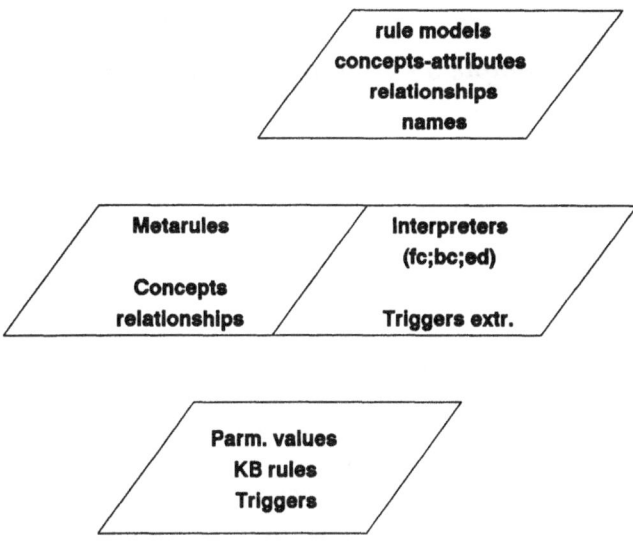

Figure 3: Three level knowledge representation.

- it did not seem reasonable to develop a great amount of work in the area of natural language because the quantity of information is reduced (one phrase at a time), and on the other side, there is a relatively restricted dictionary;
- it was necessary to evaluate the coherence of information introduced, not allowing any ambiguity in the "input language".

On the next page, an example of an interactionwith ARCA is given (Example 3).

Explanations

Any explanation module, worth its name, should not only be able to provide information about the way inferences have been made. It should also indicate the specific reasoning method used, based on a deep model supporting derived conclusions.

The traditional possibilities of "why" and "how" explanations, enriched with declarative knowledge included on the model, are also provided.

We also provide "why not" explanations that are used to answer questions such as 'why did rule number X not succeed' or 'why did rule which diagnosis is Y not succeed'. These explanations are useful to explain why a particular deductive path did not succeed.

As it is possible to determine, a priori, the kind of user who is using the system, it can adapt its explanations complexity. Therefore, it is possible that the same question may have different answers, taking into account the deepness of the presented knowledge and the type of language used, considering the users's degree of expertise.

Clinicians are well aware that good medical practice depends on keeping up to date with clinical literature. To use this literature most effectively, a physician must

---

Example 3 - volunteer information:

```
Input concept (or type 'help')
>help
Concepts are:
      dominant run
      heart rate
      ...
      ...
Input concept (or type 'help')
>dominant run
Input value of attribute existence (or type 'help')
>help
Possible values to attribute existence are
      exists
      not exists
Input value of attribute existence (or type 'help')
>exists
Input value of attribute type (or type 'help')
A
You had introduced
      Dominant run exists and is of type A
Correct?
Y
```

---

critically assess these studies in the context of a particular patient and decide in what ways the experimental trial is relevant to the case in hand (*Rennels et al 1989*).
In order to make it easier, the system provides extracts of different studies concerning same context of those under analyses, thus allowing a quick review of existing experimental evidence.

Learning

A Data Base with a number of significant cases will be explored to provide information about a priori probabilities of different pathologies, of some symptoms and classes of diagnosis. Furthermore, diagnosis and associated therapies are saved together with their specific proof tree to be exploited later.

A new program will compare different paths, leading to the diagnosis. It will try to detect singularities which permit the extraction of triggers, as well as intermediate facts which point to a possible more direct way to reach a certain conclusion.

Triggers, extracted in this way, will be tested in following sessions as long as certain pre-conditions are established. An event driven inference mechanism is activated by these "triggers", allowing a by-pass in systematic inference.

Knowledge Acquisition

Together with the acquisition of triggers from traces and statistical information from data base, another module of ARCA gives the expert the possibility to input new rules in a formal but friendly language. Entered rules are semantically and syntactically checked before being automatically translated to PROLOG rules (with inexact reasoning calculation formulas included if applied) and added to the knowledge base.

It is important to notice that the acquisition of new rules intends to be very easy. Great help is offered during the acquisition process, not only to validate the rule "syntactically", but also "semantically", e.g. to guarantee database coherence and consistency regarding the established model of the theory.

As we have a Selfknowledge module it is possible to check for consistency on the acquired knowledge or rules.

At this moment this is done in two steps:

- first, a comparison is made between the new rule and the existing ones to check if they are contradictory (e.g. the same diagnosis is reached by two opposite and not simultaneously valid paths);
- secondly, the new rule is fired and the path leading to a solution is conveniently checked to see if there is any contradiction in the deduction.

If any contradiction arises, the expert who is introducing the rule is warned and is expected to solve the problem as well as to maintain the Knowledge Base consistency.

Graphic Capabilities

To enable on-line visualization of the ECG that is being analysed, the system is able to present the trace of the ECG on a screen.

It is also possible to view an individual QRS complex, with the presentation of all calculations made up by the system (for example PR interval, QRS interval, P wave amplitude, etc).

Evaluation

Here remains an arduous amount of validation work to be done once the prototype has been finished. A confrontation between the expertise exhibited by the system and that of different, well accepted experts is foreseen at an expert conference during several sessions. Various cycles of evaluation/correction have to be done before the system will be accepted by the medical community.

First level evaluation is being done with the help of Prof. C. Abreu-Lima from Cardiology Services of Hospital S. João - Porto. It consists of comparing ARCA's diagnosis with physician's diagnosis made in several patients and covering all ARCA's domains.

The next step (to start next October after the complete integration of different modules) will be a conference with five Portuguese experts to confront diagnosis.

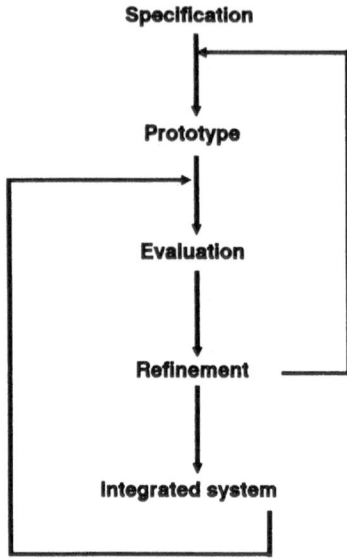

Figure 4: Evaluation/correction cycle.

Evolution

A great amount of work can be done to improve ARCA's performance. We think it will be necessary to incorporate a greater amount of knowledge, referring to other areas of cardiac diseases, but still keeping the internal structure of the system. New rules must be introduced not only concerning the diagnosis, but also the knowledge itself. This can be done using the acquisition module referred above.

In this way it is possible to extend from a small subset of cardiac diseases (in our case, arrhythmias) to a larger system concerning different subjects in related areas. Connection with other databases could lead to a more general overview about patient's pathologies, thus focussing the physician's attention to more critical problems.

It is also important that the acquisition and processing subsystem could interact with the expert system to make the processing of new parameters possible when they are needed.

Although our subsystem has a good performances in waves and QRS complexes detection, which can be inferred from its use in Oporto's S. João Hospital for the last 3 years, some work could be done in order to improve the detection of P waves. The approach we will use to advice on therapeutic prescription is not based on rules. We intend to implement a planning algorithm, using a paradigm of node expansion followed by critics or possible mutual interaction in order to prescribe a coherent set of actions, leading to an acceptable treatment.

Lists of drugs, their utilization preconditions and previewed effects are inspected to select candidate "nodes" to be submitted to this strategy in order to reach the final plan.

Conclusion

Different from other ECG diagnostic programs, ARCA arrives at a diagnosis (and aims to plan a therapeutic prescription) using not only the ECG parameters classification, but also more complex expert heuristics. Moreover, our project aims to develop a complete integrated system from the ECG recording to the final treatment plan.

ARCA is capable of providing "why", "how" and "why not" explanations as well as on-line graphical visualization of the ECG and individual waves.

It allows volunteering of information and inclusion of new rules/knowledge acquisition.

It is also possible to obtain concept descriptions and explanation, metaknowledge description and tutorial information concerning all known concepts.

Some elementary learning capabilities are under test and could be a valid and useful improvement.

Including several pre-existent databases with ARCA, which contain relevant information about patients, will allow the evolution of a growing integration of medical information into the hospital.

Acknowledgements

We would like to thank "Fundação Luso-Americana para o Desenvolvimento - FLAD", "Instituto de Engenharia de Sistemas e Computadores - INESC", "Junta Nacional de Investigação Científica e Tecnológica - JNICT" and "Hospital de S. João - Porto" for their collaboration.

References

Abreu-Lima C., Marques de Sá J. P., "Novos aperfeiçoamentos do Sistema de Electrocardiografia Computadorizada do Porto". BioEng'88, Porto 1988, pp. 112-113

Barnett, G. Octo, "The Computer and Clinical Judgement" in New England Journal of Medicine, 1982, pp. 307:493-494

Oliveira, E., Rocha, J., Cunha, P., "Model Based Expert System for Diagnosis of Cardiac Arrhythmia" in Proceedings of Computer in Cardiology, Leuven, Belgium, September 13 - 16, 1987, pp. 639-642

Rennels, Glenn D. et al, "A Computational Model of Reasoning from the Clinical Literature" in AI Magazine, Spring 1989, pp. 49-56

Shibahara, T., "On using knowledge to recognize vital signals: knowledge based interpretation of Arrhythmias" in Proceedings of International Joint Conference on Artificial Intelligence, Los Angeles, L. A., 1985, pp. 307-314

Wartak, J., "Processing of electrocardiograms by a computer", 1978.

Questions from the discussion:

Wyatt: It seems that you have got a model based knowledge acquisition tool. Is this approach general enough that it can be applied to other domains as well?

Oliveira: Our acquisition tool is well suited to gather different kinds of knowledge from the expert.
- first it asks for all concepts involved together with their attributes and relationships. A kind of semantic net is then automatically built;
- then, rules in a flexible, though concise, input language are accepted from the expert and, immediately, codified into the new Knowledge Base.

We think that our program reflects a general approach only depending on what kind of specific functions each of the rules need. If these functions are too specific and domain dependent, then, of course, they must be codified to support high level rules.

PC-based Multistep Infusion Regimens and On-line Control of Four Infusion Devices[*]

A.A. d'Hollander[1], F. Cantraine[2], E. Coussaert[2] and L. Barvais[1]

1 Department of Anesthesiology, CUB Erasme Hospital, Brussels, Belgium

2 Department of Data Processing, Faculty of Medicine, Free University of Brussels, (U.L.B.), Brussels, Belgium.

Abstract

An IBM PC based system was built up to control on line one to four commercially available infusion devices (ID) with RS-232 serial port. The multistep infusion regimen of each drug can be preprogrammed using pharmacokinetic simulations. These simulations are facilitated by the use of resident or on line updated pharmacokinetic model data bases. The feasibility of the preparation of the i.v. drug reservoir and the composition of the multistep infusion regimen is checked according to the weight of the patient and the duration of the infusion session. For each infusion step, the precision obtained with the ID selected from the ID data base is calculated and displayed. The final solution elaborated by the user in interaction with the different software possibilities is stored and constitute an infusion sheet (IS). Several infusion sheets can be pooled to form a drug administration session (DAS). Each DAS can be retrieved for immediate execution. Preprogrammed or on line coordinated actions between IDs are available according to external events or any calculation made from the IS parameters. Due to a local communication net, the PC use for other tasks can be ruled out during a DAS execution but the full control of each ID remains under the clinician's supervision for immediate interaction.

---

* This study was partly supported by the F.N.R.S. (Fond National de la Recherche Scientifique; contract nr : 3.4570.87 F) and by the fellowship SWIFT to the "Erasme Foundation".

Introduction

Intravenous anesthetic drugs are to be delivered according to posological[*] schemes adapted by the anesthetist to the patient's age, biometry, pathology and to the scheduled surgery. These posological schemes consist generally in a loading dose followed by repeated injections with or without a continuous maintenance infusion rate. Ideally, during intravenous anesthesia, drug delivery should be constantly adjusted by bolus administration and/or by raising or lowering the infusion rate to obtain the wanted pharmacodynamic effect (*Revesetal, 1984; Alvis et al, 1985*). Hence, the preoperative knowledge of the theoretical plasma drug concentration obtained after different infusion steps is of sustained clinical interest to organize the drug infusion session preoperatively.

Simulation of Plasma Concentration

A basic question is how to simulate the plasma concentration generated with a multistep infusion scheme from a multicompartment pharmacokinetic model? This goal is fulfilled by the software SPINA allowing to simulate the theoretical drug distribution and the theoretical infusion rate according to bi- or tri-compartment mamillary pharmacokinetic models. To permit the selection of the most appropriate pharmacokinetic models for a patient with a given pathology, SPINA contains a database of pharmacokinetic model records retrieved from the literature. This program is written in LOTUS 1-2-3 (version 2.1) commands and macros and is run on an IBM personal computer or compatible with 640 Kbytes of random access memory, operating under MSDOS 2.1. The models are classified according to different keywords: age, biometry, pathology and indication, to accelerate the selection criteria.

Once the anesthesiologist has chosen one pharmacokinetic model, a pharmacokinetic simulation can be easily and rapidly performed after introducing the target plasma drug concentration. So doing, different solutions are proposed to the user to accelerate the choice of an infusion steps sequence reproducing the desired plasma concentration. On request, SPINA provides the graphs of the compartmental drug distribution and of the infusion rates which maintains the target concentration (*Barvais et al, in press*).

SPINA MENU An overview

The main menu of SPINA is divided into four functions: the pharma-**DATABASE** management, the pharmacokinetic **SIMULATION**, the **RESET** and the **EXIT** function.

- **DATABASE** : This function permits the management of the pharmacokinetic model records stored in the Lotus worksheet. Each record is issued from a published pharmacokinetic compartment study. The bibliographical research

---

[*]   We use the term posology to identify an infusion regimen, possibly containing several successive IV steps.

was partly carried out with the help of the database "Medlars". All the selected models are mamillary models with elimination from the central compartment. Selection of the models depends upon the presence of the values of the turnover rates (kij) and of the central compartment volume (V1) in the original work. On each record, the code, the authors' names, the title of the study and the bibliographical reference are reported as well as the values of the various pharmacokinetic parameters. Underlying comments give information on the number of patients, their sex, the method of dosage used and the study conditions. The subsequent commands of the database menu : **List, Choice, Installation, Modification** and **Deletion** are used to manage the pharmacokinetic model records. The records retrieved from the literature and provided with the software are protected. All the modifications of the database are saved automatically.

● **SIMULATION** : this function performs the pharmacokinetic simulation. Its seven submenus offers the opportunity to the user to select [**List, Choice**] and visualize [**View**] the parameters of a model, to simulate one sequence of succeeding infusions [**Posology**], to display the solutions graphically [**Graph**] and to archive [**Archive**] the simulation.

● **RESET** : This command reinitializes the worksheet of **SPINA**.

● **EXIT** : This function permits to leave **SPINA** and to return to MSDOS.

First the anesthetist preoperatively simulates and adapts the IV drug administration protocol to the patient's profile and the presumed time schedule of the surgery. The next step is to check whether the prepared infusion scheme can effectively be executed during the surgical procedure with the infusion device available in the O.R. or in the I.C.U. Furthermore, the most economical way to prepare the drug reservoir solution is determined. This sequence of checks require repetitive and time consuming arithmetical operations. The physician, obliged to use a given infusion device with fixed minimal and maximal flow rates and a prefixed maximal reservoir volume -seringue or iv bag-, must calculate the total volume needed for the duration of the surgical procedure. Eventually he has to define the most appropriate drug concentration in the infusion device reservoir to have enough anestetic drug for the patient's mass and pharmacokinetic profile. It is also justified to determine the concentration of the reservoir and the total amount of drug needed requiring the minimum drug package units proposed by the hospital pharmacy. As numerous anesthetists prefer to titrate the amount of drug to be administered in μg/kg/min and because the flow rate units of the selected infusion devices, are defined in volume per time units -ml/hour or μl/min for example-, the final calculations remain the conversion of each step of the prescribed infusion regimen into the flow rate units of the selected infusion device. Without computer support, these manual arithmetic conversions can often be confusing.

Feasibility and Precision of Multistep Infusion

One has to check the feasibility and the precision obtainable with one infusion device in case of multistep infusion. For this purpose, **CINA** has been developed (*Barvais et al, in press*). This software verifies the compatibility of any infusion regimen with the technical features of the selected infusion device according to the drug packaging available from the pharmacy and to the syringe volume or to the selected IV bag of the infusion pumping device. To reduce the errors coming from the conversion of μg/kg/min into an integer value : ml/h, e.g., CINA also suggest drug concentration to reduce eventual bias. Finally, CINA converts the prescribed infusion scheme into the flow rate units of the selected infusion device according to the patient's weight and the chosen drug concentration. All this information is saved in a disk file, called "infusion sheet" (IS) which can be printed or stored on a floppy disk.

CINA Menu An overview

The main menu of CINA has 4 functions : **DATABASES, COMPOSITION, RESET, EXIT.**

- **DATABASES** : This function is divided into three sections : **in fusion device DB, IV drug packaging DB, posology record DB**

    a) **Infusion device DB** contains a list of several models of commercialized infusion devices, with built-in RS-232 serial port and some information concerning essential technical features. For each infusion device, the flow rate unit, the minimum and maximum flow rates and the conversion factor of the flow rates in ml/min are noted.

    b) **IV drug packaging DB** provides the list of the IV packagings available from the hospital pharmacy. Several drugs may have more than one packaging. For the computation of the IS, CINA selects the most appropriate packaging of the database according to the drug requirement. Any new drug or packaging may be introduced, modified and added.

    c) **Posology record DB** : contains, for each drug the record of IV infusion regimen that we have called posologies. Each posology is identified by a code, composed by 7 characters, which reminds information about the proposed infusion sequence. Each posology record may contain a list of several successive IV steps which may be expressed either in μg/kg or in μg/kg/min. Time is defined in minutes and seconds. The number of steps is not limited. For each drug, the different posologies already included in the database are classified according to keywords for five selection criteria concerning the patients of the reference study (age, biometry, pathology, indication and user). The user keyword allows the user to identify each posology specifically. These keywords help the user to select the appropriate posology record among those of the database. Many posology records are coming from the literature.

    On each posology record, the code, the authors' name, the title of the study and the bibliographical reference are reported. Comments specify the particular conditions of the reference study.

    The commands of the database menu allow to insert new posology records and to modify or to delete any information about existing posology records.

- **COMPOSITION** : This function of the infusion sheet contains 6 commands : **NAME, DEVICE, POSOLOGY, MODIFICATION, VERIFICATION, INFUSION SHEET.** These commands allow the anesthetist to complete the information needed to optimize the composition of infusion sheets adapted to the prescribed posology and the selected infusion device.

For any IV bag drug concentration, CINA is able to compute :
* the mode of preparation of this IV bag drug concentration
* the minimum volume of the bag needed
* the minimum and maximum flow rates
* the minimum delivery time for the induction and the bolus steps
* the maximum relative error between the prescribed and delivered flow rates

If the anesthetist does not impose the concentration of the IV bag, the CINA selects automatically the drug concentration generating the maximum flow rate of the selected infusion device for the higher prescribed flow rate.

● **RESET** : This function reinitializes the worksheet of CINA.

● **EXIT** : This command memorizes the modifications of the three sections of the database function and finally allows to leave CINA and to return to MSDOS.

Cathecholamines, vasodilators, antihypertensive agents, antiarrhythmic drugs, i.v. anesthetic compounds are very active molecules which require continuous IV administration to assume a better control of their pharmacodynamic effects. Consequently, more than one infusion device is sometimes required simultaneously for the same patient.

Simultaneous Control of four Infusion Devices

How to install and control four infusion devices simultaneously with one PC? The development of microcomputers and the commercialization of infusion pumps with serial ports has enabled the design of a computerized system for the monitoring and the simultaneous control of IV drug infusions administration. MINA has been developed for driving 4 infusion devices simultaneously (*Cantraine et al, 1989*).

MINA ensures accurate drug titration, informs the user about the current and future status of the multistep infusion sheet, records the successively delivered flow rates and, eventually, coordinates the 4 pumps to external or internal events.

MINA : An overview
Pre Drug Administration Configuration Procedure
The user has to enter the patient's name and weight. There after, the user verifies the connection of the infusion devices to the corresponding port of the communication controller. An error message is displayed by the system in case of inappropriate connection.

For each infusion device, MINA allows the composition of the one IS either de novo - directly from the keyboard - or by the retrieval of residential IS previously composed with CINA. Each IS is a specific ASCII file corresponding to one drug and one in fusion device.

With the de novo composition procedure the user must enter the drug name, the concentration of the drug reservoir, the flow rate (μg/kg/min) and the duration (minutes) of each of the infusion steps. As with CINA, MINA gives notice of any incompatibility between the prescribed flow rates and the performances of the selected infusion device, according to the concentration of the reservoir. Then, the program computes the prescribed flow rates into the specific flow units of the selected infusion device. A bolus step of predetermined size related to the body weight may also be introduced.

Drug Administration Session (DAS)

During drug delivery, MINA provides the control of the 4 IDs via the keyboard. The control of an ID is organized either manually via the keyboard by selecting a number from 1 to 4 associated with that ID or, depending of the DAS, the control of each ID is organized directly via the coordination table (see the display commands). In the general screen, which provides information about the 4 IDs, a blinking label indicates which ID remains under the direct control of the keyboard for the immediate execution of the different function keys.

MINA menu : the essentials

Each function key (F1 to F10) is associated with a specific command, the meaning of which is displayed on the bottom line of the general screen.

F1: START

This command starts an infusion step of the IS.

F2: BOLUS

The bolus command allows to stop temporarily the active infusion step and to insert the predefined bolus step. Thereafter the F1 command is automatically reactivated once the bolus administration has been performed.

F3: STOP

This commands stops the selected infusion device. Its submenu allows to select one of the options :

⤶: this option permits a stop period of undetermined duration.

s: this command acts as the ⤶ option but, before a new F1 restart is allowed, the new volume of the ID reservoir is to be entered via the keyboard.

e: this option permits a general emergency stop for the 4 IDs.

a: resumes the DAS and saves all the commands executed.

F4: CATAlogue

This command displays information about the IS file names of the current directory according to its submenu

F5: LOAD

This key loads the information of the selected IS.

F6: MSDOS

This command gives direct access to the DOS commands. All IDs remain under the control of MINA but the keyboard and the screen are available to execute any program which does not use the serial port of the PC. Striking "EXIT" results in a return to MINA general screen.

F7: MODIFication

This command allows the modification of fields of one IS or of the coordination table. Moreover, this command permits free text - event marker or comment - to be inserted into the PRN archive file.

F8: DELetion

This function deletes completely the selected infusion step. If this deletion concerns an active infusion step, **MINA** takes immediate control over the ID at the next infusion step.

F9: INSERTion

This function permits the introduction of a new infusion step and the creation of a new IS by typing the different parameters which compose the IS.

F10: VIEWS

This function selects the type of screen to be displayed. Its submenu is composed of 4 options: a, c, p, ↵

a: ARCHIVE page. This option displays the last page of the disk archive file of the successive flow rates carried out by the 4 in fusion devices and the time these flow rates were initiated and stopped.

c: COORDINATION table. This screen is displayed from one of the four ID and presents the coordination table of this ID.

p: displays the PREPARATION screen.

↵: toggles between the "GENERAL" and the "COMMANDS" screens.

The "GENERAL" screen displays the information about the delivery of the 4 drugs:
- type of infusion device
- drug name
- elapsed time from the start of the infusion
- forecast infusion period before the end of the reservoir flow rate and remaining time of the active infusion step
- cumulative administered dosis
- "alert" messages for abnormalities detected by the ID logic control: empty reservoir, occlusion of the infusion line, air in line,... .

The "preparation" and "command" screens provide information about the mode of preparation of the ID reservoir, the prescribed flow rates of the IS and their respective duration.

Discussion

Up to now, no computer processing system allowing the simultaneous control and surveillance of 4 IV infusion devices from a personal computer has been proposed. The main problems encountered during the preparation of the system presented in this document were : the lack of standardization of the infusion devices, the diversity of the drug packaging, the variability of the posological schemes, the complexity of the different commands which have to be executed during critical care therapy, the necessity to act rapidly on any infusion program, to control of successive flow rates and the coordination of the different in fusion devices. **MINA** tries to meet all these problems.

Finally, the **MINA** communication net allows to preserve the computer for other clinical tasks and to retake the manual control of the ID.

References

Reves JG,Spain JA, Alvis JM, Ritchie RG: Continous infusion of fentanyl during cardiac anesthesia : An automated system (abstract). Anesth. Analg. 63 : 266, 1984.

Alvis JM, Reves JG, Govier AV, Menkhaus PG, Henling CE, Spain JA, Bradley E: Computerassisted Continous Infusions of fentanyl during cardiac anesthesia: Comparison with a manual method. Anesthesiology 63 : 41-49, 1985

Barvais L, Coussaert E, Cantraine F, d'Hollander A: The pharmacokinetics of intravenous anesthetic drugs given by infusion: SPINA a sofware program. Eur J Anaest.(in press)

Barvais L, Coussaert E, Cantraine F, d'Hollander A: CINA : a software designed to compose infusion sheets for anesthetic intravenous drugs. Int J Clin Monitoring and Computing.(in press)

Cantraine F, Barvais L, d'Hollander A, Coussaert E: MINA: monitoring of intravenous anesthesia: A system to monitor the infusion of four intravenous drugs under the control of a personnal computer. Int J Clin Monitoring and Computing.(in press)

Question from the discussion:

Talmon: What kind of man-machine interface has your system and how long does it take for someone to learn to use the system?

d'Hollander: This system has no sophisticated man-machine interface for economical reasons first but also to restrict the use of the full system to a "trained for the system" user. Nevertheless, adequate use of the MINA part of the system to control a DAS execution can be teached in less than 15 min even for physician unaware about the software once the schema of the MINA menu has been explained.

MINA MENU OVERVIEW

F1 = START

F2 = BOLUS

F3 = STOP   ↵

                    s = syringue replacement

                    a = DAS stop (save all commands executed)

                    e = emergency stop of all IDs

F4 = IS file names catalogue

F5 = IS display and loading

F6 = MSDOS

F7 = MODIFICATION (infusion steps or coordination table)

F8 = DELETION (infusion steps)
F9 = INSERTION (infusion steps or immediate IS composition)
F10 = SCREENS   p = preparation of drug reservoir
                c = coordination table
                a = archive
                ↵ = toggle general(4 IDs)/1 ID screen

One prototype of the described system has been in use for more than two years in unselected patients scheduled for cardiac adult surgery. To day, more than 300 patients have been anesthetized with the help of this system.

A System for Interactive Knowledge-Based Simulation With Application in Management of the Critically Ill

Torgny Groth and Mikael Hakman

Unit for Biomedical Systems Analysis (BMSA), Uppsala University, Uppsala, Sweden.

Abstract

The following paper describes an interactive knowledge-based modelling & simulation system (KBSIM) providing some new means for designing and developing decision support for the management of the critically ill patient. It combines quantitative simulation with symbolic reasoning techniques, using a relational data base management system for data storage and inter-process communication.

A flexible User Interface Management System controls the activities of the various subsystems and their interaction with the user. Graphical, dynamic and interactive user interfaces can easily be designed and evaluated. The KBSIM system is shortly described and illustrated as applied to the design of fluid resuscitation of traumatized patients.

Introduction

Computers may be used in various ways to support human decision making. Database management systems provide the basic facilities for entry, storage, retrieval and presentation of data.

Packages for spread-sheet calculations, statistical analysis, graphical display and so called knowledge-based expert reasoning have made computers even more useful in this respect.

In engineering, and science in general, computer modelling & simulation has for a long time been recognized to be a very powerful technique for studying and controlling complex systems, which are not tractable by traditional mathematical and statistical analyses (*Groth, 1983*). In clinical medicine modelling & simulation has also great potentials for representation and processing of the vast amount of detailed physiological and biochemical knowledge available, and for providing the means to evaluate various diagnostic or treatment alternatives as a basis for medical decision making (*Groth, 1980; 1984*). Even though knowledge-based expert system technology is also concerned with management of complex systems, the need for computer modelling & simulation has not diminished with the appearance of the 'artificial intelligence' techniques. By combining the two approaches a new type of system for 'knowledge-based simulation' can be built, which provides complementary facilities of great potential value for developing decision support for management of highly dynamic systems. Numeric modelling & simulation may then be used to describe and predict the dynamic behaviour of underlying processes, and symbolic reasoning techniques may be used to represent empirical experience and to make prescriptions.

The present paper describes the architecture and functions of a system for interactive knowledge-based simulation as implemented on a Hewlett-Packard 9000/350 workstation under the UNIX-operating system. For illustration it has been applied to the design of fluid resuscitation of traumatized patients.

System Description

The architecture of the KBSIM-system is outlined in Fig 1. It is composed of four major software modules:

- A Package for Continuous System Simulation (CSSP);
- A Relational Database Management System (RDBMS);
- A System for Symbolic Reasoning; and
- A User Interface Management System (UIMS).

The KBSIM system contains three knowledge-bases, of which the 'Model Description' represents the detailed knowledge about the processes of the system of interest; in this case an extensive pathophysiological model of traumatized patients. The 'Rule Description' represents the clinical heuristic knowledge about fluid therapy administration, and the 'User Interface Description' reflects the knowledge about the intended users, their abstractions and preferences.

The User Interface Management System

The User Interface Management Systems (UIMS) is used for the design and control of the user-interface (see Fig. 2). It consists of four parts:

- A User Interface Description Interpreter
- A Diagram Manager
- A Forms Manager
- An Event Manager

All parts are written in the C-language and use the facilities of the HP-UX operating system (UNIX) to the largest possible extent.

The 'Interpreter' reads the 'User Interface Description' (see Fig 3 for an illustration) and controls the other parts of the system. The interpreter itself is built with use of two well-known UNIX tools: the lexical scanner generator, **LEX**, and the parser generator, **YACC** (yet another compiler-compiler). Therefore the UIMS allows not only for a description of the user interface (in terms of windows, diagrams,

Interactive Knowledge-Based Simulation

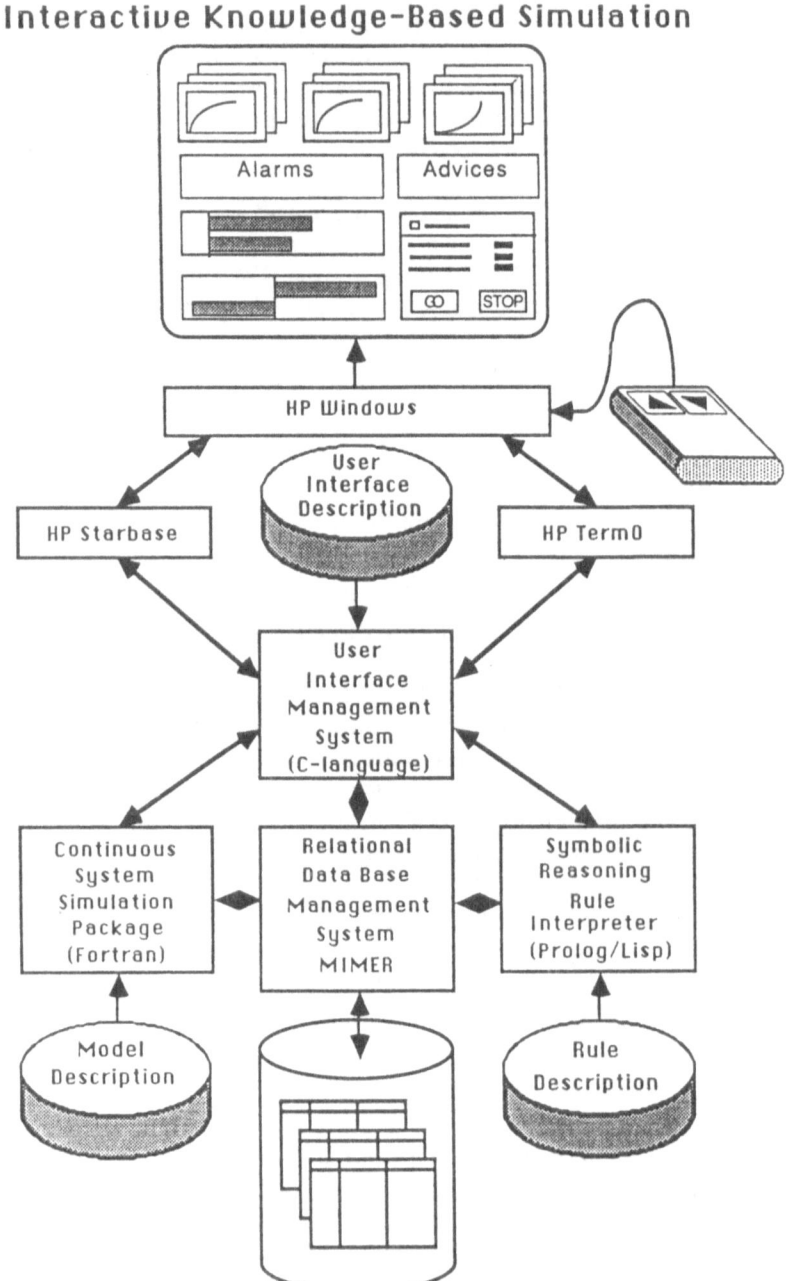

Figure 1: KBSIM architecture.

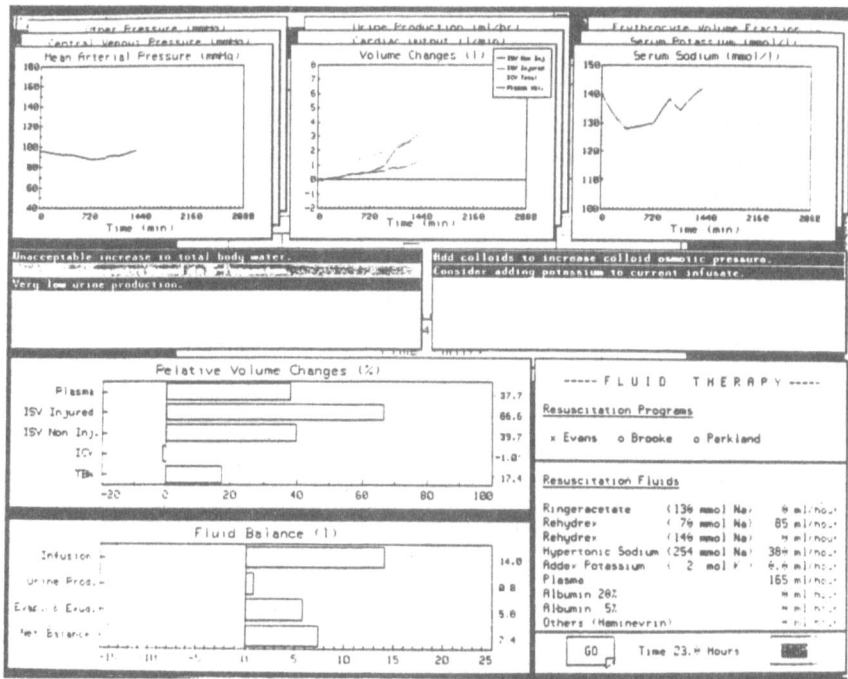

Figure 2: KBSIM's User Interface Management System.

forms, various widgets and gadgets etc.) but the specification language itself may also be redefined or modified at will.

The 'Diagram Manager' maintains a set of "living diagrams" like XY-charts, Bar-charts etc. It uses the HP Starbase Graphics Library and the HP Windows package to produce and control the diagrams on the screen (see Fig. 2).

The 'Forms Manager' controls the appearance and behaviour of a set of forms. Each form is a collection of a number of different input elements: Radio Button, Push Button, Entry Field, Menu etc. (See Fig. 2 lower right for an illustration).

The 'Forms Manager' performs its tasks through the HP TermO interface and the HP Windows package.

The 'Event Manager' is responsible for managing incoming events. Events are sent by HP Windows as a result of user operation of the mouse but also by the Continuous System Simulation Package and the 'Inference Engine' as a result of computations and symbolic reasoning, respectively.

All parts have a direct access to the Relational Database Management System. This is used for storage of long-term data, temporary data (the rewind function etc.) and for inter-process communication.

User interface description

XY CHART "Pressure"
    POSITION X 209 Y 64
    DIMENSION WIDTH 600 HEIGHT 350
    FOREGROUND BLACK
    BACKGROUND WHITE
    TITLE "Mean Arterial Pressure (mm Hg)"
    SCALE XMIN 0 XMAX 2880 YMIN 40 YMAX 180
    XAXIS
      NAME "Time (min)"
      TICS DELTA 60 MAJOR 12
    YAXIS
      TICS DELTA 10 MAJOR 2
    VARIABLE "pa"
      PATTERN COLOR RED

INPUT FORM "Programs"
    POSITION X 600 Y 400
    DIMENSION WIDTH 40 HEIGHT 7
    TEXT "Resuscitation Programs" AT X 1 Y 3 VIDEO UNDERLINE
    FIELD "Evans"
      PROMPT "Evans" AT X4 Y 5
      VALUE AT X2 Y 5 LENGTH 1
      TYPE RADIO BUTTON FOR
        TABLE "FPLAH"
        TABLE "FRDXH"
    FIELD "FRHDLH"
      PROMPT "Rehydrex (70 mmol Na)" AT X 1 Y 6
      VALUE AT X33 Y 6 LENGTH 4 DECIMALS 1
      TYPE REAL MIN 0 MAX 1000 STEPS 5
    FIELD "STOP"
      PROMPT "STOP" AT X 33 Y 7
      VALUE AT X33 Y 7 LENGTH 4
      TYPE LOGICAL PUSH BUTTON
      ACTIVE VIDEO REVERSE COLOR RED

Figure 3: Example of the User Interface Description.

The Continuous System Simulation Package

The package for modelling and simulation of continuous systems (CSSP) contains three parts:

- A Model Description Editor
- A Model Description Translator/Compiler, and
- A Simulator Engine

The 'Model Description Editor' is used to describe the model of the system to be simulated, in a language based on the Continuous System Simulation Language (CSSL) Specification (see Fig. 4 for a short example). Systems are represented by a set of ordinary differential equations and algebraic equations when required.

Model description

```
********************************************************
*
*                    VOLUME MODULE
*
********************************************************
*
*                  -----WATER FLOWS-----
*
FTIN. = FINV
VECV. = FINV + FWMA - FUW - (FEVP + FEVPS + FEVPL)
VICV. = FDRC - FOSM


FINV = FRDX + FRHDL + FPLA + FALB + FNACL + FNABI + FHEM +
       + FRHD + FADNA + FHYP + FADK


FDRCN = 0.04 * FDRC
*
*                  ......VOLUME DISTRIBUTION .........
*
OSME = (0.937*QENA + 250)/VECV
OSMI = (0.833*qCK + 0.937*qCPNA)/VICV
FOSM = 431*(OSME - OSMI)/10
VTBW = VECV + VICV
```

Figure 4: An example of a simulation written in CSSL.

The notation used is very close to ordinary mathematics; a name of a variable followed by a dot represents the first derivative of that variable.

A Macintosh with the Stella modelling and simulation package may be used to build models in terms of a graphical model description editor. Such Stella-models can then be translated into a CSSL-description and up-loaded to the HP workstation.

The 'Translator' translates the model description into compiled FORTRAN code, which is executed by the 'Simulator Engine'. The simulator calls various subroutines from a Run Library, e.g. for numerical integration of the differential equations, etc. The simulator then stores the calculated values of selected state variables in the system database at specified time intervals. The simulator also reads initial values of state variables and descriptive parameters from the system data base. Some of these values have been entered via special input forms describing the actual case studied, while others are derived by symbolic reasoning and mathematical transformation. A PC station with dynamic input forms written in MS-Windows is used for entry of data describing patients to be simulated.

The Data Base Management System

The system data base is managed by selected modules of a 4th generation Relational Data Base Management System, MIMER (*Savant Enterprises 1984; MIMER Software AB, 1987*): MIMER/DB is used to store and retrieve (i) patient data which have been entered from the PC-station via input forms; and (ii) simulation results produced by the Simulator Engine.

MIMER/DB is also used for inter-process communication; some processes write data in the data base while other processes read these data. The management of all semaphores, signals and other data in shared memory is done internally in MIMER/DB.

The System for Symbolic Reasoning

The system for symbolic reasoning consists of three parts:
- A Rule Description Editor
- A Rule Interpreter, and
- An Inference Engine.

The 'Rule Description' follows a syntax illustrated in figure 5 with a rule of the sample application.

Variables from the 'Model Description' (e.g. CPLK and CPLNA) are mapped into the user's terminology (S-Potassium and S-Sodium in this case). The rules are "if-then" type of rules with 'actions' made up of e.g. ALERT or ALARM and ADVICE-messages, and acoustic 'Beep' signals.

The 'Rule Interpreter' interprets the 'Rule Description' and provides the interpreted knowledge-base to the 'Inference Engine'. The inference engine reads values of relevant variables from the system database as soon as they are generated and stored there by the 'simulator engine'. Then the inference engine performs one whole cycle of symbolic reasoning and fires specified actions. Both the 'rule interpreter' and the 'inference engine' were written in Z-Prolog. Z-prolog is a symbolic list-processing language with many aspects strongly inspired by Common Lisp. (Z-prolog has been developed by ZYX AB of Sweden and is marketed by Hewlett-Packard). The communication between Z-Prolog programs and the rest of the KBSIM-system was performed in HP-LISP.

Sample Application

The KBSIM system description above has been illustrated with examples from an application to fluid resuscitation of traumatized patients. This application has

Rule Description

S-Potassium is "CPLK"
S-Sodium is "CPLNA"

if
    S-Sodium > = 130
and
    rate_of_change S-Sodium < (130 - S-Sodium)/6
then
    alert "Significant negative trend in S-Sodium"
    advice "Consider increase of sodium content in the infusate"
    set alert_S-Sodium_falling
    beep 2 high short

if
    alert_diuresis
and
    alert_MAP
and
    Hct_normal
and
    alert_S-Sodium_Falling
then
    alert "Suspect aldosterone effect on diuresis."
    advice "Consider increase of hypertonic sodium."

Figure 5: Example of a rule from the sample application.

been developed in collaboration with A. Hedlund, B. Zaar and G. Arturson at the Burn Center, Department of Plastic Surgery, Uppsala University Hospital, and will be described in more detail elsewhere (*Groth et al, 1989*).

General Description

Shock-preventing fluid therapy following trauma has, for a long time, been a matter of discussion with respect to composition, volume and infusion rate.
The pathophysiology of a tissue trauma with various leakage rates is very complex. In the clinical situation there are limited possibilities to measure important patient state variables, such as e.g. organ blood flows.
"Patient-Simulators" may then be very useful by providing indirect model-based measurements of such variables, and by providing possibilities for interactive generation of treatment alternatives, as a basis for decisions on the 'best choice' (*Artursson et al, 1984; 1989*). The simulation model used here is an extensive pathophysiological

model (*Hedlund et al, 1988*). It was designed to describe fluid shifts and the hemo-dynamics in connection with fluid therapy of traumatized patients. The administered fluids of various composition with regard to electrolytes and colloids form the 'forcing inputs' to the model. The model includes 6 modules with detailed descriptions of the systemic circulation; the water and protein transfer between plasma and interstitia in muscle and intact skin, viscera, and injured skin; the influence of fluid-, and electrolyte-regulating hormones; the renal function; the distribution of sodium, potassium, urea and proteins; and finally the distribution of water in the intra-, and extracellular spaces. The model consists of about 150 state variables, some of which are of direct clinical interest in monitoring fluid therapy, e.g. arterial and central venous blood pressures, cardiac output, organ blood flows, fluid shifts, urine production and fluid distribution. The knowledge-base of the reasoning system in this application to crisis management of burned patients is made up of about hundred rules (*Wiener et al, 1989*). This system is here implemented as a 'Fluid Therapy Watchdog'. Different knowledge-bases may be loaded for different types of patients (*Wiener et al, 1989*).

System Operation
The user operates the KBSIM/FLUIDTHERAPY system as follows:

- Patient to be studied is defined and described via input forms on a PC-station connected to the HP Workstation.
- Predefined 'Resuscitation Programs' may be activated by moving the mouse pointer (an arrow) to the radio-button in front of the selected program (e.g. 'Evans') and by clicking the mouse-button (lower-right window in Fig. 2).
- The simulation is then started by clicking the GO push-button (and stopped temporarily by using the corresponding STOP-button). All the diagrams, charts and values shown on the screen start 'living', and simulated time is displayed in between the two push buttons.
- The user may then
  * sit back and watch the effect of the selected fluid therapy program on 'Relative Volume Changes' (plasma, interstitial fluids in injured and intact tissue, intracellular spaces, and total body water), and also keep an eye on 'Fluid Balance' (cumulated infusion, urine production, evaporation and exudation, and net balance).

    These results are continuously displayed in barcharts in the lower-left windows of Fig. 2.
  * consider alerts, alarms and advice generated by the reasoning system and displayed in different signal-colours in the two windows in the second row from the top.
  * interact with the system and change fluid inputs by pointing with the mouse on the input fields of the different fluids on the menu and by clicking or pressing the left or right mouse-button to increase or decrease the rate of infusion in defined steps. The numerical values of the changed fluid rate are immediately shown in the corresponding field.
  * During a simulation run the user may at any time inspect the graphical windows where the time-course of selected state variables are continuously displayed; pressure variables in the upper-left stack of windows, fluid flows and volumes in the middle stack,

and laboratory variables in the right stack. After a simulation run (or during as well) the user can display the rates of the administered fluids in a time-plot.

Discussion

Computer modelling and simulation are efficient techniques for increasing insight and understanding of dynamic behaviour of complex systems. It may also have a bearing on clinical decision making by helping (i) to detect 'wrong conceptual models'; (ii) to formulate clinical 'rules of thumb' and 'production rules'; and (iii) to optimize the design of measurement procedures and treatment programs.

Some examples from critical care medicine are given in *Groth, 1980, Arturson et al, 1984, Hedlund et al, 1988* and *Wiklund et al, 1986.* In combination with so called 'expert system' techniques we obtain a new type of system for knowledge-based simulation, which has great potentials in designing decision support for management of dynamic processes. Numeric simulation and symbolic reasoning may be integrated in various ways: One approach is to enhance an expert reasoning system by embedding mathematical models which are automatically processed under the control of the reasoning system (*Shamsolmaali et al, 1988, Hara et al, 1986*). Another approach, as used here, is to enhance the simulation procedure by embedding 'Expert Watchdogs' assisting the user by providing 'intelligent alerts, alarms and advice' on how to proceed in various situations during an interactive simulation session, in order to achieve defined objectives. This approach has certain advantages during a design process and in training, by giving the user a possibility to evaluate his measures by direct feedback from the system (cf. flight simulators).

This feature of the system, to assist in evaluation of alternative procedures (e.g. treatment), should also be useful as a means for decision support.

The KBSIM system shortly described in this paper also has great potentials as a testbed for

- evaluation of 'expert system modules' which are developed to ultimately control or assist in management of a real-time process (e.g. procedures for intelligent alarming, closed-loop control etc.); and for
- design and evaluation of user interfaces for different purposes.

Acknowledgement

This work was performed within the Nordic R&D Project on Knowledge-Based Systems in Medicine (KUSIN-MED). The support of the Nordic Fund for Technology and Industrial Development, and participating companies (Hewlett-Packard Sweden AB, Pharmacia AB and MIMER Software AB) is gratefully acknowledged. Our thanks are also due to Armin Seidel for his work on the system for symbloic reasoning.

References

Artursson G, Groth T, Hedlund A and Zaar B: Potential use of computer simulation in treatment of burns with special regard to edema formation. Scand J Plast Reconstr Surg 18:1984, 39-48.

Arturson G, Groth T, Hedlund A and Zaar B: Computer simulation of fluid resuscitation in trauma. First pragmatic validation in thermal injury. Burn Care Rehab, 1989, in press.

Groth T: Modelling and simulation in medicine--Present state and future trends. In Proceedings of MEDINFO 83, eds. van Bemmel, Ball and Wigertz. IFIP-IMIA, North-Holland, Amsterdam 1983, pp. 859-862.

Groth T: Pathophysiological models as information processing elements in clinical decision making. In Proceedings of MEDINFO 80, eds. Lindberg, Kaihara. IFIP-IMIA, North-Holland, Amsterdam 1980, pp. 819-822.

Groth T: The role of biodynamic models in computer-aided diagnosis. In Computers and Control in Clinical Medicine. eds. Carson and Cramp. Plenum Press, New York and London 1984, pp. 27-46.

Groth et al: KBSIM/FLUIDTHERAPY. A system for optimized design of fluid resuscitation in trauma. In preparation 1989.

Hara S, Tanaka H, Furukawa T: Fluid therapy consultation system (FLUIDEX). Automedica, 7: 1986, 1-16.

Hedlund A, Zaar B, Groth T and Arturson G: Computer simulation of fluid resuscitation in trauma. Description of an extensive pathophysiological model and its first validation. Comp Meth Progr Biomed, 27:1988, 7-21.

MIMER: The Software Machine. Concepts and Facilities. Savant Enterprises, Carnforth 1984.

MIMER/DB: Database Manager and Program Interface. MIMER Software AB, Uppsala, Sweden, 1987. ISBN 91-7878-012-8.

Shamsolmaali A, Carson E, Collinson P and Cramp D: A knowledge-based system coupled to a mathematical model for interpretaton of laboratory data. IEEE Engineering in Medicine and Biology Magazine, June 1988, 40-46.

Wiener F, Hedlund A and Groth T: A knowledge-based information system for advice in the crisis management of the burn patient. Submitted for publication, 1989.

Wiener F, Wiklund L and Groth T: A decision support system for fluid management of the surgical patient. Submitted for publication, 1989.

Wiklund et al: Kinetics of carbon dioxide during cardiopulmonary resuscitation. Crit Care Med 14: 1986, 1015-22.

Question from the Discussion

Beneken: How many parameters do you need to match the patient in your fluid therapy model good enough? As it seems to be quite a lot, is the effort to do the matching justified in an efficient approach to decision support?

Groth: The total number of variables and parameters in the model is about 150. Most of these are given standard values from handbooks of physiology. Some selected quantities are adjusted to obtain a patient-specific model, e.g. distribution volumes, renal functional mass, heart-strength, modifiers for drug effects and parameters describing trauma. These quantities are set at values derived from data entered via screen input-forms, e.g. body mass, heart function (impared or reduced), medication and burn surface area (dermal and/or subdermal). It remains to be investigated how far we have to go further in "tuning" the model to the individual patient, and whether it is justified or not in terms of improved care. For comparison one could look at computer-aided radiotherapy where the doseplanning is performed by numeric simulation in the individual case before treatment.

Decision Support In Patient Monitoring By Interactive Information System Including Knowledge-Based Components

G. Rau[1], Th. Schecke[1], H. Kaesmacher[2], G. Kalff[2]

1 Helmholtz-Institute for Biomedical Engineering, Aachen University of Technology, West Germany.

2 Clinic of Anesthesiology, Aachen University of Technology, West Germany.

Abstract

The anesthesiologist can be considerably supported, if information about the patient's parameters and recent therapeutic actions is displayed in a clear and comprehensive way. The anesthesia information system AIS, developed for this purpose, is described.

Furthermore, additional support can be obtained by providing so-called intelligent alarms and therapy recommendations. These functions are provided by the knowledge-based system AES-2, which is currently under development. AES-2 is integrated in the information system AIS and draws its conclusions solely on the information assembled by the information system. AES-2 requires hybrid knowledge representation schemes that include adequate modeling of uncertainty.

Introduction

Creating an information system that assists the anesthesiologist in his tasks of patient monitoring, record keeping, and decision making is a particular challenge, as such a system must be both efficient and manageable in an operating room environment (Rau 1979). Therefore, emphasis of our anesthesia information system AIS (Rau, Trispel 1982; Klocke et al. 1986) is placed on the design and improvement of the human-computer interaction. The principles for designing the user interface and for designing the integrated decision support components of AIS can be adapted to other applications in patient monitoring.

Anesthesia Information System AIS

Information is displayed on a high resolution color graphics monitor. According to a careful task analysis, diagnostic and therapeutic information is organized in pages, thereby maintaining a consistent display structure. The patient's vital parameters, which are automatically registered, are permanently visible on each "working page"; more specific information, e.g. drug administration or events, is displayed on demand by selecting the appropriate page. Interaction is performed via touch input, which facilitates "direct manipulation" of the corresponding information elements: "virtual keys" are activated by touching the screen and analogue data (e.g. amount of medication) is input by adjusting "virtual sliders" on the screen. User interaction both for controlling information display and for recording data items is based on the same simple and consistent interaction sequence. In addition, the user is guided by appropriate color coding. A digital plotter provides an on-line hardcopy documentation of all assembled information (anesthesia record).

Anesthesia Decision Support System AES-2

AIS provides a considerable decision support to the anesthesiologist by displaying the required information in a clear and comprehensive way. This function of AIS is being extended by a knowledge-based decision support component, the system AES-2 (Anesthesia Expert Assist System). AES-2 provides (1) intelligent alarms and (2) therapy recommendations. It is currently focussed as an example on the assessment of hemodynamics during aortocoronary bypass surgery after completion of extracorporeal circulation.

The design of an alarm system for patient monitoring has been a severe problem since many years - both for patient monitoring in intensive care and for perioperative patient monitoring during anesthesia. Currently, an alarm is generated if the value of a patient parameter exceeds a threshold determined separately and independently for each signal (Fig. 1a). Thus, a certain deficiency of the patient's state can lead to divers alarms all related to one single cause. Therefore, the combination of several signals to yield a condensed information about a deficiency of the patient's state ("intelligent alarm") is an important component of our decision support system AES-2. In our approach, we base the assessment of a situation on the decision process of an experienced anesthesiologist. He relates the values of different signals to each other, watches for trends and considers the context, e.g. the patient's age or recent medications, (Fig. 1b). The aggregation of these information leads to the decision, whether any alarm and which alarm must be generated.

The intelligent alarm function of AES-2 aggregates all information recorded by AIS, i.e. values of the patient's vital parameters, their trends, drug administration and preoperative patient data, to five so-called state variables: myocardial contractility, heart rate, vascular tone, anesthetic level and blood volume. This aggregation process is specified by formalized rules such as:

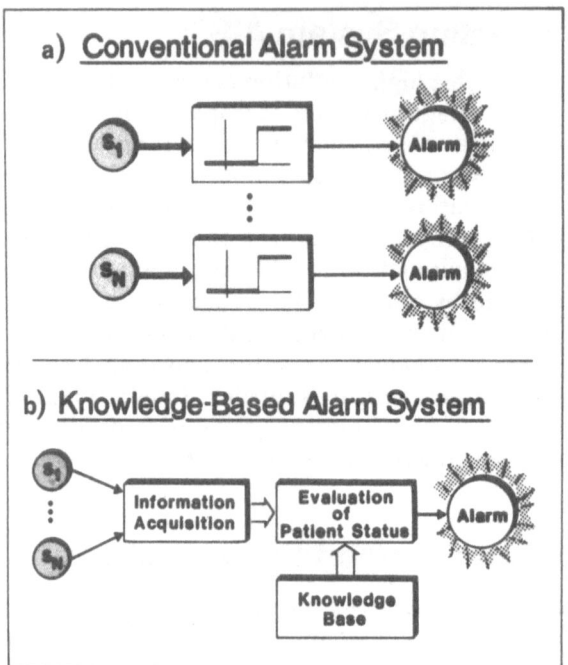

Figure 1:   Alarm Function: Conventional(a) Versus Knowledge-Based(b) Approach (**From Schecke et al. 1988a)**

> "IF systolic blood pressure is below normal
> and left atrial pressure (LAP) is increasing
> and systolic blood pressure is not increasing,
> THEN myocardial contractility is too low."

Recording of a certain data item triggers appropriate rules to update the assessment of the state variables (forward chaining).

These rules contain concepts that can not be defined exactly; therefore we need appropriate methods for representing aspects of uncertainty. For instance, the definition of systolic blood pressure being "normal" should reflect the gradual transition of blood pressure values from a range characterized as normal to a range of e.g. "below normal" (Fig. 2a). We apply a fuzzy set approach to model this type of uncertainty (Schecke et al. 1988b, Zimmermann 1987).

According to this approach a concept that can not be defined adequately by crisp boundaries, e.g. the concept of "normal systolic blood pressure", is represented by a so-called membership function (Fig. 2b). For each pressure value this function yields a value between 0 and 1. This "grade of membership" characterizes the grade of compatibility of a given pressure value with the concept of "normal". Logical relationships between fuzzy concepts, i.e. AND, OR, are modeled by applying certain

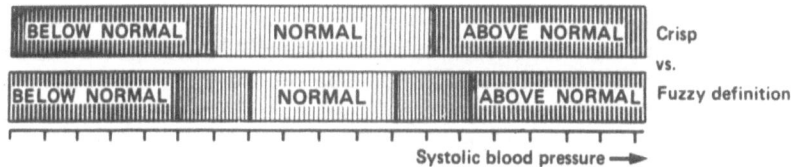

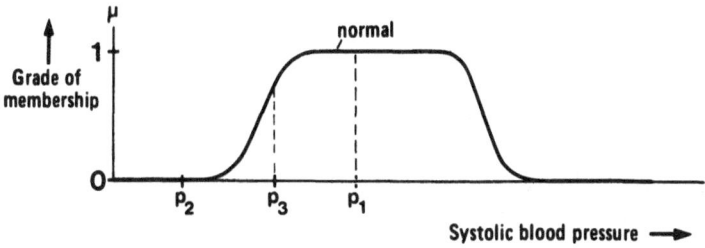

Figure 2: a) The Problem of Defining "normal".
           b) Grades of Membership: The Basic Concept of Fuzzy Set Theory (From
           Schecke et al. 1988b)

mathematical operators on the corresponding membership grades or membership functions. Empirical results indicate that selection of appropriate operators for this purpose depends on the individual application (Zimmermann 1987). We are currently investigating which operators, in particular which triangular norms and conorms, are appropriate for our application.

Whereas knowledge about assessment of the patient's state is represented by rules, we consider an object-oriented approach most adequate for representing knowledge about drug properties and therapy strategies. Thus, all knowledge about a certain drug, e.g. initial dosage (which may depend on patient's weight) or duration of effect, is combined in the slots and slot functions of a certain object representing this drug. Therapy strategies are represented by a 3-level-hierarchy of plans (therapy plan level, medication plan level, dosage plan level) which is described in more detail in Schecke et al. 1988b. This representation is supported by the known features of object-oriented programming, such as grouping objects together in classes and multiple inheritance of methods and functions.

The user interface of AES-2 is consistent with the user interface of AIS. It supports a hierarchical information structure based on subsystems (e.g. hemodynamics), state variables (e.g. vascular tone), and primary information (e.g. left atrial pressure). It was designed with respect to known cognitive models from process control and adapted to the monitoring and decision making task of the anesthesiologist (Schecke et al. 1988c).

Evaluation

Field testing of the anesthesia information system AIS was performed in parallel to the conventional procedure of anesthesia record keeping by a member of the medical staff standing beside the principal anesthesiologist. Experiences from these experiments lead to many improvements of display and interaction design. They also show that manual data input by a touch input facility in combination with automated recording of patient variables allows exact and rapid record-keeping (Rau et al. 1988).

Validation of the decision support component AES-2 in the OR is difficult. For instance, a knowledge engineer who permanently asks the anesthesiologist to comment on the output of AES-2 would distract the anesthesiologist's attention from the patient. Therefore, we intend to preoptimize AES-2, i.e. validate its knowledge base, as far as possible before field testing in the OR. We have designed a special production environment for this purpose that includes several simulation components (Schecke et al. 1989). Simulation is mainly based on anesthesia records assembled by AIS. Similar to playing back a video tape, the recorded patient data and the recorded actions of the anesthesiologist can be played back in the laboratory and input into AES-2. Differences in situation assessment between AES-2 and an anesthesiologist can be analysed and discussed. An additional simulation component comprises a physiological model of the circulatory system (Popp et al. 1989). This model enables us to reproduce both typical and extreme clinical situations and predispositions (like heart insufficiency, hypertension etc.).
Initial results from a retrospective study (Fick 1989) support the design principles of AES-2 (information structure, uncertainty modeling) but also show the requirement for further refining the knowledge base, especially for incorporation of trend analysis.

References

Fick, M.: Aufbereitung von Wissensgrundlagen fuer eine rechnergestuetzte Entscheidungsfindung zur Beurteilung der Haemodynamik bei kardiochirurgischen Operationen. Med. Thesis, Aachen University of Technology (in german), 1989.
Klocke, H., Trispel, S., Rau, G., Hatzky, U., Daub, D.: An Anesthesia Information System for Monitoring and Record Keeping During Surgical Anesthesia. J Clin Monit, vol. 2, 246-261, 1986.
Popp, H.-J., Schecke, Th., Rau, G., Kaesmacher, H., Kalff, G.: Einsatz eines interaktiven Kreislaufmodells bei der Entwicklung eines wissensbasierten Systems in der Anaesthesiologie. 23. Jahrestagung der Deutschen Gesellschaft fuer Biomedizinische Technik, August 31 - September 2, Kiel (in German), 1989.
Rau, G.: Ergonomische Ueberlegungen bei der Gestaltung komplexer medizinischer Instrumentierung unter Einsatz von Mikroprozessoren. Biomedizinische Technik (Ergaenzungsband), Vol. 24, 10-15 (in German), 1979.
Rau, G., Trispel, S.: Ergonomic Design Aspects in Interaction Between Man and Technical Systems in Medicine. Med Prog Technol, 9:153-159, 1982.

Rau, G., Klocke, H., Schecke, Th., Daub, D. Kalff, G.: First Evaluation of a Highly Interactive Anesthesia Information System. Abstracts, Computing in Anesthesia and Intensive Care, J Clin Monit, Vol 4 No 2, 156-157, 1988.

Schecke, Th., Rau, G., Klocke, H., Fick, M., Kaesmacher, H., Hatzky, U., Kalff, G.: Knowledge-Based Decision Support in Anesthesia: Toward Intelligent Alarms and Beyond. Abstracts, Computing in Anesthesia and Intensive Care, J Clin Monit, Vol 4 No 2, 159, 1988a.

Schecke, Th., Rau, G., Klocke, H., Kaesmacher, H., Hatzky, U., Kalff, G., Zimmermann, H.-J.: Knowledge-Based Decision Support in Anesthesia: A Case Study. Proc. IEEE Int. Conf. Systems, Man, and Cybernetics, August 8-12, Beijing and Shenyang, 962-965, 1988b.

Schecke, Th., Langen, M., Rau, G., Kaesmacher, H., Kalff, G.: Knowledge-Based Decision Support for Monitoring in Anesthesia: Problems, Design and User Interaction. in: O. Rienhoff, U. Piccolo, B. Schneider (eds.), Expert Systems and Decision Support in Medicine, Berlin: Springer, 256-263, 1988c.

Schecke, Th., Popp, H.-J., Thull, G., Rau, G., Kaesmacher, H., Kalff, G.: Design of a Knowledge-Based Decision Support for Anesthesia Using Simulation Tools for Knowledge Acquisition and Validation. 2nd European Conference on Artificial Intelligence in Medicine, London, 29th-31st August (to appear), 1989.

Zimmermann, H.J.: Fuzzy Sets, Decision Making, and Expert Systems. Boston: Kluwer Academic Publishers, 1987.

Questions from the Discussion

Beneken: In your system you are using and displaying reference values for the critical parameters during the monitoring. Are these values fixed or established anew for each patient?

Rau: Most reference or normal values are situation dependent. The knowledge-based approach enables us to model these dependencies. This can be demonstrated by the following rule:

```
IF   patient is older than 65 years,
THEN define as normal for 'syst. blood pressure':
        80 -- 0,
        90 -- 0.65,
        115 -- 1.0,
        150 -- 0.2,
        165 -- 0
```

which specifies the membership function of the concept "normal systolic blood pressure" (represented in polygonal form). The condition part of this rule reflects the fact that blood pressure assessment must consider the patient's age.

Andreassen: You have reduced the manual input of observations during the surgery virtually to zero. This means that things that are normally available to the anesthesiologist like muscle tone, reflexes, etc. are not recorded. How much do you feel that you have lost by not including this information?

Rau: After many discussions with our medical partners and their colleagues we have come to the following conclusion: We must accept as part of the problem definition that we can not require the anesthesiologist to input additional information. In those situations when he really needs decision support he has no time for this additional interaction. Therefore, we look at the problem from the other side: "How much support for the anesthesiologist can be achieved, if we restrict information processing to only those information items that can be recorded automatically in clinical routine or that must be documented anyway."

The construction of AES-2 is our method to investigate this problem.

As far as we know by now, knowledge-based decision support can be provided only for a restricted set of problems in anesthesia. We think that the assessment of hemodynamics belongs to these topics. We will be able to say more about this problem after some experiences with AES-2 in the OR.

Computerized Monitoring And Decision Support During Anaesthesia

Carsten Eckhart Thomsen[1], Kurt Nørregaard-Christensen[2], Annelise Rosenfalck[1]

1 Department of Medical Informatics and Image Analysis, Aalborg University, Denmark.

2 Department of Anaesthesiology, Aalborg Hospital, Denmark.

Abstract

Changes in the electroencephalogram were studied during anaesthesia for three different agents. For each agent ten healthy women (ASA group I) were examined during a non-critical surgical procedure. Two channels of EEG were stored simultaneously with F_ACO_2, F_IO_2, MAP, ECG and temperature. Signal processing was made off-line. Each 2 second long EEG segment was characterized in a set of spectral features extracted by autoregressive modelling. Hierarchical clustering was used to define a common set of basic patterns for each anaesthetic agent. With reference to the set of basic patterns, the EEG was classified and the result represented in a class probability histogram. For each group of patients the basic patterns were related to the clinical depth of anaesthesia and assigned colours accordingly. Using this colour code, the class probability histogram showed a highly simplified interpretation of the anaesthetic depth. Another effort to provide decision support to the anaesthesiologist is an expert system for anaesthesia, where the first prototype is limited to the respiratory system. The knowledge representation and inference mechanism in the expert system are based on a causal probabilistic network.

Introduction

The aim of the study was to correlate changes in the electroencephalogram (EEG) to the depth of anaesthesia (*Klein and Davis 1981; Pronk et al, 1987*), and to evaluate the performance of the EEG compared to more commonly used physiological parameters in intensive care units. This evaluation was done by investigating changes in the EEG in thirty women scheduled for simple hysterectomy. In all patients, there was no history of neurological disorders, and tranquilizers and analgesics were not administered routinely previous to operation. The EEG has hitherto not been clinical useful for monitoring the level of anaesthesia because the changes were agent specific and dependent on the critical state of the patient (*Editorial/Lancet, 1986*). To overcome this problem only patients belonging to ASA group I were selected and each anaesthetic agent was analyzed individually. The anaesthesia was controlled by the same experienced anaesthesiologist in all patients according to clinical signs indicating adequate anaesthetic level for surgical needs. Three different anaesthetic agents were used: ten women were anaesthetized with halothane, ten with isoflurane (both volatile agents) and ten were anaesthetized with etomidate/fentanyl (intravenous agent). For the two volatile agents the anaesthesia was induced with thiopentone 5mg/kg body weight, and maintained with isoflurane 1.0-2.5% or halothane 0.5-1.75% in oxygen nitrousoxide 1:2. The group of patients anaesthetized with etomidate/fentanyl was induced with 94-169mg/450-875μg and maintained with 0.5-1.2mg/1.7-3.9μg/min. To study the changes in the EEG according to different anaesthetic levels, a 50% increase in anaesthetic loading was established for 20 minutes, when the clinical condition was stable. Approximately 20 minutes after return to maintenance level a slight hyperventilation was induced corresponding to an End Tidal carbondioxide concentration of 4.0-4.5 vol%. After 20 minutes hyperventilation was discontinued. During surgery the EEG from both hemispheres (P3-F_{p1} and P4-F_{p2}) were recorded on magnetic tape together with the traditional physiological parameters ECG, mean arterial blood pressure (MAP), End Tidal carbondioxide concentration (F_ACO2), inspired oxygen concentration (F_IO2) and temperature.

Signal Processing

The signals were analysed off-line using an INTEL 310 computer system equipped with a high resolution colour graphic display and analog to digital converter (12 bit resolution in 8 ch.). Hard-copies of the displayed parameters were made on a Tektronix 4696 colour-graphic jet-ink printer. The EEG was filtered with a 25Hz 4th order anti-aliasing filter, sampled at 100 Hz and preemphasized digitally with a first order high-pass filter at 4.5 Hz (fig. 1).

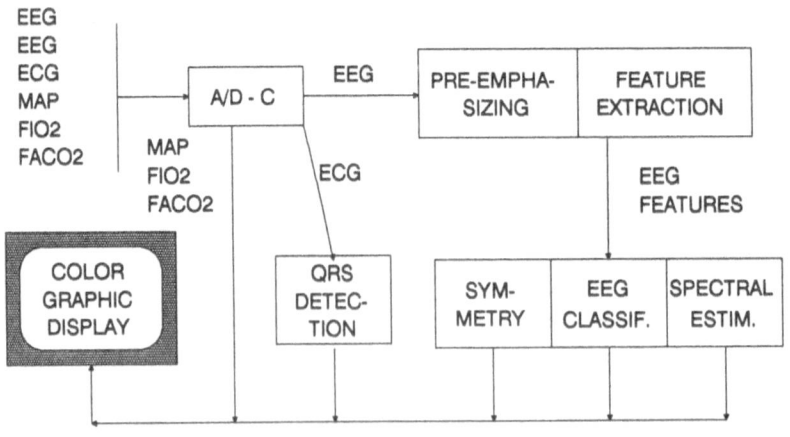

Figure 1: Signal processing pathway through the system.

From each 2 sec. segment 11 parameters were extracted (10 normalized autocorrelation coefficients and RMS amplitude) These features can easily be transformed into frequency spectra using techniques from AutoRegressive (AR) modelling (*Makhoul, 1975; Jansen, 1985; Jansen et al, 1981*). Based on this feature vector the pattern recognition was performed by a probabilistic classifier (Bayes' decision theory) expressed in a set of linear discriminant functions (*Duda and Hart, 1973*). The classifier used a learning set of patterns defined by off-line hierarchical clustering analysis on data from patients anaesthetized with the same agent.

During learning we selected a set of approximately 1000 EEG segments from each patient representing typical EEG patterns from different levels of anaesthesia. During hierarchical clustering (7) the two most similar segments were merged step by step starting with the initial number of segments ending with one. The segments were as in pattern recognition characterized by 11 parameters containing spectral information and amplitude. Euclidean distance between feature vectors was used as similarity measure. The clustering sequence was represented graphically in a dendrogram (fig. 2).

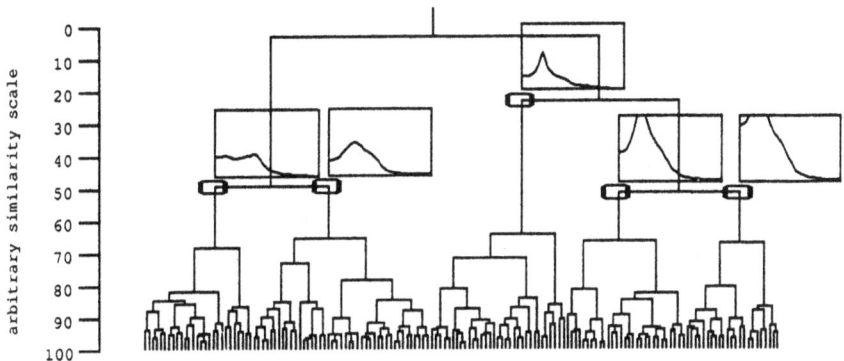

Figure 2:   An example of a dendrogram - a graphic description of the result from hierarchical clustering. The dendrogram illustrates merging of clusters as a function of similarity (ordinate). The small spectra are mean values for subtrees at the lower left corner of each spectrum. This particular dendrogram is a smaller part of the dendrogram for the group of patients anaesthetized with isoflurane.

By interactive inspection of nodes in this dendrogram, guided be meanspectra for subtrees below nodes where the similarity measure decreased rapidly, a representative set of 10-15 classes were defined. To generate a common learning set for a specific anaesthetic agent, data from 5-10 patients were included in the clustering sequence using "linked" clustering analysis (fig. 3).

From the individual dendrograms we selected a level, where 50 clusters were represented. By merging the 50 clusters from each of the ten patients anaesthetized with the same agent, we gathered 500 EEG patterns representing a <u>common</u> EEG subset.

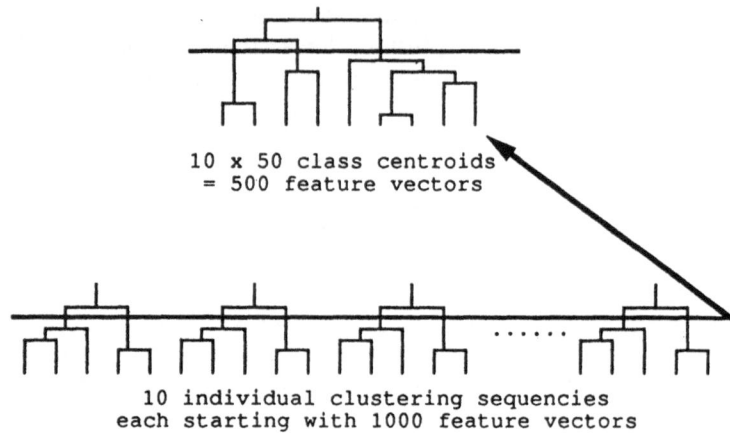

10 x 50 class centroids
= 500 feature vectors

10 individual clustering sequences
each starting with 1000 feature vectors

Figure 3:   An illustration of "linked" or stepwise clustering analysis to include data from a
            number of patients in the learning process.

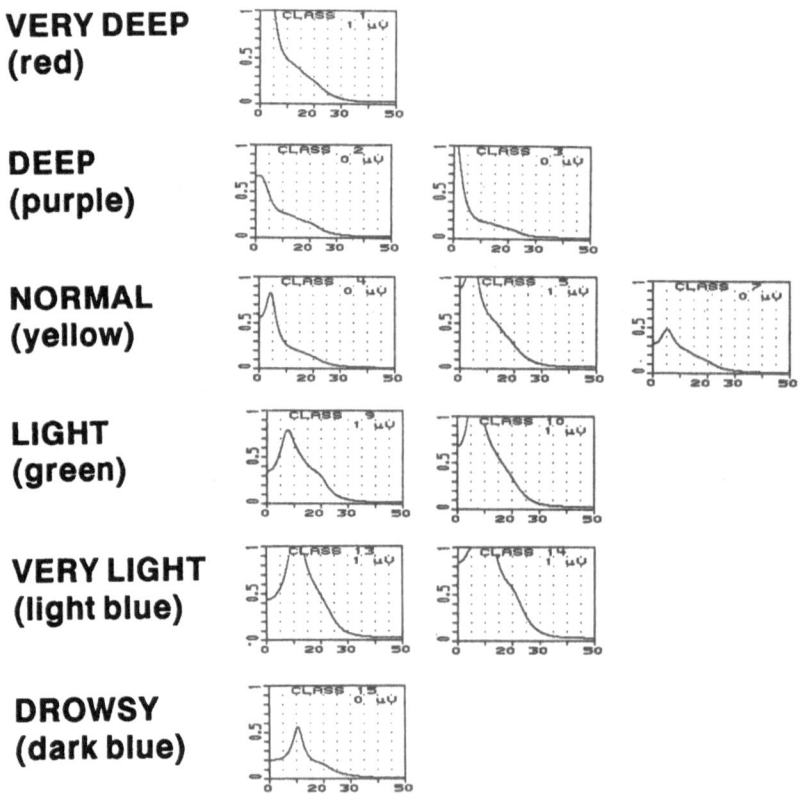

**VERY DEEP
(red)**

**DEEP
(purple)**

**NORMAL
(yellow)**

**LIGHT
(green)**

**VERY LIGHT
(light blue)**

**DROWSY
(dark blue)**

Figure 4:   The set of basic EEG patterns from the isoflurane group correlated to the depth
            of anaesthesia and colour coded to give descision support to the anaesthesio-
            logist about the anaesthetic level.

After an additional clustering procedure, a set of classes could be defined, which was used as learning set in all patients anaesthetized with that particular agent.

The occurrence of each class was then related to clinical statements and assigned colours according to the level of anaesthesia (fig. 4) for each anaesthetic agent (e.g.: blue = "drowsy", green = "light anaesthesia", yellow = "normal anaesthetic level" and red = "very deep anaesthesia").

Results

The peak frequency was found to be the dominating feature, but the whole configuration of the spectrum plays an important role in classification of anaesthetic level. A peak frequency of 10-12 Hz was found during light anaesthesia for isoflurane. The medium clinical level of anaesthesia was characterized by a peak frequency of 4-6 Hz and deep levels of anaesthesia by a peak frequency of 1-3 Hz.

The three set of classes and colour codings were used during on-line pattern recognition, where parameters from the EEG were displayed as a function of time:

- as [colour] density spectral array plots (fig. 5 left column) (*Bickford et al, 1971; Bickford et al, 1973; Flemming and Smith, 1979*), where each plot/line represents the averaged amplitude spectrum during the last 10 sec.
- as the asymmetry between the EEG from the two hemispheres(fig. 5 2nd column from the left).
- as class probability histograms (fig. 5 middle column), where each line represents the relative occurrence of any class in percent.

In addition the trend curves for F_IO_2, F_ACO_2, MAP and heart rate (HR) were displayed (fig. 5 the two right columns). In all patients investigated these parameters were kept within normal limits. The class probability histogram reflected in all patients the level of anaesthesia when the concentration of the anaesthetic agent was adjusted either based on clinical signs or according to the protocol. In addition towards the end of surgery when pain stimuli were less intense the class probability histogram often appeared as if the concentration of the anaesthetic agent had been increased. During clustering analysis on data from the three groups of patients we experienced the importance of having a learning material without outliers. In the group anaesthetized with isoflurane, all recordings were very "clean" and contained practically no artefacts, which gave a good and reliable set of basic patterns, and a well defined anaesthetic scale. In the two other groups the set of basic patterns based on data from all ten patients in each group gave some inconsistency in the class probability histogram. Furthermore a number of classes could not be assigned colours according to the anaesthetic level. This problem was investigated by reducing the number of patients from each group to five to be included in the clustering process. Otherwise the learning process was similar. The two new sets of basic patterns were then used for all ten patients in each group respectively. The result was a better consistency and a more reliable configuration of the class probability histogram during on-line analysis. The improvement was not isolated to patients inside the learning group, but was also observed for the five patients not involved in

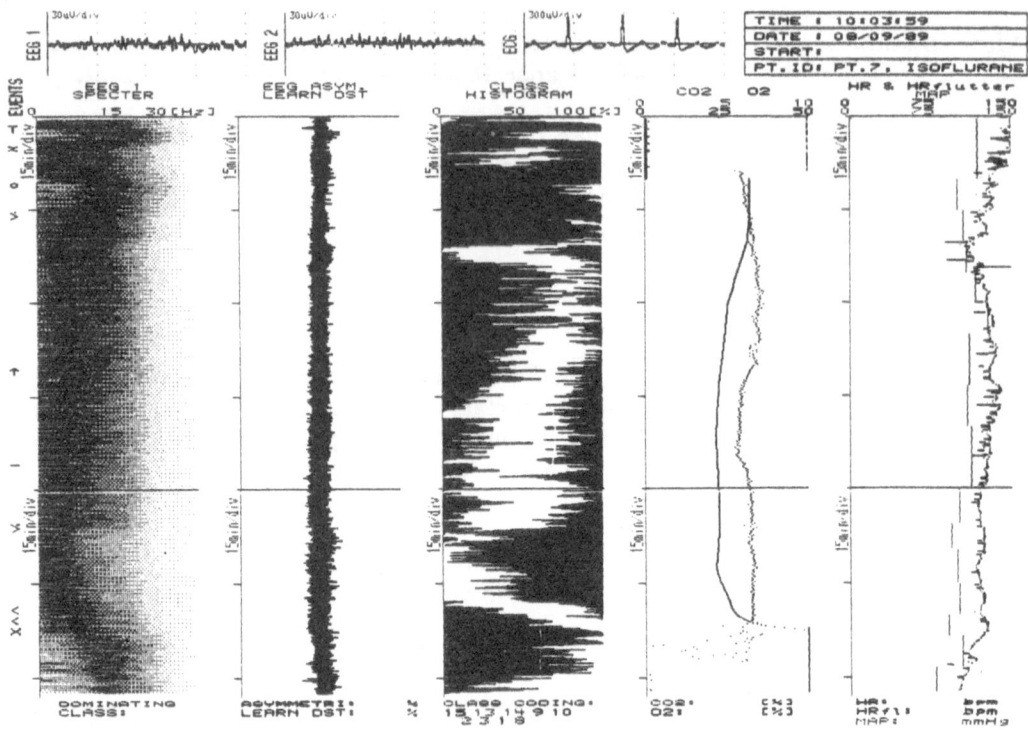

Figure 5:   An example of a hardcopy from a patient anaesthetized with isoflurane. Vertical
axis is time and the total duration is 1 hour 30 minutes. Data from the EEG
processing are displayed in the three columns to the left and trend curves from
the traditional physiological parameters are displayed in the two right columns.
Events are marked along the time axis at left: (T) Thiopentone; (x),(X) start and
stop of anaesthesia; (o) start of surgery; (^),(-) start and stop of hyperventilation;
(>),(<) in- and decreased induction of anaesthesia.

the clustering analysis. This indicates that the method will perform well on a larger
population not included in the learning process.

Conclusion

Within this year the technique is going to be evaluated in clinical practice. The
"run-time" version of the program will then be implemented on an INTEL
PC-120 system (80386, 16Mhz Personal Computer), and an increased effort will be
paid to the human interface. In addition the raw signal will be stored by the system,
to maintain the control of visual inspection during evaluation. We expect that on-line
intelligent decision support systems are going to be the key issue for management of
patients during anaesthesia, and that signal processing and display techniques are
the basis for this kind of systems.

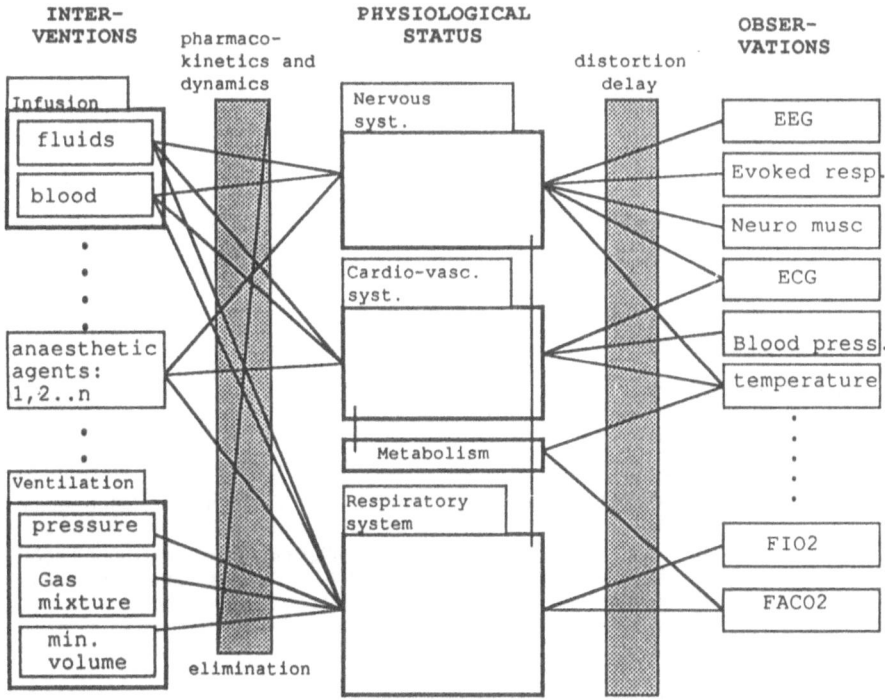

Figure 6: The basic structure of a knowledge based system for anaesthesia. In the left part of the figure we have interventions controlled by the anaesthesiologist, and in the right part we have either clinical observations or outputs from monitoring devices. In the middle the human physiology, divided into the main physiological subsystems.

Knowledge Based System

At present we are working on an expert system for anaesthesia. The knowledge representation and inference mechanism are based on a causal probabilistic network (*Pearl, 1988; Lauritzen and Spiegelhalter, 1988*). A preliminary version of the structure of this system is outlined in fig. 6.

We have concentrated our effort to one of the physiological subsystems - the respiratory system. The aim was to establish a causal net, where essential physiological variables and interconnected relations were represented (fig. 7). This model was the first attempt to establish causal relations between "interventions" and "observations" structured from domain specific knowledge, but it is still far from being complete. In the first prototype for the network representing the respiratory system each node have three possible outcomes: reduced, normal and increased. We have limited the complexity of the prototype in the following manner: Patient - male, 30 years, 70 kg body weight and no chronic disorders, Anaesthetic agent - only halothane and metabolism is postponed to later prototypes. In the sense of handling knowledge from the treatment (interventions) as well as the observations, the anaesthesia

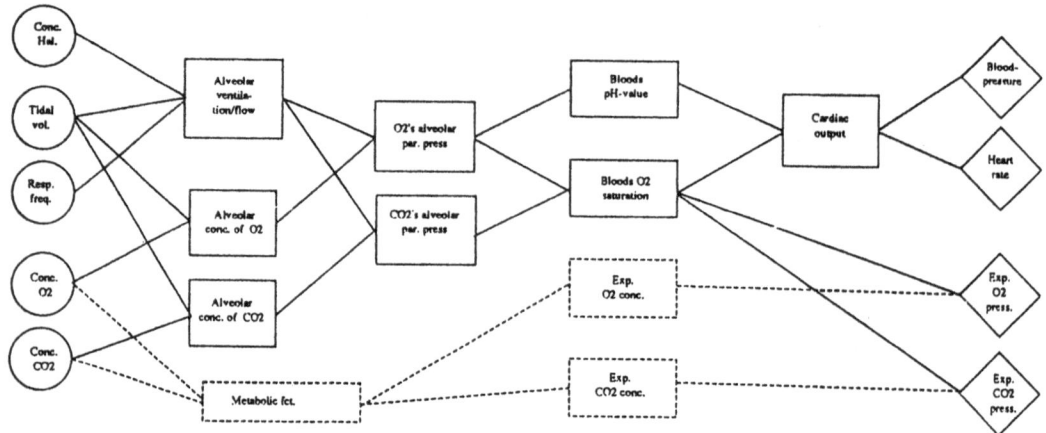

Figure 7:   Configuration of the causal net for representation of domain knowledge within the respiratory system. Rectangles are internal physiological variables, circles represents interventions from the anaesthesiologist and the rhombs in the right part of the figure are monitored/observed parameters. In the figure the following abbreviations are used: resp. = respiration, conc. = concentration, exp. = expiratorical, hal. = halothane, vol. = volume and freq. = frequency.

situation differs from the diagnostic situation, where the inference machine based on observations sets up the most probable diagnose. In anaesthesia we have both the observations and interventions from the anaesthesiologist as input to the system. The fundamental idea is then to detect a conflict between these two types of information to obtain an early warning for a situation where the patient reacts abnormal. To enable the system to give advises to the anaesthesiologist it must detect where in the physiological system the abnormality is located. It may thus be necessary to handle some of the parameters in the physiological models as random variables in the same way as other physiological parameters.

REFERENCES

Bickford R G, Flemming N I, Billinger T W. Compression of EEG data by isometric power spectral plots. Electroencephalography and Clinical Neurophysiology 1971; 31: 632.

Bickford R G, Brimm J, Berger L, Aung M. In: Kellaway B, Petersen I, eds. Application of compressed spectral array in clinical EEG, in Automation of clinical elctroencephalography. New York: Raven Press1973: 55-64.

Duda R O, Hart P E. Pattern classification and scene analysis. New York: John Wiley & Sons Ltd.,1973.

Editorial. Lancet 1986; i: 553-554.

Flemming R A, Smith N T. Density modulation: A technique for the display of three-variable data in patient monitoring. Anesthesiology 1979; 50: 543-546.

Jansen B H. Analysis of biomedical signals by means of linear modelling. CRC Critical Reviews in Biomedical Engineering 1985; 12: 343-392.

Jansen B H, Bourne J R, Ward J W. Autoregressive estimation of short segment spectra for computerized EEG analysis. IEEE Transactions on Biomedical Engineering 1981; 28: 630-638.

Klein F F, Davis D A. The use of time domain analyzed EEG in conjunction with cardiovascular parameters for monitoring anesthetic levels. IEEE Transactions on Biomedical Engineering 1981; 28: 36-40.

Lauritzen S L, Spiegelhalter D J. Local computations with probabilities on graphical structures and their application to expert systems. The journal of the royal statistical society series B (methodological) 1988; 50: 157-224.

Makhoul J. Linear prediction: A tutorial review. Proceedings IEEE 1975; 63: 561-580.

Pearl J. Probabilistic reasoning in intelligent systems. San Mateo: Morgan Kaufmann, 1988.

Pronk R A F, Simons A J R, Ackerstaff R G A, Boezeman E H J F. Intra-operative EEG monitoring. Proceedings of the Ninth Annual Conference of the IEEE Engineering in Medicine and Biology Society 1987; 3: 1250-1251.

Questions From The Discussion

Talmon: Can you explain why the performance of the system was better when it was trained on only 5 cases rather than on all 10 both for the cases included in the learning set and those not included?

Thomsen: When the system was trained on data from only 5 patients, these patients were carefully selected with respect to the absence of disturbances of all kinds - not only artefacts but also disturbances from an abnormal patient reaction to the anaesthetic agent. As a result, we got a set of basic patterns closely related to the depth of anaesthesia rather than to any other interventions from the surgical procedure. Even when this set of patterns are used on patients outside the learning group, the classification result gave the best fit to the set of patterns related to the anaesthetic depth, although the individual EEG recordings includes patterns, influenced by small variations in the ventilation, body movements, pain stimuli etc.

Wyatt: How did you perform an evaluation of you method and what was the result of that?

Thomsen: The first preliminary part of the evaluation was a complete analysis of the 10 patients included in the training process, which confirmed that it was possible to extract patient independent characteristics from the EEG related to the depth of anaesthesia. Comparing the clinical evaluation from the anaesthesiologist with the EEG analysis, it was obvious that, in some instances, the anaesthesiologist adjusted the induction of the anaesthetic agent, without knowing the result of the signal processing. In these cases the EEG analysis "agreed" with the treatment of the patient. The second part of the evaluation was related to the reduction of the training set from 10 to 5 patients, where the class probability histogram from the 5 patients not included in the training set confirms that the method can handle data which has not been presented to the system previously. The third part of the evaluation will be an on-line evaluation in clinical practice primarily based on patients from ASA group I.

Talmon: You proposed a method for monitoring the anaesthetic level. Others, like R. A. F. Pronk, have tried to monitor whether the brain was compromised during surgery. Aren't these objectives not interfering with each other? And how sensitive is you method when the brain gets compromised?

Thomsen: We have too little knowledge to give a proper answer to this question. Related to the previous question the evaluation of the method so far has only involved patients from ASA group I scheduled for hysterectomy where the brain is not compromised. If the evaluation in the future shows problems related to this question, a possible solution could be parallel running classification processes - one related to anaesthetic depth and one or more related to different types of "brain warnings". To the last part of the question, we expect that our method may be very sensitive to changes in the EEG pattern, as reported by Pronk, when the brain is compromised. The reason is probably that we use a set of features, which can describe small and/or complex changes in the frequency spectrum.

SIMPLEXYS Real Time Expert Systems in Patient Monitoring

J.A. Blom

Medical Electrical Engineering Group, Eindhoven University of Technology, Eindhoven, the Netherlands

Abstract

The SIMPLEXYS real time expert systems toolbox has a compact linear time inferencing algorithm. It allows the construction of very fast real time expert systems for applications such as patient monitoring and clinical control systems that must run in compact and inexpensive computer hardware.

Besides speed, features of SIMPLEXYS are: a powerful but simple, understandable knowledge representation language that enforces comprehensible knowledge bases; checks of the logical consistency of the knowledge base; an intuitive interface to the "external world" (Pascal 1code); an ability to handle dynamically changing contexts and data; temporal reasoning; predictable response times; and extensive debugging facilities.

One application, an "intelligent" clinical control system for controlled hypotension, is described in some detail.

Introduction

When the rate of information presented to them is too great, humans have a tendency to overlook relevant information, to respond inconsistently or too slowly, or to panic; the cognitive load overwhelms them, and problem solving capabilities degrade dramatically. If the cognitive burden is above all due to a too short period of time to finish tasks, a real time expert system could provide assistance. In a recent article, *Laffey et al, 1988* give an excellent overview of the current state of the art in real time expert systems. They introduce the problems that SIMPLEXYS addresses as follows:

---

1   For its better readability, this paper takes Pascal as the language that SIMPLEXSYS interfaces with. A SIMPLEXSYS Pascal version is not available for distribution, however. Licenses can be obtained for a version that interfaces with the C. language. This version is about 3 to 4 times faster than the Pascal version.

A knowledge based system operating in a real time situation (for example, crisis intervention or threat recognition) will typically need to respond to a changing task environment involving an asynchronous flow of events and dynamically changing requirements with limitations on time, hardware, and other resources. A flexible software architecture is required to provide the necessary reasoning on rapidly changing data within strict time requirements while it accommodates temporal reasoning, non-monotonicity, interrupt handling, and methods for handling noisy input data.

Real Time Expert Systems Are Different

Most expert systems ask questions and expect answers. A consultation session to solve a particular problem often takes a lot of time at the computer keyboard, and timing is not an issue. A real time expert system is essentially an instrument. Instruments do not ask questions, they must stand alone, require minimal interaction with the user, and be fast. In patient monitoring, the quantity of data to be analyzed is overwhelming, and the results of the analysis must be available with minimal delay. *O'Reilly and Cromarty, 1985* discuss the notion of real time. The most common connotation is "fast": a real time system is a system that processes data quickly. Also: "perceptually fast", or "faster than a human can do it". A better definition is: "fast enough", or "the system responds to incoming data at a rate as fast or faster than it is arriving". We adopt the following more formal definition: A system exhibits real time behavior if it is *"predictably* fast enough for use by the process being serviced" [*Marsh and Greenwood, 1986*; italics ours]. Under all possible conditions, the system's response time should be adequate. At best, a real time expert system should guarantee an upper limit for the time it needs to analyze the data, whatever their values and whatever processing is required: a "worst case processing time".

A real time system is different, in that the data to be analyzed are not static. Incoming sensor data are not durable or have a decay in validity with time or cease to be valid because events have changed the state of the system. Two approaches to the processing of real time data are possible.

In the first approach, a complete new set of data is processed whenever an event occurs; an event could be clock tick or a (significant) change of one or more of the input data. This is the familiar expert systems approach: each data set resembles a filled out form that has to be analyzed, and an event is just a message that a new form has arrived for analysis. The new form probably has most of its data in common with the previous one, and consequently much of the data processing time may be "wasted". That, however, will not be a problem if the analysis is fast enough. SIM-PLEXYS uses this approach.

The second approach does not reevaluate conclusions based on unchanged data. An event only retracts those conclusions that were based on the data that have become outdated, and only recalculates those same conclusions, now employing the new data. This approach is called truth maintenance, a process that always keeps the conclusions in line with the data. Truth maintenance, however, is a complex process, and this approach may be even less efficient than the former. Moreover, truth maintenance and retraction of earlier conclusions is possible only, if the system is purely logical, not if conclusions can have unretractable "side effects" such as firing a missile or applying a drug.

With either approach, the system's operation should be continuous: partial or complete failure of one or more parts of the system, especially temporary failure of one or more of the sensors, should not necessarily imply that the system stops functioning. Missing data may be common, and the validity of some of the data can decay with time, e.g. due to a degradation in sensor performance.

Events may be either synchronous or asynchronous. If the events occur synchronously with some clock, the time available for analysis is constant. The time necessary for an analysis of the data may depend on the data, however. If the time necessary is on average longer than the time available, the load is of course too heavy for the system. If the time necessary is only sometimes longer than the time available, buffering the data may be a solution, if this does not degrade the worst case response time too much. In case of a more permanent system overload, another option may be to decrease the rate of the analysis.

Selecting a system cycle time greater than the worst case processing time of course guarantees a worst case response time smaller than the system's cycle time. In a patient monitoring context, this robust approach is recommended. If necessary, an increase of the system's cycle rate can be realized through more powerful computer hardware.

Asynchronous events are events that do not conform to an a priori known schedule; the time available for analysis now depends on the time between events, which may be completely unpredictable. There is a large probability that some events will succeed each other so fast that the available processing time for some of these events will be too short. Temporarily buffering new data may again be a solution, but even if a worst case processing time is known, computation of a worst case response time will not be easy since it depends on the statistics of the event's occurrences. Since events can vary in importance, it is also an option not to process an event as long as more important ones demands processing time. Other "focus of attention" heuristics exist as well.

Current Problems in Real Time Expert Systems

affey et al, 1988 review several real time expert systems; they mention applications in aerospace, communications, medicine, process control, and robotics. They also give an overview of existing real time expert system tools. Some of the most important current problems are considered to be:

- the slow execution speed of rule-based systems (90% of the time is spent in searching);
- production systems that use forward or backward chaining are exponential time (*O'Reilly and Cromarty, 1985*); worst case analysis probably results in unacceptable response times;
- frame languages using only simple inheritance are suitable (searching is then limited to linear lists); most frame languages are more complex, however, resulting in exponential searching times.

Currently existing real time expert systems are far from satisfactory. *Laffey et al, 1988* conclude that, although "considerable effort is being put into developing real time systems, a much more difficult area than traditionally has been approached using expert systems", the results so far are disappointing: "trying to apply current shells to real time domains is like trying to use Prolog for a number-crunching application or FORTRAN for a symbolic processing application". And "no one seems to be considering the ramifications of using exponential-time algorithms in a real time application". SIMPLEXYS specifically solves this problem.

SIMPLEXYS Design Goals

SIMPLEXYS (*Blom, 1987*) grew out of the need to implement real time expert systems such as "intelligent" patient monitors and clinical control systems. Besides the obvious attention to efficiency (we wanted our applications to run on small machines such as PCs), the design of SIMPLEXYS was guided by two more considerations: safety and understandability of the knowledge base code.

Real time expert systems must of course be fast enough. They must also be safe. In a real time expert system errors are less likely to be discovered in time than in a typical expert system, because it may run without much interaction with a human for extended periods of time. Without much regard for the current AI fashions (but see *Hajek, 1988*), we have designed a set of tools that are geared to both. Although to the knowledge base developer SIMPLEXYS expert systems appear to be rule based, internally the knowledge is represented as a semantic network, a directed graph. A semantic network provides speed because it can be exploited in a way that abolishes searching. And it provides safety because it allows many checks of the consistency of the stored knowledge, for instance to detect circular reasoning. Most other expert system tools don't offer such checks.

Documentation is also important. To make a patient monitoring system smarter, more and more medical knowledge has to be incorporated into its software. That type of knowledge is difficult to embody into a FORTRAN or machine language program, and when done, it is difficult to show exactly which knowledge is stored and how it is used. In a well designed expert systems language it ought to be easy to ascertain which knowledge is implemented and how. A related problem is the maintenance of the knowledge, keeping it up to date, adapting it to new demands. The format of the SIMPLEXYS knowledge base is an attempt to resolve these problems.

The SIMPLEXYS Toolbox

The SIMPLEXYS expert systems toolbox consists of the following components:

- A language, designed to encode knowledge. A program written in this language is called "a knowledge base" or "a knowledge program".
- A compiler that translates the knowledge base into an efficient internal representation.
- A knowledge consistency checker that performs several correctness checks on the knowledge base.

- A program that allows a number of run-time debugging options to be incorporated into the expert system.
- An inference engine, the expert system's reasoning mechanism. Linking the inference engine with the internal representation of the knowledge base produces a ready to run expert system.
- A debugger/tracer that analyzes the expert system's results either at run time (when non-time-critical debugging is possible with stored or simulated data) or off-line, from data stored during the expert system's operation.

SIMPLEXYS has several features that do not often exist in other expert systems:

- SIMPLEXYS was designed to be as efficient as possible in order to be able to implement real time high data flow applications such as process control and process supervision/monitoring.
- SIMPLEXYS incorporates a tool to check for several types of semantic errors in the acquired knowledge. Real time expert systems such as "intelligent" patient monitors must be safe. The acquisition of the knowledge to be implemented is not a simple process, and errors are to be expected. The error checker can assist in the acquisition and implementation of logically error-free knowledge. Other tools can analyze the expert system's derivation of conclusions once it actually runs, and help find and trace more profound failures.
- Real time systems cannot do without some form of temporal reasoning. Time is an important variable, and reasoning about past, present and future may all be equally important. Reasoning about sequences of events is necessary as well. In contrast with most expert systems, which can only handle a "static environment" where the information to be processed is not time-varying, SIMPLEXYS expert systems can efficiently handle both static and dynamic environments.

Implementation of Knowledge

Expert systems frequently make a distinction between "long term knowledge", which is stored in eg. rules, and "short term knowledge", which consists of measurements, results of computations, answers to questions etc., stored in "working memory". Due to its real time nature, SIMPLEXYS refines this distinction. It has four types of knowledge:

- Case-independent fixed knowledge about the application. This knowledge is implemented as

  a. rules: among the rules are the goal rules; the conclusions to be derived;

  b. the script or protocol: the description of the dynamics of the case;

  c. procedures: actions to be performed, e.g. to acquire data or to display results;

  d. storage locations for data that must be collected, stored, computed, displayed.

- Case-dependent fixed knowledge, i.e. knowledge about the case which does not change during the case. This knowledge is implemented as

  a. fact rules: fixed facts about the current case, such as the patient's age category.

- Medium term knowledge, which is available once acquired, but may be updated. This knowledge is implemented as

a. state rules, which remember the context;

b. memo rules, which remember earlier results, such as complications that have arisen.

● Short term knowledge, which is to be re-acquired in each run (e.g. the data to be analyzed). This knowledge is implemented as

a. ask rules, which ask questions from the user;

b. test rules, which test data;

c. evaluation rules, which store higher level intermediate or final conclusions;

d. externally supplied data values, e.g. patient measurements.

The Logic of SIMPLEXYS

SIMPLEXYS implements a propositional logic comparable to boolean logic. Expressions consist of two types of entities, propositions and operators. Propositions are indicated by "names", such as tiger, heart_rate_normal, etc. Operators are indicated by the "special symbols" not, and, or, etc. Operators are monadic (one argument, eg. not p) or dyadic (two arguments, eg. p and q). Parentheses can be used to form sub-expressions.

Normally, formal logics are two-valued. In the type of three-valued logic that is implemented in SIMPLEXYS, a logical value can be either TR (true), FA (false) or PO (possible, maybe, unknown). Three-valued logic is a better approximation of human reasoning, because in many practical situations it will neither be possible to decide that a proposition is true nor that it is false, e.g. because some data may be unavailable. If p is any proposition, we can distinguish these three truth values:

p = TR: p has been proved to be true;

p = FA: p has been proved to be false;

p = PO: p can at this moment neither be proved to be true nor proved to be false; we lack the knowledge to decide that p is true and we lack the knowledge to decide that p is false; p is "possible", unknown.

Internally, invisible to the user (except when debugging), a fourth "truth value" exists:

p = UD: p is undefined, i.e. the value of p has not yet been evaluated; accessing a rule with value UD automatically leads to its evaluation, which returns TR, FA or PO, never UD.

Operators have their intuitive interpretation. They are evaluated through table look-up. An example is the definition of AND (see table on next page).

AND	TR	FA	PO
TR	TR	FA	PO
FA	FA	FA	FA
PO	PO	FA	PO

An Informal Introduction to the SIMPLEXYS Language

The following very incomplete informal exposure will try to develop some feeling for the way in which knowledge is implemented in SIMPLEXYS. The first example is taken from a small "animal farm" knowledge base and is very simple: acquire an item of knowledge by asking the user.

> BLACKSTRIPED: "the animal has black stripes"
> ASK
> THEN FA: BLACKSPOTTED

ES terminology is not quite standardized. For want of a better name, and in agreement with *Fagan, 1980*, the "knowledge chunk" combined in the above three lines is called a rule, although it resembles a frame as well.

The first line assigns a symbolic name to the rule, by which it can be referenced in other rules, and a text string that is used in formulating questions and providing explanations. In common ES parlance, BLACKSTRIPED itself is called a variable or parameter, because after evaluation it will obtain a logical value.

The second line states the rule's type, the method by which its value can be computed (in frame language: the if needed part); in this case it is an ASK rule, a rule that obtains its value by asking a question. ASK rules should, of course, not exist in a real time system, but they have shown to be indispensable during the system's design stages.

The third line states extra knowledge that becomes available as well, as soon as the answer is given. In this case we know that if an animal has black stripes, then it will not also have black spots. These so-called THELSEs (short for THENs and ELSEs; an ELSE applies if the rule evaluates to FA) generalize the notion of implication. They have two purposes. First, they improve knowledge base maintenance by grouping together all knowledge having to do with a concept. Second, they improve efficiency by allowing multiple conclusions from a single evaluation. In more common ES terminology, THELSEs would be called associated assertions or side effects; they are not merely "side effects", however: they have an exact logical interpretation.

> TIGER: "it is a tiger"
> MAMMAL AND CARNIVORE AND TAWNY AND BLACKSTRIPED

This evaluation rule can be read in two ways. First, semantically, as a definition: "a tiger is a blackstriped, tawny, carnivorous mammal". Second, syntactically, as a sequence of tests: "if it (an animal) passes the tests for MAMMAL, CARNIVORE, TAWNY and BLACKSTRIPED, then it will be considered a TIGER".If there is a discrepancy between these interpretations, the rule is in error or incomplete, i.e. the definition is either incorrect or implemented incorrectly.

The evaluation of the ANDs is conditional. If MAMMAL evaluates to false, TIGER will immediately return false; the remainder of the expression need not be evaluated.

The most approximate "standard rule format" of the above SIMPLEXYS rule would be:

> IF
>
>> MAMMAL AND CARNIVORE AND TAWNY AND BLACKSTRIPED
>
> THEN
>
>> TIGER

This rule format belongs to two-valued logic, however, where default values are false: it is "known" not to be a tiger unless it can be proved that it is one. The SIMPLEXYS logic is "richer"; the default value is PO, unknown, and inferencing tries to establish both that it is and that it is not a tiger (it is of course a contradiction, and detected as such, if it is and is not a tiger). This distinction has been characterized as "closed world" (as in Prolog) versus "open world" (as in SIMPLEXYS).

TEST rules provide an interface with the "external world", i.e. a "normal" computer language. The SIMPLEXYS language can be considered a super-set of Pascal, as is shown in this example:

> HRNORMAL: "the heart rate is normal"
> BTEST (HR > HRLO) and (HR < HRHI)

The keyword BTEST (Boolean TEST) indicates that the Pascal Boolean expression that follows it should assign a value of either TR or FA to the rule. Similarly, the keyword TEST allows the assignment of either TR, FA or PO.
This rule compares HR (a Pascal variable, presumably a measurement) with limits HRLO and HRHI. These limits may be Pascal constants or (context dependent) variables that are possibly (re-)defined by another rule. The Pascal code, that is interfaced with, may be arbitrarily complex.

Memo rules serve as an internal memory. Any rule can give a value to a memo rule. This value remains in effect until replaced.

> NORMAL: "the patient has no known problems"
> MEMO
> INITIALLY TR {true unless subsequently redefined}

DIABETES: "the patient has diabetes"
MEMO
THEN FA: NORMAL {if the patient has diabetes, he/she is
not a normal patient}

CHECK_DIABETES: "the records show a history of diabetes"
BTEST db_search (diabetes) {interface with a data base}
THEN TR: DIABETES {and, through chaining, FA: NORMAL}

An example of a rule using another rule's history is:

CAN_EXTUBATE: "extubation is allowed"
ASSIST > (15 * minutes) AND RESPIRATION_STABLE
THEN DO writeln ("consider extubation")

In this rule, "minutes" is a Pascal constant with value 60 (used for better readability; a rule's history is numerically stored as a number of seconds). This rule should be read as: "extubation must be considered if the patient's ventilation has been in ASSIST mode for more than 15 minutes and if his RESPIRATION is STABLE". The third line attaches an action to the rule, in this case to be executed when it is true.

Scripts or protocols are implemented using STATE rules and state transition statements; the internal representation of a script is a Petri net. The function of a STATE rule is to provide an anchor, a starting point, for the inferencing process, i.e. to define which conclusions should be derived, i.e. to define a (partial) context. If a STATE rule has the value TR, it is said to be part of the currently active context.

In the following example, STATE rules ASSIST and EXTUBE denote contexts. Associated with either STATE rule is, in this example, one goal rule. During consecutive analyses, this goal rule is to be evaluated, and that as long as its context is active, i.e. as long as the STATE rule that it is anchored to has value TR. In context ASSIST the goal is ASSIST_ANALYSIS, in context EXTUBE the goal is EXTUBE_ANALYSIS. Rule EXTUBATE is called a state transition rule; as soon as it evaluates to TR, context ASSIST is left (rule ASSIST obtains value FA) and context EXTUBE is entered (rule EXTUBE obtains value TR). Schematically:

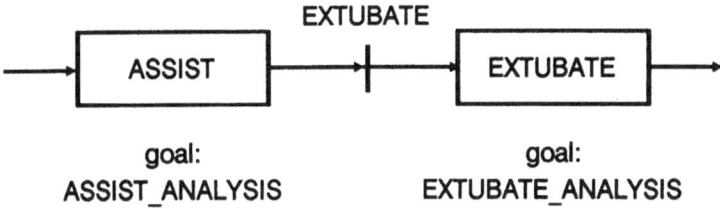

In this example, two STATE rules denote contexts:

>ASSIST: "ventilation is currently in assist mode"
>STATE
>THEN GOAL: ASSIST_ANALYSIS
>
>EXTUBE: "the patient is currently extubated"
>STATE
>THEN GOAL: EXTUBE_ANALYSIS

One state transition rule, a rule of any type, denotes the condition, that should lead to a state transition or context switch:

>EXTUBATE: "extubation is performed"
>TEST ... {detect extubation}

And one state transition statement describes which state transition rule controls the progress of the active context:

>ON EXTUBATE FROM ASSIST TO EXTUBE

Usually protocols are, of course, much more complex.

Semantic Networks: Speed and Safety

Quillian, 1967 developed the idea of the semantic network, consisting of nodes to represent concepts and associative links between those nodes to represent meaning in some way. His nodes were dictionary entries, and the "meaning" of such a node was the collection of nodes that could be reached through one or more links. In most practical cases, such a definition is unmanageable. The "first order meaning" is the collection of all concepts pointed to by links of length one; the equivalent, but more expanded "second order meaning" is the - usually much larger - collection of all concepts pointed to by links of length two; and so on in ever expanding circles. The ultimate "meaning" of a concept would probably include most dictionary entries. Such definitions are essentially circular.

Semantic networks became much more manageable, when "primitive" nodes were introduced: nodes which themselves are obvious in some sense and need not be defined in terms of other nodes. Primitives seem to be possible in "micro-worlds" only, such as *Winograd's, 1972* blocks world, where the blocks and the operations on them are primitives. This is not much of a limitation in expert systems, since necessarily expert systems can be concerned only with some small aspect of the real world, which itself is considered uncoupled from the rest of the world, and where all concepts that are frequently referenced can be primitives. The advantage is obvious: possibly with some effort, non-primitive nodes can now be expressed in (expanded to) primitives only; hence, if the (values of the) primitives are known, all nodes can be explicitly "evaluated".

Speed aspects

Currently, most rule based expert systems work interactively and allow rules to be added, deleted and edited. This necessitates dynamic storage of rules, in lists. In many applications, this type of interaction is unnecessary: the program "stands alone" and runs without supervision.

Another reason for inefficiency in current expert systems is the fact that most are glorified pattern matchers: they do little but searching. LISP is the core of many expert systems; in LISP, everything is stored in one huge complex list, so to find a particular entry, on average half the list has to be traversed (breaking the list up into a set of smaller lists is therefore a good way to increase performance - *Kary and Juell, 1986*). Surprisingly, many current expert systems use even worse searching strategies.

In many cases searching can be avoided completely. If the knowledge base (the rule set) is fixed, and if it is also known beforehand, which conclusions are to be derived (which rules must be evaluated), it is possible to use this knowledge to advantage. When all rules and all links between rules are known and available for analysis, they can be built into a semantic network, "compiled" and assigned known memory locations, such that when a rule is evaluated, no searching is necessary to locate a sub-rule (in "backward chaining") or a "next" rule (in "forward chaining"). Similarly, data can be stored in known memory locations.

Efficiency can be increased even more if we realize that the context in which the rules are evaluated, can usually be forced to be static. This is most easily seen in a forward chaining system, in which all data are gathered (e.g. on a form) before the expert system run is started. Since now the data are fixed, so are the possible conclusions about the data (the rule values after evaluation). It is not necessary for the form to be fully completed before the analysis starts; in fact, the analysis itself will indicate which items must be provided. Replacing (correcting) an item must be forbidden, however. Now it is only necessary to evaluate each rule once (once at most, in fact: only if its value is required), saving the rule's value for re-use whenever it is needed again. This realization resulted in a linear time inferencing algorithm and is the fundamental reason for the efficiency of SIMPLEXYS. Thus the usual "combinatorial explosion" of the number of evaluations is effectively prevented and very efficient expert systems can be built, even if they have a large number of rules. Compilation of the rules, and especially the checking of their consistency, takes more than linear time, of course, but at compile time waiting is much less a problem.

Evaluation/acquisition of a rule's value proceeds as follows:

- step 1: If the rule's value is TR, FA or PO, take that value and exit. Step 1 is all that is ever needed in the retrieval of FACT, MEMO and STATE rule values; in the case of ASK, TEST and evaluation rules, step 1 is all that is needed if the rule has been evaluated before in the same run.

- step 2: The rule's value is now UD, i.e. it has not been evaluated before. Ask a question if it is an ASK rule, perform a test on data if it is a TEST rule, or evaluate the rule's expression if it is an expression rule. The rule's value will now be either TR, FA or PO; if it is TR or FA, go to step 4.

- step 3: At this point, the rule's value is PO, but not all available knowledge may have been used yet. Try to get a TR or FA value by evaluating those rules that have as a consequence a THELSE TR or a THELSE FA to the current rule, until the current rule's value becomes TR or FA or until no more such rules exist.
- step 4: The rule has now been evaluated for the first time, and its value is TR, FA or PO; store this value.
- step 5: Execute the appropriate THELSEs of the rule, if any. THELSE TR/FA/POs will assign values to other rules, THELSE GOALs will evaluate other rules, and THELSE DOs will perform actions.
- step 6: Take the rule's value and exit.

Safety aspects

The development of expert systems is difficult and time consuming. This is due not only to the difficult nature of the task but also to the lack of sophisticated and refined knowledge engineering tools to assist in the acquisition, documentation and debugging of knowledge.

The acquisition of the domain knowledge, i.e. the process of extracting the knowledge from a human expert, is by far the most difficult part of building an expert system, because the human expert has no ready access to his own store of knowledge. Support in this area is most needed. One of the most wanted tools is generally considered to be a program to check the correctness of the knowledge as it is implemented in the expert system: a knowledge base checker/debugger. Not many of these tools are available, and when they are offered as part of a support facility their quality is not always adequate. In the process of verifying that a system is accurate and reliable, a major task is checking that the knowledge base is correct and complete (*Suwa et al, 1984*). Unfortunately, since no formal mathematical methods are available, knowledge base debugging usually involves testing and refining the system's knowledge. This is necessary because many errors can arise in the process of transferring expertise from a human expert to a computer system. Three types of errors exist: the knowledge base can contain errors because the expert's knowledge is incomplete or incompletely transferred; because the knowledge engineer's interpretation of the expert's knowledge is erroneous; or because of an erroneous implementation (transcription) of the knowledge into the support language's syntax and semantics.

The standard way of debugging the knowledge base is by observing the system's behavior in a great number of test cases. Although this is an essential part of testing the consistency and completeness of a knowledge base, it will never guarantee that the knowledge base is completely debugged. A better way to achieve reliability is to try to design a program that checks the knowledge base for completeness and consistency during the system's development. Some work in this field has been reported, such as TEIRESIAS (*Davis, 1976*), a program that provides aids for debugging an EMYCIN knowledge base. Besides that, step-wise development of the knowledge base is usually a good idea; catching errors is almost always easier in the early development stages.

No program can offer full-proof checking, because no program has a deep understanding of the domain knowledge. Some aspects of the knowledge base, however, can systematically and mechanically be checked: its logical completeness and consistency. Semantic networks are ideally suited for such checks, and SIMPLEXYS incorporates a number of them, such as tests for circular reasoning and conflicting implications.

Applications

Thus far, SIMPLEXYS has been employed in three projects. A first project, a feasibility study, was a paper re-implementation of VM (Ventilator Manager, *Fagan, 1980*), a well-documented real time expert system that monitors patients in an intensive care unit. This implementation of VM, which was originally written in LISP, was uneventful. The SIMPLEXYS implementation has 118 rules, of which 65 TEST rules, and a user interface to enter data from the keyboard and print results to the screen. Its MSDOS .exe file has a size of 55 kilobytes, and the worst case response time was estimated to be about 0.2 seconds on a 10 MHz 8088 system. The logical correctness of the knowledge base was verified and several simulations, but no tests with real patient data, were performed.

In a second project, a SIMPLEXYS program analyzes three automatically acquired signals from an anesthesia machine (respiratory pressure, respiratory flow, carbon dioxide concentration) to provide "smart alarms" about the functionality of the equipment. It provides diagnostics like "stuck inspiratory valve" and "leak in endotracheal tube". The system runs on an IBM PC AT and has a cycle time of 5 seconds, most of which is necessary to maintain a sophisticated graphics display.
This project intends to add an "intelligent" analysis software module to an anesthesia machine, possibly part of a future anesthesia work-station (*Beneken and Blom, 1983*).

In a third project, SIMPLEXYS is being used to implement a clinical control system to stabilize the mean arterial blood pressure at an artificially lowered value through an infusion of the drug sodium nitroprusside. This is a difficult control problem, which has kept many researchers, ourselves included, busy over many years without much progress. The problems are many: an often poor signal quality due to frequent artifacts in the blood pressure signal, a large "dead time" in, and a pronounced non-linearity of the response, reflexes that oppose the pressure decrease, and, in general, a huge variability of the patient's characteristics, both between patients and for the same patient at different times. Worst case simulations indicate that an expert system based controller may solve the problem (*den Brok, 1986; den Brok and Blom, 1987; Bierens, 1987*).
Thus far, automatic controllers can handle some 95% of all patients. That is not good, however, for those are also the patients that are easiest to manage manually, i.e. those whose infusion flow rate is allowed to remain constant over extended periods. It is the difficult 5% that needs to be tackled, the difficult-to-manage patients who now require far too much attention. But the controller is necessary for all patients, not for only 5% of the population, since initially it is not known whether an individual patient is a difficult case or not, or if he will become one later on.

Simulation run normal sensitivity

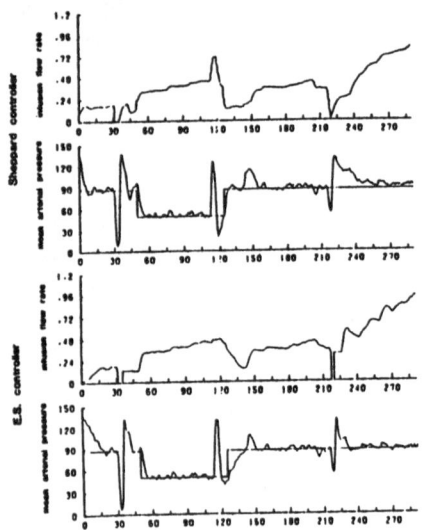

Fig 1.

Simulation run very high sensitivity

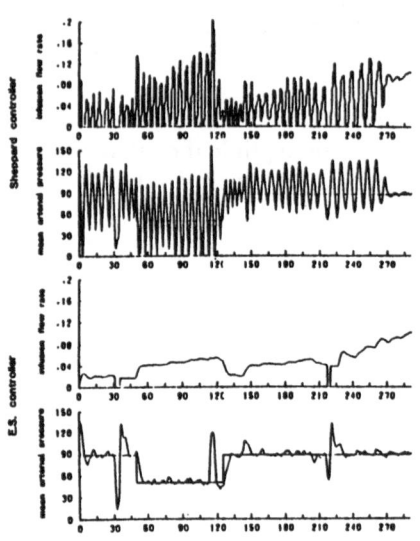

Fig 3.

Simulation run very low sensitivity

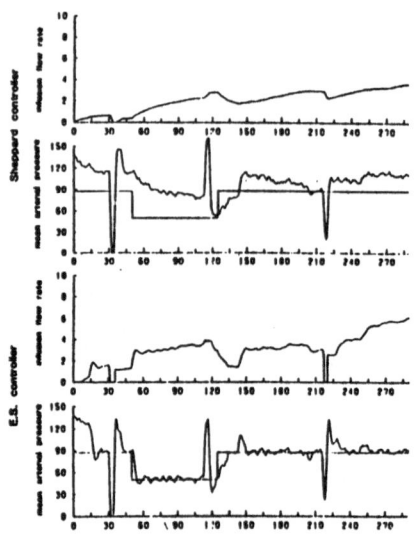

Fig 2.

Fig. 1.
A simulation run with a normal sensitivity "patient", comparing Sheppard's controller with the new Expert System controller. Times are in minutes. Setpoint changes occur after 50 and 125 minutes. Negative artifacts occur after 30 and 220 minutes. The ES controller has the knowledge that these are dangerous situations (shock?); it shuts off the infusion flow immediately and waits till the pressure returns to the setpoint. A positive artifact occurs after 110 minutes. The Expert System controller has the knowledge that this situation is not dangerous (incision?); it keeps the infusion flow rate constant for a while, waiting for a "spontaneous" return of the pressure. Note that in this "patient" more and more SNP is needed to keep the pressure near the setpoint.

Fig.2.
A simulation run with a "patient" having a sensitivity 9 times less than in figure 1; otherwise there are no differences. Note the change in scaling of the infusion flow rate. Sheppard's controller is far too slow. The ES controller initially needs some extra time to learn about the very low sensitivity.

Fig.3.
A simulation run with a "patient" having a sensitivity 9 times greater than in figure 1; otherwise there are no differences. Note again the change in scaling of the infusion flow rate. Sheppard's controller is unstable. Now the ES controller needs no time to learn the sensitivity, because initially it assumes the worst case: an extremely sensitive patient.

Thus far, we have only done simulations in order to compare the performance of our controller versus another (the one that *Sheppard, 1976* designed years ago, and that as far as we know is still in use in his surgical intensive care unit). The design of our expert system based controller was based on simulated "worst cases" that originate from animal studies (*Blom and de Bruijn, 1982*).

In a comparison of the two controllers for patients with a normal SNP sensitivity, the results are almost identical. If the patient has a very low SNP sensitivity, Sheppard's controller is too slow: for much too long, the blood pressure remains far from the value it should be at; this is an indication that manual control must take over. The performance of our controller is as good as before. If the patient's SNP sensitivity is very high, Sheppard's controller becomes unstable; thus manual control is required again. Our controller still works adequately.

The system has about 125 rules, runs on an IBM PC AT, and has a cycle time of 5 seconds, most of which is necessary to scroll the displayed trend graphs of SNP and pressure.

Another advantage op the expert systems approach was demonstrated in this clinical control system: it was easy to combine knowledge on signal analysis, control theory, pharmacology, anesthesiology and surgery, as well as general medical knowledge.

Conclusions

SIMPLEXYS was designed for real time applications, where fast performance is of primary concern. The fact that each rule is evaluated once at most, guarantees a linear time algorithm and a worst case response time, which can be estimated rather well: evaluate, for each active context, all its goal rules, and return the maximum time required; or, faster but more roughly: return the time required to evaluate all goal rules, irrespective of context.

Execution speed of the current version has been estimated as about 1000 rule evaluations per second when running on a standard IBM PC. Currently operational small prototype expert systems show that standard data processing and input/output operations (data acquisition, extraction of the necessary features from the signals, scrolling of graphics displays) need much more time than the inferencing process.

SIMPLEXYS was also designed to be safe. The currently implemented consistency checks must be considered a first attempt to ensure the logical consistency of a knowledge base as much as possible. SIMPLEXYS allows better consistency checking than most other expert system languages, most of all because the relations between rules are explicitly expressed.

References

Beneken JEW, Blom JA. An integrative patient monitoring approach. In: An integrated approach to monitoring, eds. Gravenstein JS, Newbower RS, Ream AK, Smith NT, p 121-131. Butterworths, 1983.

Bierens EJJ. Preliminary study for an expert system based blood pressure controller (in Dutch). Master's Thesis, Eindhoven University of Technology, 1987.

Blom JA, Bruijn NP de. Peroperative estimation of sodium nitroprusside sensitivity. Proc. IEEE Southeastcon, 564-566. Sandestin, Florida, 1982.

Blom JA. SIMPLEXYS, a real time expert systems tool. Proc. IASTED Intl. Conf. on Expert Systems Theory and Applications, p 21-25, Geneva, 1987.

Brok NWNM den. A rule based adaptive blood pressure controller (in Dutch). Master's Thesis, Eindhoven University of Technology, 1986.

Brok NWNM den, Blom JA. A rule based adaptive blood pressure controller. Proc. 2nd European workshop on fault diagnostics, reliability and related knowledge-based approaches, Manchester, 1987.

Davis R. Applications of meta level knowledge to the construction, maintenance and use of large knowledge bases. Report STAN-CS-76-552, Stanford AI Laboratory, Stanford University, Stanford, Calif., July 1976.

Fagan LM. VM: Representing time-dependent relations in a medical setting. Dissertation, Dept. of Computer Science, Stanford University, Stanford, Calif, June 1980.

Hajek J. A knowledge engineering logic for smarter, safer and faster (expert) systems. Eindhoven University of Technology (EUT) Computing Center Note 41, 1988.

Kary, D.D., Juell, P.L. TRC, an expert system compiler. SIGPLAN Notices, vol 21, no 5, May 1986.

Laffey TA, Cox PA, Schmidt JL, Kao SM, Read JY. Real-Time Knowledge-Based Systems. AI Magazine, 27-45, Spring 1988.

Marsh J, Greenwood J. Guide to defense and aerospace systems. Pasha Publ., Arlington, Va. 1986.

O'Reilly CA, Cromarty AS. "Fast" is not "Real-Time" in designing effective real-time AI systems. Appl. of Artif. Intell. II, 548 249-257. Intern. Soc. of Optical Engng, Bellingham, Wash. 1985.

Quillian MR. Word concepts: a theory and simulation of some basic semantic capabilities. Behavioral Science 12, 410-430, 1967.

Sheppard LC. Correlation analysis of blood pressure responses to vasoactive drugs, with particular reference to clinical surveillance of the post-surgical cardiac patient. Ph.D. Thesis, University of London, 1976.

Suwa M, Scott C, Shortliffe EH. Completeness and consistency in a rule-based system. In: Rule-based expert systems; eds. Buchanan BG and Shortliffe EH. Addison-Wesley, 1984.

Winograd T. Understanding natural language. Academic Press, 1972.

Questions from the Discussion

Fox: Your controller of the mean arterial pressure worked remarkably well. Can you explain why it works so well and where it deviates from the better known controllers based on standard control theory concepts?

Blom: Some of the knowledge that we collected about the properties of the drug's effect (significant dead time, non-linearity, upward drift and especially a large and unpredictable variability in time of the patient's sensitivity) indicated that this would be a difficult control problem, if we wanted a full-proof solution. First we tried out other approaches, such as several adaptive control strategies, but in the clinic the signal quality frequently was too bad to obtain a reliable estimate of the patient's sensitivity. So in this case none of the well known control methods was appropriate, nor some more obscure ones that we tried.

But doctors do it all the time. They heuristically "adapt" their control actions to what they learn from the patient's reactions, but only very globally, and only if its necessity is obvious; no "fine tuning" here. That is quite acceptable: there is no well defined optimality criterium. So basically we took a very simple but robust controller, and adapt it approximately the way a doctor would his strategy. That proved to work. Besides that, more heuristics were added to handle abnormal conditions. No well known control method is well suited to exception handling, either. This application just seems too complex for standard solution methods.

EVALUATION

EVALUATION

The Evaluation of Medical Decision Support and Expert Systems: Reflections on the Literature

Rory O'Moore[1] and Rolf Engelbrecht[2]

1 St. James's Hospital, Dublin 8, Ireland.

2 The G.F.S. Medis Institute, Munich, B.R.D.

Introduction

Over the past ten years there has been an increasing number of publications on the evaluation of medical expert systems parallel to the increase in theoretical papers on the evaluation methodology itself. A brief perusal of the most relevant European conference proceedings over the past two years is shown in Table 1. (*Fox et al 1987, Serio et al 1987, Hansen et al 1988* and *Rienhoff et al 1988*).

	AIME 87	MIE87	MIE88 & Peter Reichertz Memorial Conference 1988
Number of Contributions	26	19	29
On Diagnosis	16	12	19
On Treatment or management	5	5	7
Independent clinical evaluation	2	2	1

Table I.: Papers on Medical Expert Systems presented at recent European Conferences.

These figures are similar to those reported by *Potthof et al, 1988,* and *Engelbrecht et al, 1987,* which included North American data. The small number of systems (c.a. 6%) subjected to independent evaluations is small considering the large amounts of research time and money currently being spent in this field. Furthermore, less than 40% of the systems described had even a rudimentary 'in house' evaluation. Several well controlled evaluations are known to be in progress and many of the initiatives have been purely research orientated and therefore not appropriate for formal evaluation. Other systems may not yet have reached the stage where evaluation is warranted. Nevertheless the apparent reluctance to test a system's potential may be contributing to some scepticism on the future role of decision support systems (*Teach & Shortliffe 1981, Gremy 1988, Van Bemmel 1988a,b* and *Shortliffe 1989*).

Problem of Acceptance

Shortliffe, 1989 recently reemphasised that physician fears play an important role in the problem of acceptance. Firstly the fear that the use of computers will lead to a loss of rapport with their patients. The second fear is loss of control. They believe the computer could take over, eliminating the challenge of independent problem solving which is so important to the practice of medicine. Some already perceive this to be under threat from governmental controls, (*Melhorn 1979*) medical audit and malpractice litigation. Shortliffe considers this is the major block. Decision support systems are not seen just as tools but as 'dogmatic agents removing all management prerogatives from physicians. There are also fears that their professional status would be reduced, they would become subservient to the computer programmer or even worse to Hospital Administrators.

Another fear is of legal liability. This has undoubtedly constrained the commercial development of such systems and may well be a major deterrent to progress (*Brannigan 1987, Young 1987, Kilian 1988, Campbell 1984*). However as *Norris and Szabo, 1982*, and *Cannataci, 1988*, point out physicians could be liable for patient injuries caused by the absence of a medical computer while on the other hand liability for injuries caused by defective medical computer programs could also be considerable.

Suspicion of Artificial Intelligence is also widespread. The need to augment decision support systems with ad hoc human expertise is seen as a major weakness. *Shortliffe, 1989*, believes there is a need to convince physicians that 'a computer based decision support tool can provide enhanced access to a form of knowledge (on which they already act without realizing it) particularly when its performance is coupled with emphasis on the users ability to make the ultimate decisions by either accepting or rejecting the advice given. Thus it should provide "just another test" or as *Gremy, 1988*, hopes "the democratization of knowledge".

Evaluations of Decision Support/expert Systems

It seems to us that the most likely way to overcome the negative feelings of fears is to involve more clinicians in the development and realistic evaluations of decision support/expert systems. As *Wyatt, 1987*, states "Doctors notorious for their distrust of computers will need convincing that such systems can offer anything other than an assault on their integrity and clinical freedom".

It is not our intention to describe in detail the many different methodologies which have been proposed and sometimes even tried. They have been classified and listed alphabetically in the reference section under the three broad headings.

- EVALUATIONS.
- THEORETICAL PAPERS ON EVALUATIONS.
- VALIDATION OF THE KNOWLEDGE BASE.

The crucial items on the evaluation process have been summarised by Clancey and Shortliffe (194). They believe that several points should be satisfactorily demonstrated:

- The NEED for the system.
- Expert level performance.
- System usability (Human interface).
- Impact on patient management.
- Acceptance by physicians.
- Impact on patient well-being.
- Cost effectiveness of the system.

In spite of the very different methodologies proposed, a consensus emerges on certain key points. For example most authors are agreed that the appropriate type of evaluation depends on (*Kulikowski 1988*):

- The stages of implementation.
- The domain of application.
- The clinical objectives of the system.
- How the system is to be used.

A majority of authors also agree that an evaluation should most appropriately be divided into two phases (e.g. *Miller 1985*). Firstly, the validation of the systems knowledge and advice (the Reliability) and secondly the evaluation of the clinical efficiency of the system (the Functionality) which includes measurement of the total impact of the system on health care delivery. However, *Shwe et al, 1989*, define validation of expert systems as "the process of proving or showing to a satisfactory degree that the behaviour of an expert system is correct with respect to the specifications made of the system". They define evaluation "as a formal study in which the performance of the system is compared to the performance of experts not involved in the development of expert systems knowledge base". These are obviously much narrower definitions that those of *Miller, 1985*, and most others. Many other similarly large discrepancies in definitions are also apparent. There is probably a need for a working group to formalize a nomenclature for evaluation methodology particularly in the context of multilingual Europe.

Factors Influencing the Success of a System

The second point which emerges from many of the reports was that perhaps the most important single factor in the success of a system is to establish the need. This by its very nature should lead to the involvement of physicians, nurses, primary care doctors in the ongoing development of the systems. The point stressed in many of the papers was that the development of a decision support/expert system should be iterative with continuous cycles of development and evaluation taking place. Thus the evaluations should commence at the very beginning of a project. In this way strong interdisciplinary links would be established between the computer scientists, medical informaticians and physicians involved in the development of the systems. Few of the systems described have been built in this manner.

The final important factor to emerge was the choice of domain. *Blois, 1980,* pointed out that computer based medical decision aids were inherently limited in their ability to assist clinicians in reaching decisions about undifferentiated patients. That is those patients for whom an initial high level general classification had not already been made. To be useful the domain should be narrowed by the clinical acumen of the physician. A good example of this is the process which the thoughtful physician utilizes before requesting radiological or laboratory investigations. It is therefore not surprising that the majority of decision support systems currently in use contain a large element of laboratory data (*McDonald 1984, Pryor 1983, Kendall 1984, Richardson 1984, Tierney 1987, 1988*). There are many reasons for their relative success:

- The fulfill a practical and perceived need to help control the increasing spiral of laboratory usage and cost (*O'Moore 1988a,b* and *Spackman and Connolly 1987*).
- They have been shown to help alleviate one of the major problems of modern medicine that of information overload (*O'Moore 1988a,b*).
- They fit well into the clinical process with an accepting target group of users (e.g. Junior Hospital Doctors, General Practitioners) (*Lavril et al 1988, Botti 1987*).
- The laboratory staff save time (*Kendall 1984, Aitkins 1983*).
- The experts (laboratory consultants) do not feel threatened by the system as it increases their productivity and,as each report is read and signed by them, possible legal problems are avoided. This process also provides an iterative evaluation/modification cycle. (*Aitkins 1983, Kendall 1984*).
- The laboratory data is less 'fuzzy' than purely clinical data. A further advantage of such relatively simple decision support systems is that it is possible to evaluate the impact on patient care by decision analysis and cost benefit analysis (Beck 1986) or even more simply by observing the improvement of the variables measured following the introduction of the system (*Richardson 1984, Pryor et al 1984, McDonald et al 1984*).

A more complex extension of such systems is in the area of patient monitoring of both long-term illness and acute illness in intensive care. This area which depends largely on laboratory data forms one of the best test beds for the realistic evaluation of decision support systems in medicine. There are numerous tasks for multi-disciplinary teams to undertake. For example the optimum combinations of clinical and laboratory data required to manage patients in different situations have yet to be determined. The use of such data for temporal reasoning is in its infancy and offers exciting prospects (*Tusch 1989*). There are also realistic prospects of embedding decision support systems within existing patient management data bases (*Lavril 1988, Nolan et al 1989*).

Summary

In summary we strongly support the suggestion (*Gashnig 1984, Lundsgaard 1987, Wyatt 1987*) that an increase in well planned and carried out evaluation studies will be major factors for both the present and future progress of knowledge based systems. They form a key route by which clinical credibility for decision support systems may be achieved.

References

Books

I *Barber. B., Cao Dexian, Quin Dulie, Wagner, G.* (Eds) MEDINFO 89'. North Holland (1989).

II *Fox, J., Fieschi, M., Engelbrecht, R.* (Eds) AIME 87'. Lecture Notes in Medical Informatics, 33 (1987). Springer Verlag.

III*Hansen, R., Solheim, B., O'Moore, R.R., Roger, F.H.* (Eds) MIE '88. Lecture Notes in Medical Informatics 35, Springer Verlag pp 1-764 (1988).

IV*Rienhoff, O., Piccolo, U., Schneider, B.* (Eds) Expert Systems and decision support in medicine. The Peter Reichertz Memorial Conference. Lecture Notes in Medical Informatics, 36, pp 1-591 (1988). Springer Verlag.

V *Serio, A., O'Moore, R.R., Tardini, A., Roger, F.* (Eds) Proceedings MIE 87'. Vol I-III, EDI Press Rome, pp 1-1644 (1987).

General

Arborelius, E., Timpka, T. Study of the Practitioner's knowledge need and use during Health Care consultations. Part 2: The Dilemma Spectrum of the GP. In I. 101-105 (1989).

Beck, J.R. Laboratory Decision Science applied to Chemometrics: Strategic testing for thyroid function. Clin. Chem. 32, 1707-1713 (1986).

Brannigan, V. The regulation of medical computer software as a 'device' under the food, drug and cosmetic act. Computer Meth. Prog. in Biomed. 25, 219-229 (1987).

Campbell, J.A. The expert computer and professional negligence: Who is liable? Ed. Yazdani, M., Narayanan, A. In Artificial Intelligence: Human Effects. Pub. Ellis, Horwood, Chichester U.K. (1984).

Cannataci, J.A. Liability and responsibility for expert systems. Complex No. 588. Norwegian Research Centre for Computers and Law. Univ. Oslo 2, Norway (1988).

Gremy, F. Persons and computers in medicine and health. Meth. Inform. Med. 27, 3-9 (1988).

Kilian, W. Liability for deficient medical expert systems-keynote address. Expert systems and decision support in Medicine. 33rd Annual Meeting of G.M.D.S. Hannover (1988) (Available G.M.D.S.).

Melhorn, J.M. Current attitudes of medical personnel towards computers. Comp. Biomed. Res 12, 327-334 (1979).

Nolan, J., Brosnan, P., Murnane, L., Boran, G., Breslin, A., Grimson, J., Cullen, M., O'Moore, R.R. A PC based decision support/patient management system for thyroid disease. In AIME 89' Lecture Notes in Medical Informatics. 38, Ed. Hunter, J. Cookson, J., Wyatt, J. 189-198 (1989).

O'Moore, R.R. The effectiveness of decision support systems in clinical chemistry. In Progress in Biological Function Analysis. Ed. Van Bemmel, J., Michel, J. & Willems, J. 269-276 (1988a). North Holland.

O'Moore, R.R. Decision support based on laboratory data. Meth. Inform. Med. 27, 187-190 (1988b).

Spackman, K.A. & Connolly, D.P. Knowledge based systems in laboratory medicine and pathology. Archiv. Pathol. Lab. Med. 111, 116-119 (1987).

Teach, R.L., Shortliffe, E.H. An analysis of physician attitudes regarding computer based clinical consultation systems. Comp Biomed Res 14, 542-558 (1981).

Tusch, G., Bernauer, J., Gubennatis, G., Rading, M. Knowledge acquisition using syntactic time patterns. In AIME 89' Lecture Notes in Medical Informatics, 38. Ed. Hunter J., Cookson, J., Wyatt, J. 315-324, (1989) Springer Verlag.

Van Bemmel, J. Systems evaluation for the health of all. In III. 27-34 (1988a).

Van Bemmel, J.H. Decision support in Medicine: Comparative methodology and impact on the medical curriculum. In IV 3-19 (1988b).

Young, F.E. Validation of medical software: Present policy of the food and drug administration. Annals of Internal Medicine 106, 663-667 (1987).

Evaluations

Adams, I.D., Chan, M., Clifford, P.C., Cooke, W.M., Dallos, V., De Dombal F.T., Edwards, M.H., Hancock, D.M., Hewett, D.J., McIntyre, N.M., Somerville, P.G., Spiegelhalter, D.J., Wellwood, J., Wilson, D.H. Computer aided diagnosis of acute abdominal pain: A multi centre study B.M.J. 293, 800-804 (1986).

Adlassnig, K.P., Koarz, G., Scheithauer, W. Present state of medical expert system - CADIAG.2 Meth. Inform Med 24, 13-20 (1985).

Adlassnig, K.P. The application of ROC curves to the evaluation of medical experts systems. In V, 951-957 (1987).

Aitkins, J.S., Kunz, J.C., Shortliffe, E.H., Fallat, R.J. PUFF: An expert system for interpretation of pulmonary function data: Comp. Biomed. Res. 16, 199-208 (1983).

Akhavan-Hedari, M., Adlassnig, K.P. Preliminary results on Cadiag-2/Gall: A diagnostic consultation system for Gall Bladder and biliary tract disease. In III, 662-666 (1988).

Barnett, G.O., Cimino, J.J., Hupp, J.A., Hoffer, E.P. DXPLAIN - An evolving diagnostic decision support system. JAMA 258, 67-74 (1987).

Berner, E.S., Brooks, C.M. Needs assessment for computer based medical decision support systems in Proceedings XII SCAMC Washington IEEE p 232-236.

Botti, G., Michel, C., Proudhon, D., Fieschi, D., Joubert, M., Fieschi, M. Feasibility study of the expert system Sphinx - In V, 957-966 (1987).

Botti, G., Joubert, M., Fieschi, D., Proundhon, H., Fieschi, M. Experimental use of the medical expert system SPHINX by General Practitioners: Results and analysis. In I, 67-71 (1989).

Bowen, T., Payling, L. Expert systems for performance review. J. Opl. Res. Soc. 38, 929-934 (1987).

De Bliek, R., Friedman, C.P., Blaschke, T.F., France, C.L., Speedie, S.M. Practitioner preferences and receptivity for patient specific advice from a therapeutic monitoring system. In proceedings of XII SCAMC Meeting, Washington, IEEE p 225-228 (1988).

Diamond, G.A., Staniloff, H., Forrester, J. Computer assisted diagnosis in the non invasive evaluation of patients with suspected coronary heart disease. J. Am. Coll. Cardiol. 1, 444-455 (1983).

Engelbrecht, R., Potthof, P., Schwefel, D. Expert systems in medicine: Results from a technology assessment study. In DIAC-87 Directions and Implications - Computer professionals for social responsibility, 125-133 (1987).

Engelbrecht, R., Schaaf, R., Lewis, M. Assistance in medical treatment and treatment analysis with an interactive drug consultation system. In I, 253-256 (1989).

Fox, J., Myers, C.D., Greaves, M.F., Pegram, S. Knowledge acquisition for expert systems: Experience in Leukaemia diagnosis. Meth Inform Med 24, 65-72 (1985).

Gorry, G.A., Sliverman, H., Pauker, S.G. Capturing clinical expertise - a computer program that considers clincial response to digitalis. Am. J. Med. 64, 452-460 (1978).

Habbema, J.D., Hilden, J., Bjerregaard, B. The measurement of performance in probabilistic, diagnosis V general recommendations, IV. Utility considerations. Meth. Inform. Med. 20, 80-96 and 97-100 (1981).

Hammersley, J.R., Cooney, K. Evaluating the utility of available differential diagnosis systems in Proceedings XII SCAMC meeting (1988), Washington, D.C. IEEE, p 220-224.

Hickham, D.H., Shortliffe, E.H., Bischoff, M.B., Scott, A.C., Jacobs, C.D. The treatment advice of a computer based cancer chemotherapy Protocol Advisor - Ann. Int. Med. 103, 928 -936 (1985).

Kendall, R.I., Ulinski, D.E., Richardson, L.D., Bradley, C.A., Parl, F.F. Computer assisted interpretive reporting with trend analysis of creatinine kinase and lactate dehydrogenase isoenzymes. Am. J. Clin. Path. 79, 217-222 (1984).

Kingsland, L.C. Evaluation of medical expert systems: Experience with the AI/RHEUM knowledge based consultant system in Rheumatology. In selected topics in medical artificial intelligence. Ed. P.L. Miller pp 212-221. Springer Verlag (1988).

Kingsland, L., Sharp, G., Capps, J., Benge, D., Kay, D., Reese, P. Hazelwood, S., Lindberg, D. Testing of a criteria based consultant system in Rheumatology. In MEDINFO 86 Ed. Van Bemmel J., Ball, M.J., Wigertz, O. 514-157 (1986). North Holland.

Lavril, M., Chatellier, G., Degoulet, P., Jeunemaitre, X., Menard, J., Rovani, C. ARTEL: An expert system in hypertension for the general practitioner. In IV, p 314-321 (1988).

Lemonnier, P., Adlassnig, K.P., Horak, W., Hay, U. Hepatitis serology findings. In III, 636-670 (1988).

Michel, C., Botti, Fieschi, M., Joubert, M., SanMarco, J., Casanova, P. Validation of a knowledge base intended for general practitioners to assist in treatment of diabetes. In Medinfo 86 Ed Salamon, R. Blum, B., Jorgensen, M. North Holland 122-127 (1986).

Miller, R.A., Pople, H.E., Myers, J.D., INTERNIST-I. An experimental computer based diagnostic consultant for general internal medicine. New Eng. J. Med. 307, 468-476 (1982).

Myers, J.D. The computer as a diagnostic consultant, with emphasis on laboratory data. Clin. Chem. 32, 1714-1718 (1986).

McDonald, C.J., Hui, S.L., Smith, D.M., Tierney, W.M., Cohen, S.J., Weinberger, M., McCabe G.P. Reminders to physicians from an introspective computer medical record: A two year randomized trial Ann Int. Med, 100, 130-138 (1984).

Nakache, J.P., Gueguen, A., Dougados, M., Nguyen, M. Evaluation and Validation of a Functional Index in Ankylosing Spondylitis. In II, 229-238 (1987).

Nelson, S.J., Blois, M.S. et al. Evaluating reconsider - a computer program for diagnostic prompting J. Med. Systems 9, 379-389 (1985).

Potthof, P., Schwefel, D., Rothemund, M., Engelbrecht, R., van Eimeren, W., Expert Systems in Medicine. Int. J. Technology Assessment, 4, 121-133 (1988).

Pryor, T.A., Gardner, R.M., Clayton, P.D., Warner, H.R. The HELP system. J. Med. Sys. 7, 87 -102 (1983).

Quaglini, S., Stefanelli, M., Barosi, G., Berzuini, A. Evaluating the performance of anaemia. In II,229-238 (1987).

Reggia, J.A. Evaluation of medical expert systems: Case study in performance assessment in proceedings IX SCAMC Baltimore IEEE 287-291 (1985).

Richardson, T. The effect of computer generated comments on the distribution of anticonvulsant concentrations. Ann. Clin. Biochem. 21, 184-187 (1984).

Rovani, C., Jeunmaitre, X., Degoulet, P., Sauquet, D., Aime, F., Lavril, M., Devries, C., Chatellier, G., Plovin, P.F., Corvol, P. Worst situation evaluation of an expert system in hypertension management. In V, 967-973 (1987).

Schewe, S., Scherrman, W., Gierl, L. Evaluation and measurement of benefit of an expert system for differential diagnosis in Rheumatology. In IV,36, 351-354. (1988).

Schneider, J., Renner, R., Engelbrecht, R., Piwernetz K. DIAMON: First Evaluation Results. In I, 222-225 (1989).

Shamsolmaali, A., Collinson, P., Gray, T.G., Carson, E.R., Cramp, D.G. Implementation and evaluation of a knowledge based system for the interpretation of laboratory data. In AIME 89' Lecture notes in Medical Informatics. Ed. Hunter, J., Cookson, J., Wyatt, J. 38, 167-176 (1989).

Soula, G., Thirion, X., San Marco, J.L., Vialettes, B., Guliana, J., Navez, I. A multi-centred validation of the fuzzy expert system Protis. In III, 647-651 (1988).

Spitzer, R.L. & Endicott, J. DIAGNO II: Further development of a computer program for psychiatric diagnosis. Am. J. Psychiat. 125, 12-21 (1969).

Tierney, W.M., McDonald, C.J., Hui, S.L., Martin, D.K. Computer prediction of abnormal test results. JAMA 259, 1194-1198 (1988).

Tusch, G., Bernauer, J., Gubernatis, G., Rading, M. A Knowledge-Based Decision Support Tool for Liver Transplanted Patients. In I, 131-135 (1989).

Weiss, S.M., Kulikowski, C.A., Galen, R.S. Representing expertise in a computer program: The serum protein diagnosis program. J. Clin. Lab. Auto 3, 383-387 (1983).

Wyatt, J. The evaluation of clinical decision support systems: a discussion of the methodology used in the Acorn project. In II, 229-238 (1987).

Wyatt, J. Lessons Learnt from the Field Trial of ACORN, an Expert System to Advise on Chest Pain. In I, 111-115 (1989).

Yu, V.L., Fagan, L.M., Wraith, S.M., Clancey, W.M., Scott, A.C., Hannigan, J., Blum, R.L., Buchanan, B.G., Cohen, S.N. Antimicrobial selection by computer a blinded evaluation by infectious disease experts. JAMA 242, 1279-1282 (1979).

Yu, V.L. Evaluating the performance of a computer based consultant. Comp. Prog. Biomed., 9, 95-102, (1979).

Theoretical papers on evaluations

Bonnet, A., Haton, J.P., Truong-Ngoc, J.M., Howlett, J. Validation of expert systems. In expert systems principles and practice pp 168-183, Prentice-Hall (1988).

Brender, J., McNair, P. Watch the system. An opinion on user validation of computer based decision support systems in Clinical Medicine. In I, 275-279 (1989).

Cohen & Howe. How evaluation guides AI research. A.I. Magazine Winter: 35-43 (1988).

De Dombal, F.T. Towards a more objective evaluation of computer aided decision support systems - in MEDINFO 83'. Ed Van Bemmel, J., Ball, M.J., Wigertz, O. 436-439 (1983).

Fieschi, M., Joubert, M. Some reflections of the evaluation of Expert Systems in Medicine. Meth. Inform. Med. 25, 15-21 (1986).

Gashnig, J., Klahr, P., Pople, H., Shortliffe, E., Terry, A. Evaluation of expert systems. In Building expert systems. Ed. Hayes Roth et al. Pub. Addison Wesley pp 241-280 (1983).

Gjorup, T. The KAPPA coefficient and the prevalence of a diagnosis. Meth. Inform. Med. 27, 184-196 (1988).

Gottinger, H.W. Technology assessment and forecasting of medical expert systems (MEST) Meth Inf. Med. 27, 56-66 (1988).

Grant, A., Parker Jones, C., White, R., Cramp, D., Barreiro, A., Mira, P., Artal, A., Montero, J. Evaluation of knowledge based systems from the user perspective. This volume, 312-324 (1991).

Kulikowski, C. Medical expert systems: Issues of validation, evaluation and judgement in policy issues. In Information and communication technologies in medical applications IEEE, 45-56 (1988).

Liebowitz, J. Useful approach for evaluating expert systems. Expert systems 3, 86-96 (1986).

Lundsgaarde, H.P. Evaluation medical expert systems Social Sc. Med. 24, 805-819 (1987).

Miller, P.L. Evaluation of artificial intelligence systems in medicine. Proceedings IX SCAMC, Washington, D.C. IEEE 281-286 (1985).

Miller, P.L. Evaluation of artificial intelligence systems in medicine. Comp. Prog. Method Biomed, 22, 5-11 (1986).

Miller, P.L. Goal directed critiquing by computer: Ventilation measurement. Comp. Biomed. Res. 18, 422-3 (1985).

Miller, P.L. Expert critiquing systems. Practice based medical consultation by computer (1986). Springer Verlag.

Nykanen, P. (Ed.). Issues in evaluation of computer-based support to clinical decision making - Sydpol Working Group 5. The Norwegian Computing Centre, Oslo.

O'Keefe, R.M. Balci, O., Smith, E.P. Validating expert systems performance. IEEE Expert Winter 81-89 (1987).

Pryor, D.B., Barnett, O., Gardner, R.M., McDonald, C., Stead, W.W. Measuring the value of information systems in proceedings VIII SCAMC 1984, IEEE 26-28 (1984).

Rossi-Mori, A., Ricci, F.L. On the assessment of medical expert systems. In expert systems and decision support in medicine. In IV 292-297 (1988).

Rossi-Mori, A., Pisanelli, D.M., Ricci, F.L. The Role of Knowledge Based Systems in Medicine, Epistemological and Evaluation issues. This Volume, 291-303 (1991).

Rothschild, M.A., Miller, P.L., Fisher, P.R., Weltin, G.G., Sweet, H.A. Confronting subjective criteria in the evaluation of computer based critiquing advice. In proceedings XII SCAMC, Washington, IEEE, 220-224 (1988).

Shortliffe, E.H., Clancey, W.J. Anticipating the second decade. In readings in medical artificial intelligence. Eds. Clancey, W.J. & Shortliffe, E.H. p 469 (1984). Addison Wesley.

Shortliffe, E.H. Testing reality - the introduction of decision support technologies for physicians. Meth. Inform. Med 28, 1-5(1989).

Sørgaard, P. Evaluating expert systems prototypes. In 9th Scandinavian Seminar on development of expert systems, Bastad (1986).

Spiegelhalter, D. Evaluation of clinical decision aids, with an application to a system for dyspepsia. Statistics in Med., 207-216 (1983).

Whitebeck, C., Brook, R. Criteria for evaluating a computer aid to clinical reasoning. J. Med. Philos. 8, 51-65 (1983).

Wyatt, J., Spiegelhalter, D. Evaluating medical decision aids: What to test, and how. This volume 274-290 (1991).

Validation of knowledge base

Bahill, A.T., Jafer, M., Moller, R.F. Tools for extracting knowledge and validating expert systems. IEE 857-862 (1987).

Barachini, F., Adlassnig, K.P. CONSED: Medical knowledge base consistency checking - In V, 974-980 (1987).

Butler, K.A. Application of correlation measures for validating structured selectors. In proceedings of III conference on A.I. applications. Washington IEEE 327-330 (1987).

Fontaine, D., Le Beux, P., Strauss, A., Morizet, P. An approach for maintaining the coherence in a medical knowledge base. In I, 44-48 (1989).

Gissi, P. Logical checks in a rule based medical decision support system. In V, 981-985 (1987).

Green, C.J., Keyes, M.M. Verification and validation of expert systems. In Proceedings Western Conference on expert systems Anaheim. IEEE Computer Society 38-43 (1987).

Indurkhya N., Weiss, S.M. Models for measuring performance of medical expert systems. Artificial Intel. Med. 1, 61-70 (1989).

Mars, N.J., Miller, P.L. Knowledge acquisition and verification tools for medical expert systems. Medical Decision Making 7: 6-11 (1987).

Shwe, M.A., Tu, S.W., Fagan, L.M. Validating the knowledge base on a therapy planning system. Meth. Inform. Med., 28, 36-50 (1989).

Wigertz, O.B., Clayton, P.D., Huag, P.J., Pryor, T.A. Design of knowledge based systems for multiple use truth maintenance and knowledge transfer. In V, 987-991 (1987).

Evaluating Medical Expert Systems: What To Test, And How ?

Jeremy Wyatt[1] and David Spiegelhalter[2]

1 The National Heart & Lung Institute, London and IBM Scientific Centre, United Kingdom

2 MRC Biostatistics Unit, Cambridge United Kingdom

Abstract

Few medical expert systems have been rigorously evaluated, yet some believe that these systems have great potential to improve health care. For this and many other reasons, objective evaluation is necessary. We discuss the evaluation of medical expert systems in two stages: laboratory and field testing. In the former, the perspectives of both prospective users and experts are valuable. In the latter, the study must be designed to answer, in an unbiased manner, the questions: "Will the system be used in practice ?" and "When it is used, how does it affect the structure, process and outcome of health care ?". We conclude with some proposals for encouraging the objective evaluation of medical expert systems.

Introduction

"At present, informatics research is both helped and hampered by problems of evaluation design ... it is especially important that evaluation guidelines be developed for the validation of medical knowledge-bases and decision-support systems" (*National Library of Medicine 1986*).

The increasing interest in the evaluation of medical expert systems, of which recent sessions at the SCAMC meeting in Washington, the COMAC/BME meeting in Maastricht and the IEEE/ENMBS meeting in Seattle are evidence, suggest that these systems are at last coming of age. Medical informaticians are no longer waiting for the technology to catch up with their ideas, but are identifying suitable clinical niches for expert systems, building them, and attempting to define their impact on health care.

Even so, system evaluation is still perceived by some as unnecessary, and certainly consumes time and effort. For this reason, we first consider arguments in favour of system evaluation, before describing our approaches to laboratory and field testing.

Why Evaluate ?

There are three major reasons for performing evaluations: ethical, legal and intellectual. Let us consider these in turn.

The ethical basis of medicine is that we strive to improve patients' health while attempting to "do no harm" and to use limited health care resources wisely. We must therefore ethically ask ourselves the following questions about an expert system before attempting to distribute it:

- Is it effective ?
- Is it safe ?
- Does it change the use of health care resources ?

Only careful evaluation can answer these questions.

The medical profession and the suppliers of pharmaceutical and other medical technologies are familiar with the problem of litigation, especially in America. Expert systems technology will also be subject to litigation, although it is not yet clear whether the courts will consider it as a product or a service (*Shortliffe 1987*). If the former, strict product liability laws dictate that it must be safe, no matter what precautions have been taken to avoid mishaps, although the "state of the art" defense may help to deflect some suits. If the courts consider medical expert systems to be a service, then they must reach the standard expected of an "informed and sensible body of opinion"; this can only be determined by an independent evaluation, which needs then to be published in a peer-reviewed journal (*Medical Protection Society, personal communication*).

There are several intellectual arguments for testing expert systems. We need to know, in a new area such as this, which technical advances lead to progress, and which domains are the most fruitful to pursue. A further intellectual problem is predicting the performance of a knowledge-based system from its structure: this will require detailed evaluation of actual systems. A final reason for testing systems is that measurement contributes to scientific progress and to the credibility of expert systems. If we wish to see an expansion in their use, evaluation must surely be a priority.

Sadly, only about 10% of the many medical knowledge-based systems that have been described over the years have been tested in laboratory conditions (*Lundsgaarde 1987*), while even fewer have been exposed to clinical trials. This may be because systems were built to investigate certain tools or techniques, or because of lack of resources, or it may be because of confusion about what to test, and how to test it.

Previous Work on Evaluation Methods

There is a considerable literature on the topic that should go some way to solving these problems. However, the papers are spread across several disciplines, so their advice is not always accessible to prospective evaluators. A further problem is that, although individually useful, no coherent strategy emerges that would guide a system developer through the design and management of an evaluation programme. We have therefore attempted to synthesise the points made in this literature, together with those from the literature on medical technology assessment and clinical trials, and Donabedian's insights into the evaluation of information systems (*Donabedian 1966*), to propose a structured method for the evaluation of medical expert systems. Where practical, we refer explicitly to our source; we would refer newcomers to the evaluation area to *Shortliffe 1975, Spiegelhalter 1983, Gaschnig 1983, Wasson 1985, Miller 1986* and *Wyatt 1987* for more details.

Summary of the Proposed Evaluation Method

The first component of our proposed three-stage evaluation method should be complete before any attempt is made to build the expert system itself. It consists solely of a definition phase. This should identify the exact decision problem which the expert system is to alleviate, the users, and their physical and social environment. It may not be possible to achieve a complete definition of user requirements without first building an early prototype system, and requesting users to comment on how this could be improved. Thus, stage one may prove to be an iterative build-test-refine cycle.

To achieve clinically relevant definition may require the performance of a medical audit or other structured data collection, rather than relying on the hunches of experts or prospective users. This is worth the effort, however, as it not only ensures that the expert system that is built fulfills a genuine role, but can also double as a baseline study (see later), and may assist in the definition of how to make measures for the later evaluation process.

After this definition phase, further prototype systems are built, the best selected and refined, preferably with more user input, until a promising system emerges. At this stage, formal laboratory testing can begin. There are two major groups whose interests can be served by this testing phase: the system users and the experts who sanction its use. The system should therefore be tested from these two points of view. Proposed measures which can be made are discussed in section 2.

In the same way that a pharmacologist would hesitate to predict a drug's effects on a disease from knowledge of its pharmacology without clinical testing, it would be dangerous to infer, solely from laboratory tests of an expert system, its effectiveness in the field. As such systems only affect patients indirectly, by influencing decision-takers, field trials are crucial to determining if they have value to patients or to decision-takers. Suggestions for parameters to measure and for methods of performing the measurements are discussed in section 3.

Laboratory Testing of an Expert System

What measures can be made in the laboratory testing phase ?

The first section discussed the need to identify a clear role for the expert system. We assume that a prototype system has now been developed, using one of the standard techniques. If the investigators are serious about using the system to assist in the routine care of patients, it is clearly necessary to perform a careful preliminary evaluation before it is introduced into clinical practice. This "laboratory testing" phase is necessary to show that the system is safe and has at least the potential to benefit patients. There is a close analogy here between our laboratory testing phase and the safety (Phase 1) and dose-finding (Phase 2) stages of drug development. However, there are important differences between drugs and expert systems, even under laboratory conditions. In particular, for an expert system to be successful it must be acceptable to clinicians, and hence its 'usability' is a vital aspect for study and evaluation.

We may therefore imagine two hypothetical protagonists who must be satisfied before a system should be considered for clinical evaluation. The first is the 'user', who would typically be a nurse or junior doctor, and the second is the 'expert', who is the authority who sanctions the use of the system, and would typically be a consultant. If a system is being considered for widespread implementation, an administrative authority may be more appropriate, while in the future, regulatory authorities may be involved in the accreditation of such systems.

At this stage of evaluation, whatever the final intention, the system is viewed as a 'decision-taker', in that its conclusions are judged directly. Only in the next phase of evaluation will its effects as an aid to clinical decisions be considered.

In considering both users' and expert authorities' perspectives, we exploit the language of Donabedian in distinguishing the structure, reasoning process and outcome of the system's reasoning. For a prospective user, the broad questions within these categories, together with the more specific questions that could be asked, are given in Table 1.

Table 1: Testing an expert system in a laboratory setting: user's perspective		
Aspect:	Primary question:	Specific questions:
Structure	Is it wanted?	Is there a percieved need? Can the advice be made available at the right place and time?
Process	Is it pleasant to use?	Is the HCI satisfactory: • desired options available? • clear pointers to system state? • effective screen/keyboard layout? • is system dialogue acceptable? Is it fast enough?
Outcome	Does it say sensible things?	Do its conclusions seem as sound as those of a respected authority? Are the explanations adequate?

The specific questions we suggest reflect a view that medical expert systems will not succeed unless they are wanted, are usable in the clinical environment, and draw conclusions that seem reasonable to the user. This may seem obvious, but too many systems have been developed which failed because they were too cumbersome to use, asked too many questions in an unintuitive order, took up more time than was available, or occasionally came up with answers that were clearly wrong, but for which they had no explanation. Questions that an expert authority might wish to ask of an expert system are shown in Table 2, again classified by the three aspects of the system.

Table 2: Testing an expert system in a laboratory setting: expert authority's perspective		
Aspect:	Primary question:	Specific questions:
Structure	Is it of good quality?	Is the role efinition adquate? Were users defined & involved? Is knowledge source appropriate? Is the knowledge representation appropriate? Are hardware and software adequate?
Process	Does it reason appropriately	Is the logic consistent and rigorous? Is the system control defined and clearly represented? Is the method of handling uncertainty rigorous? Is it robust to irrelevant variations in input data?
Outcome	Does it draw safe and potentially valuable conclusions?	Can it detect cases which are "odd" or beyond its margins? Does it make serious mistakes within its domain? Compared to current practice, how accurate are its judgements?

Several difficulties may arise in answering these questions, and are discussed in the next section.

How can these measures be made ?

Some of the issues discussed above are the subject of research into the validation and verification of knowledge-bases. Questions about knowledge-base structure and reasoning processes need be answered by those with insight into both the technology and the domain. For example, in a rule-based system, lack of an explicit representation of control or meta-level reasoning may make it impossible to scale-up a prototype, while the use of Certainty Factors for propagating uncertainty may lead to unexpected responses to small variations in input data (*Pearl 1988*).

Apart from these technical issues, there are two other categories of measurements to be made: the subjective responses of users, and the semi-objective judgement of a system's accuracy.

Measuring user response and other subjective measures

For evaluating the expert system from the users' perspective, we must have a means of measuring attitudes and "user satisfaction", which may be difficult to do formally, especially when the system being tested is only a prototype. In this case, one may resort to an informal study of users' attitudes and activities when exposed to the prototype (eg. *Greenes et al 1989*), perhaps using a structured questionnaire (*Oppenheim 1982*). Combining verbal scales with visual analogue scales may sometimes lead to a more valuable investigative tool. If more detailed data on the human-computer interface is required, ergonomists can advise on how to make and interpret more appropriate measurements.

Measures of accuracy: test sets & selection of cases

A central issue in the design of scientific experiments is the definition of how measurements are to be made (Gaschnig's "Principle 4" *Gaschnig, 1983*), and on what population of test cases (*Wasson 1985*).

This second point is easier to resolve: although data is precious, and it is tempting to use it both for debugging a system and for the laboratory testing of accuracy, this is a serious error. Any expert system will usually perform much better on such "training" data than on a fresh set of data, collected as part of a separate study (*Wasson 1985*). This "test set" should be reserved for this purpose only, and once it has been used, cannot be used as a test set again. A further point is that some systems are designed solely to provide assistance with difficult cases, and as these occur rarely, testing such a system on randomly selected cases may not be very valuable. It seems reasonable here to adopt Chandrasekaran's suggestion (*Chandrasekaran 1983*) of allowing an independent group of experts to choose difficult test cases from a pool, but to mix these with a proportion of randomly selected, "ordinary" cases.

Measures of accuracy: gold standards and peer review

"There is often no such thing as the correct answer to a clinical problem" (*Shortliffe 1987*).

In medicine, some measurements, such as the mortality rate of patients, pose few difficulties, but others, such as diagnoses, are less objective. This is even more of a problem when assessing systems which advise about management, rather than diagnosis, as some "correct" or "gold standard" judgement is required, and Shortliffe's comment has been confirmed in many studies (eg. *Bucknall 1988*). Assuming that one has access to true gold standards for some of the proposed measures, a means must be devised for agreeing on a "silver standard" for the rest.

The ideal method of assessing the conclusions of an expert system whose role is to replace consultations with an expert, is to conduct a blinded comparison of the system with the expert: a Turing Test (*Turing 1950*). However, such a method only compares the system with one expert, and experts disagree. A useful variant of the Turing test is the "peer review" process: in this case, the standard is derived from a process of review by multiple, independent experts, all given the same data and using the same criteria to judge it. Examples of the use of peer review to establish diagnostic or management silver standards can be found in (*Yu, 1979, Fox, 1985, Quaglini, 1988, Wyatt, 1989*). However, several precautions need to be taken if this process is to be used.

Firstly, the individuals who comprise the peer review committee must work independently, but using the same criteria and data, and must commit themselves to their decision on paper before discussing it with others. Secondly, they should use a paper form for recording their decisions that they have designed, and whose categories correspond exactly with the recommendations of the expert system. Thirdly, the data given to the peer review committee should not include any items that have been specially collected for use by the expert system (*Wasson 1985*), nor anything that could identify to members of the panel if it is the system's or a doctor's advice that they are rating (*Chandrasekaran 1983*). This implies not only blinding, but also that a small study should be carried out to check if the experts are actually able to identify the source of the opinion more accurately than would be expected by chance. As this peer review process is necessarily subjective, it is valuable to both quote the inter-expert agreement rate (eg. *Yu 1979, Quaglini 1988*), and to assess the intra-expert agreement rate by means of a repeatability study (eg. *Fox 1985*).

During the planning of such a peer review process, it may emerge that no one expert has time to review every set of case data in the study (*Shortliffe 1981*). In this case, a "round robin" type of process may be adopted (eg. *Quaglini 1988*), in which each set of data is reviewed by two or more experts, but no expert receives more than a workable fraction of all the cases.

Once some form of gold or silver standard is available, it is not necessarily adequate to consider error rates alone when assessing the system's advice. If the system uses measures of uncertainty, it is useful to check the realism of its expression of doubt by comparing this with the frequency with which the outcomes occur. Although of most importance when assessing statistical decision-aids, these issues of calibration and separation (*Habbema 1981*) may still arise with expert systems that give their advice in the form of an ordered list, or as statements hedged with uncertainty.

Defining reliable methods for making measurements may appear tedious, but it is necessary to estimate the expert system's likely usability and contribution to clinical practice. Furthermore, if an audit of the current decision-making practice has been carried out prior to constructing the system, as suggested in section 1, some or all of the difficulties of making reliable and relevant measures will have been met and resolved already.

The Field Evaluation of Medical Expert Systems

This section discusses the planning and execution of field trials to assess medical expert systems. Our starting point is the completion of laboratory tests that demonstrate that a system is appropriate to the clinical problem and is likely to be acceptable and effective, from users' and experts' points of view. The laboratory testing process can be justified by reference to the difficulty of predicting the outcome of an expert system's reasoning solely from its knowledge base and the structure of its inference engine. There is a similar gulf between knowing the outcome of the system's reasoning, and predicting the effects it will have on the structure, process and outcome of health care. However, there are several additional problems.

What are the special problems of field evaluation of expert systems ?

Medical expert systems are designed to give explicit advice about patient manage-ment or prognosis to a health professional. It would be naive, however, to imagine that they exert all their effects on the structure, process and outcome of health care by this means alone. Studies have demonstrated that there are several additional ways in which any decision-aid can exert its effects, including through feedback of performance and educational effects on health care personnel, the fact that the performance of decision-takers' improves because it is being studied (the Hawthorne Effect), an improvement in the quality of decisions because of more complete data collection (the Checklist Effect), and a potential effect on patients of receiving extra attention in the form of a computerised consultation (the Placebo Effect) These extra effects must be taken into account when designing clinical trials to evaluate the effects of expert systems on health care, and dictate not only what is measured, but also how it is measured.

What type of field evaluation to conduct, and when ?

Field trials of medical technology can be designed to check if the intervention has an effect on outcome (a pragmatic motive), or to elucidate how it exerts this effect (an explanatory motive) (*Schwartz et al 1967*). If a pragmatic trial of an expert system is carried out, and is successful, it may not be clear whether some simpler form of the system, such as a paper checklist or a placebo computer consultation, might not have had the same effect. Thus, most trials of expert systems need to be explanatory in nature.

A further influence on trial design is the identity of the organiser and their motives. The emphasis in the field trial will vary, from one conducted by the developer of the system who needs to check if it has potential outside of the laboratory, to one in which the manufacturer wishes to "accurately describe ... what the product does, including an account of its scope, limitations and reliability" (*Bundy 1985*), or one in which a government body wishes to examine the impact of an expert system on health service resources. Attention should be given to the correct timing of a field trial, to avoid premature trials that might discredit the system and dishearten the developers (*Gaschnig 1983*), and to avoid delay in implementing an effective system. The general issues of trial design, subject safety and consent, may need discussion with statisticians and approval by ethical committees before any field testing begins.

What measures might be made in field trials ?

"No generally accepted criteria exist for establishing that a program is safe and effective" (*Szolovits 1979*).

Despite a lack of consensus on measures of safety and efficacy, it again seems reasonable to follow Donabedian and to examine the effects of a medical expert system on the structure, process and outcome of the health care process, controlling for the effects of bias and of confounding variables. Which measures are of most significance will depend on the system's intended clinical role, its users and the motive behind the trial. Checklists of possible measures to assess the impact of the system on the structure, process and outcome of the health care process are given in tables 3 to 5. These address the following questions:

- Structure: does the system fit well in its intended environment, and is it perceived by its users as helpful ?
- Process: what beneficial or adverse effects does the system have on the processes of health care delivery ? - Outcome: does use of the system have a measurable effect on health outcome measures ?

Table 3: Measures of the possible effects of a medical expert system on the structure of health care

- Do users find the overall system acceptable? **Survey attitudes**
- Is adequate data available to the system? **Measure data completeness, repeatability, accuracy**
- Is the system's advice accessible to the users? **Measure usage rate and time**
- How well does the system integrate with other sources of expertise in the intended location? **Measure "acceptability" of conclusions, rate of implementating them**

Table 4: Measures of the possible effects of a medical expert system on the process of health care

- How often is the system used appropriately: what prevents this? **Measure (peer review)**
- Which parts of the system are not used or are abused, and why? **Log system usage and user problems; check case suitability**
- Does the system have an effect on the quality or completeness of data? **Measure**
- Does the system have an effect on important components of the health care process:
  - ¤ consultation time, length of stay **Measure**
  - ¤ number and types of investigations ordered, treatments used **Measure**
  - ¤ Quality of users' decisions during and after use (education) **Measure (peer review)**
- Does the system have a subjective effect on:
  - ¤ users job satisfaction, perceived responsibilities **Survey, log staff turnover**
  - ¤ patients' and administrators' perceptions of the interaction. **Survey, check patient return rates**

Table 5: Measures of the effects of using a medical expert system on health outcomes

- Does use of the system have an effect on individual patient morbidity? **Measure**
- Does use of the system have an effect on population morbidity? **Measure incidence or verity of disease in local population, demand for service**
- Does use of the system have an effect on mortality? **Establish case register; conduct prospective study**
- Are there any unexpected or significant side effects (e.g. erosion of skills)? **Provide daily contact with users; conduct ad hoc surveys**
- What are the overall cost/benefit ratios's, for the patient, the system user and the service provider, associated with the use of the system? **Establish measure of outcome; quantify benefits and costs**

How many measurements need to be made ?

Clearly, not all of these measures can or should be made in every trial. To avoid "data dredging", investigators should identify, before the start of the trial, a small number (2 or 3) of "major measures", changes in which are the aim of the trial. However, both to understand how the expert system exerts its effects, and to detect any unexpected adverse effects, "minor measures" need to be made. The number and nature of these will depend on the clinical problem, the type of medical expert system etc., but should be sufficient to answer the questions below:

- Would a simpler system have produced similar results ?
- Will the system readily transfer to another location ?

● How can the system be improved ?
● What adverse effects on patients, users and health service resources (demand for tests, use of drugs etc.) might be expected from use of the system ?

Principles of conducting field trials

Once these major and minor measures have been identified, and a reproducible means of making them are available, the trial proper can be designed. The default structure for any interventional trial is the randomised controlled trial with double-blinding, first developed in the 1940's by Bradford-Hill. Several modifications to this basic design need to be made to accommodate the unusual properties of medical expert systems.

These follow from considering the problems that can arise during trial management and data analysis. Only a brief discussion is given here; the reader is referred to *Pocock 1984* and *Armitage 1987* for further details.

The avoidance of systematic bias

There are four potential sources of systematic bias in trials of a medical expert system. Firstly, bias for or against the system (*Yu 1979*). This requires that all involved in data collection and final assessment should be blinded as to whether patients are in the expert system or control groups. The implication of this is that either the data required for judging whether management was improved or not must be extracted from case notes by a third party, or that the expert system's advice should be removed from the notes before trial staff see them. Clearly, to analyse the trial it is vital to retain a copy of the randomisation code in a secure place.

Secondly, the enthusiasm of the development team may help users at the development centre to obtain more benefit from the expert system than elsewhere, for example by providing an 24 hour telephone help-line. A simple precaution is to assess the system away from the development centre, employing staff with no vested interest in the system to run the trial. Circularity may be a problem if a medical expert system is built and evaluated by the same individual or team, or performs a classification task using the same data and criteria as assessors - for example, using published criteria to classify laboratory results. The remedy is to exclude system builders from the panel assessing results, and also to avoid using any parameter which is part of the diagnostic criteria as input data for an expert system making diagnostic decisions (*Wasson 1985*).

Two major statistical errors may arise from trials of insufficient power: Type 1 errors, which consist of falsely concluding that a useless intervention is effective, and Type 2 errors, which consist of falsely concluding that an effective intervention is useless. The usual problem is that the study is too small, which may arise by prematurely terminating a trial if it appears to show the desired result. Use of sample size calculations (*Armitage 1987, pp179-185*) to determine the required number of cases, as well as predefined termination criteria, should avoid both of these problems.

Controlling for confounding variables

Just as there is a need in drug trials to control for the placebo effect, in trials of medical expert systems the control and intervention groups must be matched in all significant respects apart from the availability of advice. Specific confounding variables that must be considered include the following:

- The Hawthorne Effect
- The Checklist Effect
- The Carry-over Effect
- Secular trends

The Hawthorne Effect, initially reported as an improvement in the productivity of relay-room workers in the Hawthorne factory when the lighting level was increased, which was repeated when the level was decreased (*Roethligsburger et al 1939*), may be quantified by means of a baseline study. This is a low-profile, apparently informal, study of the performance of the current decision-makers, before the installation of the expert system ; disguising its true intention is a necessary evil, which may take some ingenuity. After collecting sufficient data while the decision-takers are unaware of what is happening, a grand announcement is made that their performance will be scrutinised, and the randomised controlled trial of the expert system takes place. Comparing the performance of decision-takers between the control group and the baseline study gives an estimate of the Hawthorne Effect; this can then be subtracted from their performance in the expert system group to obtain the likely improvement in performance due to the system alone. A similar problem to the Hawthorne Effect may occur if the system has an audit function: this may enhance the performance of decision takers by giving them feedback about their failures and successes. This "feedback effect" can be quantified by recruiting a "feedback only" group of patients (eg. *Adams 1986*).

The checklist effect, due to more complete and structured collection of data, is recognised as being a major influence on the performance of junior doctors (eg. *de Dombal 1985*). It can either be controlled for or separately evaluated. In the former case, one simply ensures that the same data is collected in all cases before randomisation, but that the system's advice is only available in the expert system group. In the latter case, a randomly selected "data collection only" group of patients is recruited, and the measures of interest in this group collected and compared to the control group. Any improvement in performance is due solely to the effects of better data-collection.

To compensate for the carry-over effect, due to education of users by use of the expert system, two methods are available. Firstly, one may raise the size of the sampling unit (*Spiegelhalter 1983*), by randomising departments instead of doctors, or centres instead of departments. Secondly, one may conduct a study with alternating expert system and control periods. This allows any carry-over from use of the expert system to be quantified; however, it depends on the trial either being multi-centre with randomised or asynchronous periods, or there being no significant secular trends.

Secular trends are significant drifts in the measures of interest during the trial. They may affect all studies, but are particularly damaging in those that use historical controls and run for extended periods, or during which a major change in medical practice occurs. An example of this would be if an expert system for reducing mortality from head injury were assessed in a before / after study which happened to bridge the introduction of seat-belt legislation (*Murray 1986*). A further difficulty that can arise from the use of historical controls is Simpson's Paradox. In the example in Table 6 (from *Charig 1986*), there is an increase in the overall success rate in removing renal stones since 1980, associated with the introduction of percutaneous nephrolithotomy; however, when analysed by stone size, the new treatment is uniformly worse. How does this paradox arise? Quite simply, the cases have become easier, with a shift in the distribution of stone size, so that 77% of stones in the post-1980 cases are less than 2 cm, compared to 25% in the previous period. The simplest advice is to avoid historical controls.

Table 6: An Illustration of Simpson's Paradox (from Charig, 1986)			
	Overall success rate	Stones < 2cm	Stones ≥ 2cm
Open surgery (1972 - 79)	78% (273/350)	93% (81/87)	73% (192/263)
Percutaneous nephrolithomy (1980-85)	83% (289/350)	87% (234/270)	69% (55/80)

Avoiding problems due to poor cooperation

A common difficulty in trials is low recruitment rate and poor protocol compliance. Apart from prolonging the trial, this may reduce the generality of its conclusions. In trials of expert systems, poor cooperation may be a particular problem because the system is not something that can be given instantaneously, like a drug, but involves the user in a process of data collection, data entry, and consideration of the system's advice.

To avoid a low system usage rate, a trial run-in period, before the trial proper, may help; involving users in the design of the system from an early stage is also advocated. In some studies, it may be necessary to provide inducements to users to use the system, but this may reduce the generality of the trial conclusions. Educating the users about the system's role and reassuring them that it does not threaten their professionalism (*Essex 1989*) may help to improve usage rate and to avoid inappropriate use. Measurement during a run-in period of the time taken for data entry, the speed of reasoning, the ease of user access to the system, or users' perceptions of the system's consultation and explanation style, may suggest improvements to the system and thus increase its usability.

During a trial, a major worry is of excessive dropouts and poor follow-up. This requires good management, regular meetings with all involved, attention to detail and vigilance, to avoid irretrievable data loss.

Ensuring that the trial's conclusions are general and transferable

It is a tragedy if, after the effort of designing and running a field trial, its conclusions cannot be generalised from the particular group of patients studied to similar patients elsewhere. Two points may help to ensure transferability.

Firstly, the patients must be representative of all patients whose management is to be assisted by the system. This means defining and using explicit admission criteria, and ensuring that the site of the trial is appropriate. To demonstrate this, any report of the trial should give details of the patients and the centre involved

The choice of centre is influenced by the users and their organisational context, as an expert system that works in a teaching hospital, for example, may well not function in a rural clinic. As in drug trials, the ideal recipe is a multicentre trial including various types of centre. Secondly, the trial must be of sufficient power to ensure that its conclusions are statistically and medically valid. This requires that sample size calculations are used, and that any changes in the major measures due to use of the system are expressed with confidence limits. This may avoid the dissemination of a system that leads to a change in some measured parameter that, although statistically significant, is clinically irrelevant.

Miscellaneous practical points

Apart from the difficulties of persuading expert assessors to review cases, and users to take advantage of the system during the trial, other practical problems may emerge. For example, in a recent trial, it emerged that users were running the data of control patients through the system "out of curiosity" (*Wyatt 1989*), so it may be worth building password control into the consultation process. A serious problem in projects with multiple versions of the system and several testing centres is ensuring that the same version is used for tests in all centres. This may well not be the latest version; in fact, it is important to "freeze" a version of the system before submitting it to testing (*Chandrasekaran 1983*), although it may well be out of date by the time the field trial is over. One must avoid the temptation of assuming that the latest version is the best; adding new knowledge to sort out one problem may cause others, especially in poorly structured knowledge-bases.

Although it is important to define the protocol for studies before starting them, there will always be unexpected problems and new insights during the course of a trial. It is thus necessary to record and monitor problems as they arise, and sometimes to initiate sub-studies to clarify their cause and implications. Ensuring that there is someone sympathetic who keeps in close touch with the users may help to avoid trouble.

Proposals and Conclusions

Evaluations should be conducted more widely, and the results published

No-one could conclude, after reading this paper, that the evaluation of medical expert systems is simple. We do not wish to enshroud the area in statistical jargon or other mystique, but it is a process that needs to be carefully thought through, and may consume considerable time and ingenuity. We would also not wish the evaluation process to become a barrier to the implementation of promising systems, and would urge anyone who has developed a system for the prime purpose of improving patient care to submit it to the laboratory testing cycle, and to report their findings.

If favourable, an explanatory field trial should be considered, and if carried out, whether positive or negative, should be published. Only by following this path can system developers learn from mistakes made in the past (eg. *Wyatt 1989*).

A practical point, as yet inapplicable, is that, as is the case with drug testing, careful phase IV or post-marketing surveillance studies of systems in routine use (*Spiegelhalter 1983, Rossi-Mori 1987*) may reveal important further information. Measurements in these studies might include the effects on health-care providers and on population morbidity and mortality of the widespread use of a medical expert system; we are still some years away from being able to conduct these.

Proposals to encourage evaluation of medical expert systems

To encourage the evaluation of medical technology generally, and to foster research on methodologies, Jennett has suggested establishing an independent technology assessment body (*Smith 1984*), analogous to the American Office of Technology Assessment, which could have a section devoted to medical expert systems. This body could not only grant certificates of effectiveness, analogous to drug product licenses given by regulatory bodies, but could evolve a "code of practice" for medical expert system developers, perhaps modelled on such initiatives as the GEMINI (Government Expert Systems Methodology) project (*Montgomery 1989*). A further role might be to publish a list of all systems that are undergoing laboratory and clinical testing (*Rossi-Mori 1987*), and of those that have been accredited.

A further encouragement to system quality would be to give reviewers of applications papers access to a checklist of the minimum standards for evaluation, similar to the ones used by statisticians judging reports of trials for medical journals (*Anon. 1989*). This would not force those who were developing systems for academic reasons to undertake clinical evaluations, as their work could be judged by more appropriate criteria (*Cohen et al 1988*). However, it might lead all of us who are building medical expert systems to adopt a more thoughtful approach, and act as a focus to those who are attempting to define an evaluation methodology.

Acknowledgements

We acknowledge valuable discussions with Drs PA Emerson, Robin Knill-Jones & Charles Pantin, and the support of the IBM Scientific Centre, Winchester,

References

Adams ID, Chan M, Clifford PC et alii: "Computer aided diagnosis of acute abdominal pain: a multicentre study"; Brit Med J vol. 293, 1986, pp. 800-804.
Anon: Checklists for statisticians. Brit Med J vol. 298, 1989, pp. 41-42
Armitage P, Berry G: Statistical methods in medical research (2nd edition). Blackwell Scientific, Oxford, 1987.
Bucknall CE, Robertson C, Moran F & Stevenson RD: Differences in hospital asthma management. Lancet i:748-750, 1988.

Bundy A & Clutterbuck R: "Raising the standards of AI products"; Dept. of AI research paper no. 261, Dept. of AI, Edinburgh Univ. (also in proc. IJCAI-85), 1985.

Chandrasekaran B: "On evaluating AI systems for medical diagnosis"; AI Magazine Summer 1983, pp. 34-37 + p.48, 1983.

Charig CR, Webb DR, Payne SR, Wickham OE: Comparison of treatment of renal calculi by operative surgery, percutaneous nephrolithotomy and extracorporeal shock wave lithotripsy. Brit Med J vol. 292; 879-882, 1986.

Cohen P, Howe A: How evaluation guides AI research. AI Magazine Winter 1988, vol. 9, pp. 35-43, 1988.

de Dombal FT et alii: Computer-aided diagnosis of acute abdominal pain: multicentre study Phase II. Final Report, pub. DHSS, London; p. 4

Donabedian A : Evaluating the quality of medical care. Millbank Mem. Quaterly vol. 44; 166-206, 1966.

Essex B: Evaluation of algorithms for the management of mental illness (abstract). In: The validation & testing of decision-aids in medicine, eds. Wyatt J & Spiegelhalter D, pub. British Medical Informatics Society, London, 1989.

Fox J, Myers CD, Greaves MF, Pegram S: "Knowledge acquisition for expert systems: experience in leukaemia diagnosis"; Meth. Inf. Med. vol. 24, pp. 65-72, 1985.

Gaschnig J, Klahr P, Pople H, Shortliffe E, Terry A: "Evaluation of expert systems: issues and case studies"; in Hayes-Roth F, Waterman DA & Lenat D (eds), "Building expert systems", Addison Wesley 1983.

Greenes RA, Tarabar DB, Krauss M, Anderson G, Wolnik WJ, Cope L et al:"Knowledge management as a decision-support method: a diagnostic workup strategy application" Comp Biomed Res; 22: 113-135, 1989.

Habbema JDF, Hilden J & Bjerregaard B: "The measurement of performance in probabilistic diagnosis; general recommendations"; Meth. Inf. Med. vol. 20, pp. 97-100, 1981.

Lundsgaarde HP: "Evaluating medical expert systems"; Soc. Sci. Med. vol. 24, pp. 805-819, 1987.

Miller PL: "The evaluation of artificial intelligence systems in medicine"; Comp. Meth. and Prog. in Biomedicine, vol. 22, pp. 5-11, 1986.

Montgomery A: GEMINI: Government Expert Systems Methodology Initiative. In: Research & Development in Expert Systems V (proc. ES'88), eds. Kelly B & Rector A, pub. Cambridge Univ. Press, 1989; pp. 14-24, 1989.

Murray GD, Murray LS, Barlow P et alii: "Assessing the performance and clinical impact of a computerised prognostic system in severe head injury" Stats in Med vol 5; 403-410, 1986.

National Library of Medicine: Long Range Plan, report 4: Medical Informatics. pub. National Institutes of Health, Bethesda, Maryland; p. 73, 1986.

Oppenheim AN: "Questionnaire design and attitude measurement" pub. Heinemann, London, 1982.

Pearl J: "Probabilistic reasoning in intelligent systems." Morgan Kaufman, San Mateo, California, 1988.

Pocock SJ: "Controlled clinical trials: a practical approach." Wiley, Chichester, Sussex, 1984.

Quaglini S, Stefanelli M, Barosi G, Berzuini A: "A performance evaluation of the expert system ANEMIA" Comp. Biomed. Res. vol. 21, 307-323, 1988.

Roethligsburger FJ, Dickson WJ: Management and the worker. pub. Harvard Univ. Press, Cambridge, Mass, 1939.

Rossi-Mori A, Ricci FL: "Some comments on the evaluation of medical expert systems"; presented at AIM workshop 6, EEC, Brussels, 25/11/87, 1987.

Schwartz D, Lellouch J: Explanatory & pragmatic attitudes in therapeutic trials J Chron Dis; 20: 637-48, 1967.

Shortliffe EH, Davis R: "Some considerations for the implementation of knowledge-based expert systems" SIGART Newsletter no. 55, December 1975, pp. 9-12, 1975.

Shortliffe EH: Evaluating expert systems. Report STAN-HPP-81-9; (partially reproduced as Gaschnig 1983), 1981.

Shortliffe EH: "Computer programs to support medical decisions"; JAMA vol. 258, pp. 61-66, 1987.

Smith T: Taming high technology (editorial). Brit Med J vol. 289; 393-394, 1984.

Spiegelhalter DJ: "Evaluation of clinical decision aids, with an application to a system for dyspepsia"; Statistics in Med vol.2, pp.207-216, 1983.

Szolovits P & Pauker S: "Computers and clinical decision making: whether, how and for whom ?"; proc. IEEE vol. 67, pp. 1224-1226, 1979.

Turing, A: "Computing machinery and intelligence"; Mind, vol. 59, pp. 236-248, 1950.

Wasson JH, Sox HC, Neff RK & Goldman L: "Clinical prediction rules: applications and methodological standards"; NEJMed vol.313, pp.793-799, 1985.

Wyatt JC: "The evaluation of clinical decision support systems: a discussion of the methodology used in the ACORN project"; Lect. Notes in Med. Inform. vol 33, pp. 15-24 (Proc. AIME'87, Marseilles), 1987

Wyatt JC: Lessons learned from the field trial of ACORN, a chest pain advisor. In Proc. MedInfo'89, Beijing, eds. Manning P, Barber B. Amsterdam North-Holland, 1989.

Yu VL, Fagan LM, Wraith SM et alii: "Antimicrobial selection by computer: a blinded evaluation by infectious disease experts"; JAMA, vol. 242, pp. 1279-1282, 1979.

Questions from the discussion

Tusch: You mentioned the parallels with clinical trials. Don't you think that there are also parallels with quality assurance studies ?

Wyatt: Yes, there are certainly useful lessons and analogies from quality assurance; the GEMINI project is an attempt to apply these to the development of expert systems in general. A report from the Computer Services Association on quality assurance in expert system projects (CSA '87?) discusses the problems of defining specifications, goals for the various phases (prototype, deliverables etc.), and the question of documentation in expert systems projects. However, we feel that, for systems designed to assist health-care workers and patients, measuring changes in the processes or outcome of a health care encounter due to use of the system are more important.

Blom: Do you think that sufficient effort is already put into consistency checking of the knowledge-base so that the safety aspect can be addressed ?

Wyatt: By consistency checking I assume that you mean static and dynamic tests of KB validity. There has been a considerable amount of work on both, (refs), including programs which detect redundant, paradoxical or "isolated" rules (ones which can never fire) (articles in AI journal; MYCIN experts book), and systems which automatically generate sample cases to dynamically "exercise" the KB (ref. - X & Miller, '88).
Whether these can adequately explore all possible combinations of input data, or even all clinically relevant ones, is dubious. Also, the contribution of a completely "valid" knowledge base to system safety is not clear. It just takes a doctor to use the system on a case outside its limits, and it becomes unsafe.

However, I agree that the intensive exploration of a KB through such tools is helpful if one wishes to ensure that an expert system does what its designers intended. Unfortunately, we are still at an early stage in knowing how to specify the behaviour of KBS to achieve the desired impact on actual decisions.

The Role of Knowledge Based Systems in Medicine

Epistemological and Evaluation issues

Angelo Rossi-Mori[1], Domenico M. Pisanelli[1], Fabrizio L. Ricci[2]

1 Ist. Tecnologie Biomediche CNR, Roma, Italy

2 Ist. Studi Ricerca Documentazione Scientifica CNR, Roma, Italy

Abstract

We examine some paradigms for a comprehensive evaluation of Knowledge Based Systems (KBSs) in the health field to envisage a methodology for the proper design of such systems.

The physician is considered here for his function as a manager of knowledge (namely: patient's data, acquired expertise, "public" medical knowledge, common sense). The KBS technology is consequently an intellectual tool among the media available to the physician in his environment.

The aim of a KBS may be stated as to improve the performance of a professional in tackling defined health problems, by supporting him in the management of the knowledge. In this respect, the known experiences about the assessment of the performance of Medical KBSs seem rather narrow in their objectives. Therefore, more comprehensive contexts for the evaluation are recommended. Three levels are defined: i) efficiency of the system in itself, removed from its context; ii) overall effectiveness in the user's environment; iii) impact of the KBS technology on health. We suggest a cooperative effort to drive and support the evaluations: to establish detailed guidelines, to give rise to a collection of reviews about each system and to maintain a register of applications.

Introduction.

After the early experiments on Expert Systems, the health environment appeared as one of the most suitable fields for their large-scale application; however, whereas in other fields the practical results are unquestionable, in medicine they seem still limited. The computer applications to the clinical decisions seem not yet able to answer to the expectations they raised (*Friedman and Gustafsson, 1977; Williams, 1982*).

Knowledge-Based Systems (KBS) (*Harmon and King, 1985; Waterman, 1985*) claim to be the most advanced software achievement to support medical decisions (*Clancey* and Shortliffe, 1984; Szolovits, 1982), among many other "conventional" ones (*Shortliffe et al., 1979*); but also their successes are rare (*Buchanan, 1985*). Nevertheless, since the first attempts of application of computers to medicine, there is a definite evolution. The attitude is not anymore directed towards "automatic classification" (*Patrick, 1979*) or towards the substitution of the physician, but it is now clear that human judgement and peculiarly human reasoning capabilities (*Elstein et al., 1978*) are needed: the computer must be an efficient assistant to an "active" user, who maintains his full autonomy and responsibility (*De Dombal, 1983*).

The awareness that KBSs (and more generally computer applications in medicine) must be better understood and evaluated for their successful diffusion is well understood (*van Bemmel, 1988; O'Keefe et al., 1987; Putthoff et al., 1988; Engelbrecht, 1988; Wyatt and Spiegelhalter, 1989, Grémy, 1988; Ricci and Rossi-Mori, 1986; SYDPOL5, 1988; Schneider, 1987; Winograd, 1989*).

The goal of this paper is to foresee the potential scenarios on the introduction of KBSs in the health field, and guidelines for their design and evaluation. First, we examine the present drawbacks they show (section 2). Then we analyse the different frameworks and environments where they will be embedded (section 3) and we review the possible paradigms that is possible to apply to KBSs (section 4). Finally, we define some criteria for a comprehensive evaluation (section 5).

The Difficult Introduction of KBSs in the Health Field

Knowledge Based Systems show a delay in their diffusion in the health field, with respect to the first expectations. There was surely a confusion on public opinion, due to lack of awareness of the long time usually needed to bring a new - although exciting - technology from the scientific laboratory to the common usage.

This delay was perhaps facilitated by some peculiar way of stating goals and evaluating results in the early experiments that were more oriented towards scientific and cultural problems in computer science than to a broad diffusion in medicine.

Important methodological issues are to be solved to date and thus basic experiments are a necessity; however a precise priority scale might suggest a low number of narrow problems where efforts ought to be concentrated.

A very strong factor of resistance among the majority of physicians is the *lack of a perceived need*. Beyond the first enthusiasms, the field is not ready for this revolution. The informatization of structures (such as hospitals and clinical laboratories) and the spread of Personal Computers brought many professionals in contact with the computer, mainly for administrative management purposes or data processing. It is a different matter to deal with the processes of clinical decision making and the clinical management of the patient.

The *cost of development and commercialization* does not appear as a severe limiting factor in medicine. Let us consider for example the quickness of the introduction and the liveliness of the competition of new imaging instruments (such as NMR, CAT scanner). In those cases the usefulness of the machine results is unanimously recognized and the debate is not focused on absolute costs, but on their cost-effectiveness and rational distribution on the territory.

Many drawbacks are *common to most present Artificial Intelligence applications* (see table 1).

knowledge bases	few KB are available;
	no standard terminology: very difficult to merge;
knowledge representation methods	not adequate for many medical problems;
	require more ad hoc research;
architectures and reasoning models	require long term research;
hardware	not suitable for a cheap diffusion of the more relevant and powerful systems

Table 1: Common drawbacks of most Artificial Intelligence applications

Systematized terminology and semantic standards play a key role for the diffusion of compatible modular KBSs. The growing awareness is demonstrated by the presence of many projects (e.g. UMLS by the National Library of Medicine (*Lindberg and Humphreys, 1989*) and SESAME, a project within the AIM program of EEC) and initiatives (e.g. Semantics and Knowledge Representation subcommittee SKRAM in IEEE-MEDIX (*Harrington, 1989*)).

Three classes of application in medicine

In this paper we focus on the class of systems that are designed for the application in a professional environment.

In general, it is possible to classify KBSs in three classes that we may label as "genuine" from the medical point of view, to distinguish them from experiments in Artificial Intelligence or Cognitive Science (see table 2).

feature	research on medical reasoning	formalization of a medical topic	medical practice
class of medical application	research on medicine	research in medicine	practice of medicine
aim of the overall project	development of a theory	production of a formalization	consultation on a patient
owner of the problem	researcher in theoretical medicine	medical researcher	consulting physician
expected suggestions	towards new theories on medical reasoning	towards specific clinical experiments	for actions on a patient

Table 2. Three classes of KBSs in medicine: the scenarios

● A first class of projects refers to the *study of the medical decision process* in itself.

The research task involves the observation of the ability of reasoning in medical terms and explores the types of knowledge the physicians use; the ultimate goal is to identify the features of the intellectual process that a doctor uses in his clinical judgement.

The KBS is typically a prototype devoted to simulate the 'art' of using attainable information to define the proper management of the patient.

- A second class of KBSs regard the analysis, *formalization*, refinement and assessment *of medical knowledge* on limited topics; the aim is to help the medical scientists to analyze their own knowledge on specific fields.
- Finally, in the third class a system must *support the physician's daily activities* and provide a decision tool at the bedside. It may help him to identify components of complex problems (possible choices, causal relations, different scenarios, ...).

The next future

On the short term a sensible impact of KBSs on health is not within reach:

- the physician uses widely common sense, what is difficult to model in present systems;
- the reasoning process is not easily approximated by the mechanisms that is possible to implement with present AI methods;
- it is too complex to apply this technology to the small-scale, common, heterogeneous decisions of physicians;
- except for trivial cases (where the advice is less useful), there are frequent non-resolvable differences in the experts' approaches. It implies the unavailability of "gold standards" about building and evaluating systems. Moreover, the end-user maintains his responsibility and thus his view on the problems: no authority exists to impose any method of problem structuring and solving.

The solution is on the implementation of sub-systems that result integrated in the Knowledge Environment of the physician, with settled, validated knowledge and a limited scope. The support to the physician's decision will not focus on power / deepness of reasoning, but rather it will result from facilitating some activity that is conceivable to assist efficiently by computer: for example to browse a large amount of knowledge, or to interact with the computer itself.

Facing these difficulties, the field of KBSs is in competition with other media available to the physician in his environment. Let us consider this environment to understand this competition, to see how to compare these tools and how to evaluate them side by side, in order to design computer subsystems that have to integrate themselves in this existing structure.

The Integrated Knowledge Environment of the physician

How may the physician properly use and integrate the resources present in his environment, namely advanced computer systems, as KBSs are?

The physician's work consists in the **management of knowledge**, deciding for appropriate actions after an adequate diagnosis and monitoring their effects. He matches patient's data with his "private" knowledge (medical expertise and common sense), and with "public" knowledge (what he learned and what he consults).

Let us consider medicine against other professional sectors, where economical-administrative data (as bureaucracy) tend to represent all the information needs: for a physician, professional data (i.e. "soft" data and ill-defined information that he uses for clinical management) prevail over the others, although they are difficult to be managed by a computer.

Many "media" (instruments and agents, either computer based or not) are already present in the environment of the physician: *books, medical records, methodologies for decision making* - as flow charts, clinical algorithms, protocols, decision analysis - , *colleagues*, ...

In a very broad sense, we would have to include here also the "classical" methodological achievements of medical science, such as anamnesis, findings collection, and the diagnosis itself, i.e. *the tools that physicians developed to help their mind to manage clinical judgement and patient care*. It is a fact that after the introduction of a discovery or new technology (for example innovative imaging techniques), the involved management strategies may change completely.

Computer applications are often devoted to trivial administrative purposes, and are not directed to grasp clinical needs. We are at the beginning of an evolution in the use of computers, and it is necessary to understand how to design advanced systems for a real use from the physician. The ultimate aim of advanced computer tools is to help the physician in carrying out his work in a more efficient and comfortable way. The role of the computer system is therefore to offer some (more or less "intelligent") support to the decision made by the physician. It's not a substitution, but an incentive and an assistance to activities and capabilities peculiarly human. The computer must therefore be considered as any other support (like for example diagnostic tests): the final responsibility is always to the physician.

In synthesis, we deal with computers that help health operators in the management of available knowledge, in order to reach decisions about a patient, or more in general *to carry out their professional tasks in a more comfortable, sure, precise way.*

Embedded Knowledge Based Systems

The comprehensive *Knowledge Environment* contains different media, integrated with the physician's daily work; among them, also computer-based subsystems will be present, and in particular KBSs. The Knowledge Based technology is particularly suitable for embedded modular applications, to raise the level of "smartness" in the software; in the future, it will be very difficult to assess the impact of one single component of this environment, due to the synergism of all the media *and* the user.

In current research on KBSs, the focus about their potential functions is typically put on complex tasks, i.e. assisting and critiquing diagnosis and treatment, generating and ranking possible solutions.

More practical and low-level functions are possible with this technology, and a diffusion of embedded KBSs seems reasonable in the next future (see table 3).

Therefore our discussion regards also the management of Knowledge Bases (*Riccardi and Rossi-Mori, 1988*) and the "intelligent" user interfaces; on the contrary, the paper does not cover the evaluation of general purpose shells used to build applied systems, except when they show peculiar features with respect to the requirements of the medical field.

field	task
intelligent interface	avoiding computable questions
	choosing the next question
	generating default menus
	checking inconsistencies in the data
intelligent administrative assistant	writing prescriptions and certificates
	medical record management
knowledge browsers	literature search
	selection of similar cases
	management of encyclopedias and other organized knowledge
semantic conversion	selecting knowledge for transmission
transforming data from one purpose to another	generating queries to a database directly from the medical record
	summarizing the medical facts

Table 3. Potential tasks for modular KBSs, embedded in a medical Information System

Decision Support Systems versus KBSs

There are two historical approaches that brought to two different, well established disciplines: Decision Support Systems (DSSs) and Knowledge-Based Systems (KBSs) (*Nelson Ford, 1985; Humphreys, 1985*).

According to the current terminology (*Ginzberg and Stohr, 1982*), DSSs are a set of methodologies and techniques in a large interdisciplinary field ranging from operative research to psychology. They are normally applied in management science and to the industrial environment; appropriate tools used by these decision-makers range from databases and spreadsheets to mathematical simulation models. A typical DSS allows the manager to browse effectively and understand his data; the stress is on the numerical aspects (1).

$$\text{data} \leftrightarrow \text{DSS} \leftrightarrow \text{active user} \qquad (1)$$

A different approach is considered in the field of Artificial Intelligence. Here the systems follow their own reasoning lines: they are the most active tools available and tend to present to the user a "packaged" solution.

Two modalities are possible in this field:

- the "monitoring mode" (2), where the system has a direct access to some formalized data; this formalization has to be done previously elsewhere, either by a health operator or through an instrument (numerical data). This case is similar to the DSS approach, and is the more easy to be dealt with and evaluated;

$$\text{formalized data} \leftrightarrow \text{KBS} \leftrightarrow \text{user} \qquad (2)$$

- the "assistant mode" (3), where the user provides the interface between problem and computer. Here the system has no direct access to data, and the whole formalization is done by the user. He interprets the information about the problem, and feeds the system with preprocessed information.

$$\text{problem} \leftrightarrow \text{user} \leftrightarrow \text{KBS} \qquad (3)$$

It is always the user who understands the advice given by the system because of his background, and processes this advice to make it coherent with his idea on the problem. If necessary, he can go out from the previous model, using higher level knowledge and a more wide appraisal of the problem.

The management of such a variety of systems, contexts, modalities, environments makes very difficult, to establish a general theory of evaluation and a widely applicable methodology for design.

Nevertheless, it is still useful to present some different possible strategies for approaching systematically the topic and to fix some starting point for further discussions. It is what we propose in the following of the paper.

A Framework for Evaluation and Design

The Knowledge Based Systems show many advanced features that make them so peculiar that no previous model of evaluation and design is fully applicable. As a matter of fact, it is not clear how to evaluate the proper management of knowledge by a computer system, and how to measure the appropriateness of a reasoning line in the user and how it is being influenced by the system.

To state actual measurements and methods to evaluate a system (or better the *integrated behaviour of user and system*), efforts are needed on two complementary lines:

- **a-priori approach**: there is a need for a better understanding of the framework where these advanced systems have to be integrated. It must be worked out what they are and what peculiar features they show, with respect to the other decision aids and the user himself. A blended process of man-machine interaction has to be modeled, analysed, and evaluated, before it may be correctly designed in future systems. At the same time, it has to be clarified what is possible to observe and measure in this process. This is the approach we are following here.

- **pragmatic approach**: an analysis must start from the other side, i.e. from experiences of implementations and evaluations already carried out, in order to extrapolate the evaluation methodologies, and then to build realistic methodologies for evaluation and design, by critiquing and assessing these experiences in a comparative way.

If these approaches converge, the result will be an optimal, complete methodology for Medical KBSs design.

Paradigms for the definition of criteria.

The assessment of a new technology refers often to established paradigms, derived from fields with similar features. Therefore, in the determination of a comprehensive model to evaluate Medical KBSs, we may refer to various experiences in other fields and explore different paradigms. As a matter of fact, we may consider their features according to very different attitudes, keeping in mind: epidemiology, books, tutors, industrial products and so on (see table 4).

It would be opportune to examine separately single aspects of a KBS in comparison to the appropriate paradigm, in order to achieve a multiple, complete approach to all the possible points of view.

Formal and informal evaluation.

The most appropriate paradigm might be similar to the examinations and the informal tests passed by the physician himself, before as medical student, and later during his daily practice.

As a **medical student**, he may have passed several oral, practical and written examinations, dealing with his knowledge and know-how. His behaviour on single medical acts is also monitored, by several tests on his micro-decisions about the management of clinical cases (real or simulated). He has to demonstrate his **reliability** on controlled situations.

paradigm	criteria
• epidemiology • pattern recognition • classification methods	at present most evaluations of Medical KBSs refer to final results (accuracy, predictive values, false positives, false negatives, ...); they often recognize human experts on the field as a 'gold standard'
• decision support systems	KBSs claim to offer a support to a professional, to give hints and to make him avoid mistakes; following the debate in DSS field we may develop inclusive criteria that take into account the influence of the advices on the decisions of a physician or a health manager
• new drugs	four steps of validation and control
• industrial products • general purpose software	market acceptance is a determinant criterion (it assures that the product satisfies some need at the right price, but it may not apply in a public National Health System)
• textbooks • lessons	"success" is measurable in number of distributed copies, or attendance; users evaluate clarity of presentation and possible boringness
• experts • consultants • professionals	there is not a systematic formal evaluation on their expertise, even if it would be possible to test their background knowledge; they are judged on the basis of "conformity with expectations" and may provoke unsatisfaction and litigation by the client

Table 4. Principal criteria that is possible to convert for the evaluation of Medical KBSs

On the contrary, usually an **experienced physician** does not undergo a *formal review* on the *expertise* he accumulates during the practice of his work, even if this expertise is what actually makes him "an expert" (and hence what the KBSs are just trying to catch). The micro-decisions are evaluated as a whole, i.e. as the overall satisfaction of the patients, summarized in the **expected behaviour**. Only in the worst and serious cases of errors or incompetence they are evaluated on specific actions by their evident consequences.

As a matter of fact, there is an *informal way of communication* among a community (physicians and patients), not to establish what the abstract features of a good specialist must be (the benchmarks), but to comment upon the general **competence** of a given specialist and his **suitability** for a given patient. It applies also for textbooks (the products of the experts, like the KBSs): there is not a formal "test" of a book, but the criticisms and the reviews of colleagues and the satisfaction of the students build its possible success.

Three Levels of Evaluation.

Given the previous framework, we are now able to envisage a comprehensive assessment of medical KBSs. We proposed to distinguish at least three possible sizes of the evaluation scale (*Rossi-Mori and Ricci, 1988.*); they are summarized here in table 5.

First, the system's correctness must be assured, but the Knowledge Base is inherently modular and allows for frequent, smooth updates, i.e. the system *evolves*. Whereas it seems not realistic to test an (human) expert with frequent examination, it might be possible to set up a *log* of the performance of an evolving system, with the cooperation of a set of selected centers, and to have a regular summarization of the raw efficiency of the system. A quantitative measurement is often out of reach in this situation; nevertheless an analysis of errors, reasons and remedies is of value for users and designers.

A KBS must be evaluated in a more comprehensive manner than the mere correctness of final results. A *protocol* for a detailed discussion about the system performance (reasoning process and general satisfaction) must be established, and the collection of such reviews must be made available to potential users.

Other levels of evaluation are considered in table 5, to take into account the behaviour of the user (in presence or in absence of a KBS), and more in general the impact of this technology on specific health problems and on the health service.

Conclusions.

The physician's work consists mainly in the use of heterogeneous kinds of knowledge: he already uses a set of media to manage this knowledge; the KBSs are other tools that have to harmonize themselves in this environment.

The implementation of an Information System requires the combination of different design methodologies, each for a specific aspect of the whole system. Such methodologies were mainly conceived for applications in the private sector, related to the production of goods; they must be therefore deeply upgraded to catch also the decision making aspects and adapted to the medical field.

level	context	aspects submitted to evaluation
I. raw efficiency of the system in itself	the micro-decision cycle and the advice of the system	• static validation of the KB correctness; • measure of error rate (final results on typical cases vs atypical cases); • evaluation of the behaviour of the system with respect to a specific problem (dialogue and reasoning process); • ability to deal with pitfalls and cases perceived as difficult by the user (simple vs difficult).
II. integration within the environment of a single user	the cooperation of the physician with the computer	• long term effects on the user's behaviour: - the acceptance of the system in the routine work; - permanent changes in the user's organization - education and quality of collected data. • the performance of the user, cooperating with the system, considering also the co-presence of other decision aids.
III. impact on health care	the target environment: actual practice or medical research	• assessment of the KBS technology in the health field; • the effectiveness of multiple copies of a system on the specific health problem faced up.

Table 5. Aspects that must be observed within each level of growing generality

To develop such design methodologies for KBSs, further achievements are needed in the field of their evaluation.

We examined different paradigms to face the assessment of Medical KBSs, trying to catch the concepts that may express the peculiar features of this technology: it can emulate experts and thus affects the user's intellectual activities and the organization of his work environment.

An international cooperative effort must be established, to drive and support the evaluations, to facilitate the basic formal multi-center evaluation of a system, to test it in real environments, to refer the Knowledge Base problems for further updates. We propose to discuss and agree on detailed guidelines, to give rise to a collection of reviews about each system and to maintain a register of applications.

In this way it is possible to prepare the background for the cost-benefit appraisal of future diffused systems, and the comprehensive assessment of the impact of this technology on the health field.

References

Buchanan BG: Expert Systems: Working Systems and the Research Literature. Report KSL-85-37, Knowledge Systems Laboratory, Stanford University, 1985.

Clancey WJ, Shortliffe EH (eds.): Readings in Medical Artificial Intelligence: The First Decade, Reading, Massachusetts, Addison-Wesley, 1984.

De Dombal FT: Towards a More Objective Evaluation of Computer-Aided Decision Support Systems, in: Van Bemmel JH, Ball and Wigertz O (eds.), Proceedings MEDINFO 83, Amsterdam, North Holland: 436-439, 1983.

Elstein AS, Shulman LS, Sprafka SA: Medical Problem Solving: An Analysis of Clinical Reasoning, Cambridge, Massachusetts, Harvard University Press, 1978.

Engelbrecht R: Status and Research Needs for Expert Systems in Medicine, in: Rienhoff O, Piccolo U, Schneider B (eds), Expert Systems and Decision Support in Medicine, Berlin, Springer- Verlag: 361-366, 1988.

Friedman RB, Gustafsson DH: Computers In Clinical Medicine, A Critical Review, Comp. Biom. Res., 10: 199-204, 1977.

Ginzberg MJ, Stohr EA: Decision Support Systems: Issues and Perspectives, in: Ginzberg MJ, Reitman W and Stohr EA, Decision Support Systems, Amsterdam, North - Holland: 9-31, 1982.

Grémy F: Persons and Computers in Medicine and Health. (Keynote address, MIE'87, Roma 1987), Meth Inform Med, 27: 3-9, 1988.

Harmon P, King D: Expert Systems, Artificial Intelligence in Business, New York, John Wiley & Sons, 1985.

Harrington JJ: IEEE P1157 Medical Data Interchange (MEDIX) Committee Overview and Status Report, MEDIX Report, 1989.

Humphreys P: Intelligence in Decision Support, Major Paper at the 10th SPUDM Conference, Helsinki, 1985.

Lindberg DAB, Humphreys BL: Computer Systems that Understand Medical Meaning, in: Scherrer JR, Côté RA, Mandil SH (eds.), Computerized Natural Medical Language Processing for Knowledge Representation, Amsterdam, North-Holland, 1989.

Nelson Ford F:Decision Support Systems and Expert Systems: A Comparison, Information & Management, 8: 21-26, 1985.

O'Keefe RM, Balci O, Smith EP: Validating Expert System Performance, IEEE Expert, Winter 1987: 81-89, 1987.

Patrick EA: Decision Analysis in Medicine: Methods and Applications, Boca Raton, Florida, CRC Press, 1979.

Putthoff P, Rothemund M, Schwefel D, Engelbrecht R, van Eimeren W:Expert Systems in Medicine, Possible Future Effects, Intl J Technology Assessment in Health Care, 4: 121-133, 1988.

Riccardi M, Rossi-Mori A: A Background Knowledge Base to Assist Coding of Medical Documents, in: Rienhoff O, Piccolo U, Schneider B (eds), Expert Systems and Decision Support in Medicine, Berlin, Springer- Verlag: 328-333, 1988.

Ricci FL, Rossi-Mori A: Roles of Expert Systems and others Decision Aids into the Physician's Information System, in: Proceeding of the 1st International Expert Systems Conference, London, 1-3 Oct 1985, Oxford, Learned Information: 351-363, 1985.

Rossi-Mori A, Ricci FL: On the Assessment of Medical Expert Systems, in: Rienhoff O, Piccolo U, Schneider B (eds), Expert Systems and Decision Support in Medicine, Berlin, Springer- Verlag: 292-297, 1988.

Schneider W: Are Expert Systems Really Expert ? (Keynote address, MIE'87, Roma 1987) in: Serio A et al. (eds.), Proceedings MIE '87, Rome, Edi Press, 1987.

Shortliffe EA, Buchanan BG, Feigenbaum EA: Knowledge Engineering for Medical Decision Making: A Review of Computer Based Clinical Decision Aids, Proc.IEEE, 67: 1207-1224, 1979.

SYDPOL5 SYDPOL5 Working Group: Guidelines for quality assessment in the field of clinical expert systems. presented at MIE '88, Oslo, 1988.

Szolovits P. (ed.): Artificial Intelligence in Medicine (AAAS Selected Symposium 51), Boulder, Colorado, Westview Press, 1982.

Van Bemmel J: Systems Evaluation for the Health of All, in: Hansen R, Solheim BG, O'Moore RR, Roger FH, Proceedings MIE '88, Berlin, Springer-Verlag: 27-34, 1988.

Waterman DA A Guide to Expert Systems, Reading, Massachusetts, Addison-Wesley, 1985.

Williams BT (ed.) Computer Aids to Clinical Decisions, voll.1 & 2, Boca Raton, Florida, CRC Press, 1982.

Winograd T: In: Davis R (ed.), Expert Systems: How Far Can They Go?, AI Magazine, 10: 61-67, 1989.

Wyatt J, Spiegelhalter D: Evaluating Medical Decision Aids: What to Test, and How? This volume, 274-290, 1990.

Question from the discussion

Grant: The distinction between basic research, clinical research, and clinical practice is important. I see KBSs as an interface between these different domains, specifically between clinical research and clinical practice. There is of course the problem of updating the knowledge base. Can you comment on that ?

Rossi Mori: Yes, the three classes of systems use the same basic corpus of medical knowledge, at least in theory.

But the uses are different, and thus the approach to the problems: we have to consider a KBS as a man-machine whole; not only knowledge is involved, but also the main actor who manages that knowledge, namely the physician.

Let us consider for example two scenarios of the same class, clinical practice: a cardiologist and a general practitioner facing the same patient. In reality they face a completely different problem, with their different background and in a different environment. Potential actions, priorities, available resources, time scale imply a different attitude and thus earmarked details in medical knowledge and specific additional knowledge (e.g. on resources).

The flow of knowledge from one professional environment to another is very difficult and perhaps impossible. At present, automatic conversion from a Knowledge Base or a representation to another is not within reach.

Nevertheless, there is a corpus of Background Medical Knowledge that can be the common substrate (stable, validated and standardized) to build smarter Information Systems (*Riccardi and Rossi Mori, 1988*).

Even deeper is the gap among the three classes of systems; let me go a little further with the features of these classes.

It must be pointed out that a system in the **first class** cannot be considered as a decision aid: the importance is in spin-offs. In fact, it must produce a better insight into medical expertise, for a better teaching or for the production of new tools: they don't "produce" (or spread) formalized knowledge.

feature	research on medical rea- soning	formalization of a medical topic	medical practice
medicine seen as:	understanding an art	development of a science	exercise of an art
focus of the design	medical reasoning	a specific medical topic	a specific patient
potential spin-offs	methodologies to teach clinical skills	diagnostic-thera- peutic protocols	prescriptions, the- rapy management
medical knowledge to transmit	diagnostic methods	public-domain knowlege (books)	private knowledge (expertise)

Table 6. Three classes of KBSs in medicine: the goals

Nevertheless, these systems allow the realization of architectures and inference engines, earmarked for medicine (see for example ABEL and CENTAUR).

The **second class** of systems searches for some form of agreement of medical community on a new coherent and complete formalization, not necessarily delivered as a computer system (it may be for example fixed in a book).
Another possible goal for a system of this kind may be to supply "hints", to design specific experiments on areas that were recognized as not yet properly formalizable in the Knowledge Base; such a system may thus result in an appropriate framework either to fix problems occurring in the knowledge base, or to select and define topics for the experiments.
Finally, if the aim was the standardization among a group of experts or a better understanding of the different views, it will produce some by-product, as protocols, using the possibility of a systematic and deep comparison of different formalizations.

For an application project (the **third class**), we deal not only with medical knowl- edge, but one must consider the "cost" of accessible data (e.g. price, risks, availability of required resources, time spent, delay of results) and the relevance of each decision in the global process.
The medical knowledge must be up-to-date, but also enough "stable" and verified. It is important a broad coverage, and a standardization in concepts and in language, so that different knowledge bases can be merged (or one can switch from one to another) and meanings are preserved among users and systems.
The KBSs must not take the place of the right tools for the diffusion of scientific results: literature search and thorough reading of relevant papers may benefit from computer science, but not be replaced.

Validity of Systems Application

User confidence in case application

Peter McNair[1] and Jytte Brender[2]

[1] Dept. of Clinical Chemistry, Hvidovre Hospital, University of Copenhagen, Hvidovre, Denmark,

[2] Computer Resources International a/s, Birkerød, Denmark.

Abstract

Medical professionals are ultimately responsible for the consequences of applying any device, treatment or examination to patients, therein the application of knowledge-based systems. With this perspective, the validation of knowledge-based systems goes beyond that of certifying their overall validity into an ongoing validation of systems application for every particular case at hand. As a consequence, systems output must contain information that makes quality assessment feasible.

Introduction

Irrespective of application of decision support devices, the legal and professional responsibility of a decision resides with the medical professionals (*Cannatacci 1988, 1989*). Thereby decision support systems can only be meant for human support, and the systems should not possess authority themselves.

In the AIM Workprogramme (*Commission of ... 1988*) it is stated that:

"At present there are no formal rules of medical correctness for validating medical knowledge-based systems. Neither are there formal ways of handling differences in medical interpretation or updating systems with time and the increase of medical knowledge. One of the important applications for knowledge-based systems in medicine is their role in defining "normality", thereby saving staff appreciable time and effort which can be more efficiently directed to solving problems of abnormality. Correctness of medical knowledge based systems is therefore central to the development of biomedical informatics, especially as practitioners thereby know that a particular system for clinical use has been formally validated as correct."

However, the problem of quality assessment of knowledge-based systems goes beyond that of formal validation of their correctness, since even correct systems may grow into utter incompetence:
"A limitation of first-era systems is their brittleness. To mix metaphors, they operate on a high plateau of knowledge and competence until they reach the extremity of their knowledge; then they fall off precipitously to levels of utter incompetence" (*Feigenbaum 1986*).

Recently, the problems of knowledge acquisition and brittleness of systems behaviour has been further stressed (*Musen & van der Lei 1989*).

Normally knowledge based systems (KBSs) are developed to cope with inadequacies in human capability or accessibility in complex decision making circumstances.

"In principle knowledge based systems are particularly well suited to cope with this class of problems because they can accommodate human expertise, provide easy man-machine interaction and justify the advice and conclusion that they give." (*Commission of ... 1988*).

Hence, when the user of KBSs is less experienced than the level of experience embedded in the knowledge base, the system may gain indirect authority due to professional esteem. The explanatory capabilities of KBSs may further add to the persuasive power of the KBS. Though probabilistic belief statements (or alike certainty factors) are introduced to provide a context for interpretation, their presence in themselves may enforce the impression of accuracy and precision.

... it seems as if we have a Gordian knot.

The correctness of a system in use is a function of 1) the clinical problem, 2) the cases handled and 3) the knowledge embedded. A cut of the Gordian knot may be to provide the user (the responsible part) with means/measures that enables him/her to assess the applicability of the systems output.

The aim of this paper is to indicate
- some issues of importance concerning actual application of KBSs, as it concerns the users' confidence and prerequisites for utilizing them,
- some possible measures in estimating applicability and plausibility of casuistic system application,
- some research issues on which European collaboration/concertation may be fruitful for the evolution of KBSs' developmental basis.

Some Quality Measures

Usually a routinely used KBS has been both evaluated and found applicable for a set of clinical problems. This, however, does not imply that the KBS is applicable for all possible cases within these problem areas. The distinction on whether a KBS is applicable to a given case or not may be operationalized by comparing case characteristics to a set of in-/exclusion criteria. When included, the question arises on "how good or bad is the problem solving capability on cases with these characteristics?", i.e. the problem solving capability of the KBS must be described in terms of quality measures.

State of the Art for "Quality measures" concerning knowledge based systems are dual:

- Validation and verification as seen from the knowledge engineering site (*Brender et al. 1989*), and
- validation and verification as an a priori necessity for application as seen from the user site (*O'Keefe et al. 1987, O'Moore 1988, Brender & McNair 1989*).

The dimensions addressed so far in relation with dynamics of the KBS functionality are Reliability aspects (encompassing e.g. Correctness, Robustness and Sensitivity) and Confidence aspects (Belief statement, Confidence range, Conformity with assumption of methods application, Validity of underlying model). The literature regarding validation of these aspects is sparse, and the major approach is to express "Correctness" as the degree of conformity with a "gold standard" (the nominated "truth"), either by counting the percentages of answers that agree with an expert / expert panel (see e.g. *Michalski 1987*), or by means of kappa statistics (*Lavril et al. 1988*), thereby taking into account accidental occurrences of agreement and providing means for testing statistical significance.

The approaches till now have in common that they focus on evaluation[1] prior to application (epidemiological validation), while evaluation of applicability on single cases (case related validation) remains unaddressed.

Some Measures for Case Related Validation

Case related evaluation may adopt the techniques and tools that are available for epidemiologic evaluation. The challenge is that for the interpretation of validity in case application each of these techniques has to be used in the reverse direction.

It may be illustrated as follows:

- As regards the applicability of systems, i.e. can we rely on using the system at all?: The epidemiologic validation aim at measuring and deciding on whether the system's model of the real world conforms with the given population. In a case related validation the aim is to elucidate whether the case at hand match with

---

1   "Evaluation" is "the judging or measuring of system characteristics", i.e. putting value to object characteristics with reference to an established set of criteria. "Evaluation" is "the judging or measuring of system characteristics", i.e. putting value to object characteristics with reference to an established set of criteria. "Verification" is "the act of proving whether an object is in accordance with specifications".

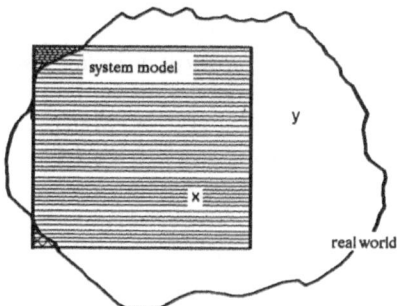

Figure 1:   The figure illustrates the extension of the system's model of the world in comparison with that of the real world. The case marked "x" lies within the system's
model, while that of "y" lies beyond, i.e. the system is applicable for "x", but not
for "y".

the system's model (figure 1), or in other words, to which extent does the case in
question resemble the "experience base"?.

● As regards the plausibility, i.e. what level of thrust can be given to the system's
conclusion(s)?: The epidemiologic validation serves to test whether the system's
belief statements conform with the distribution of classifications as observed in
the real world. The case related validation of plausibility has the purpose of
indicating the extent to which a case at hand belongs to the different classifications of the systems model (figure 2).

● As regards the confidence ranges, they comprise a frame of reference for interpretation of the above two aspects, reflecting the variance in these, e.g. 1) their
95% confidence limits (when probabilities are used) or 2) latent alternative
output statements that may be inferred when pure stochastic variation in input
variables is considered.

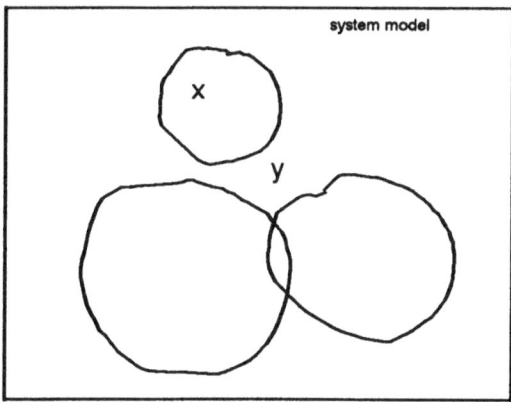

Figure 2:   The figure illustrates the extension of different culsters within the system's model
of the world. The case marked "x" obviously belongs to a well-defined cluster,
whereas the case "y" may belong to several or none of the defined clusters.

Examples for plausibility estimation may be:

- The PV_{pos} and PV_{neg} descriptors (*Gerhardt & Keller 1986*) provide measures on the Technique's/technology's predictive values in diagnosing. When used in case related interpretation of results, belief statements (probability of correct interpretation) for interpreting the output as positive (disease) resp. negative (normal) may be deduced by calculating PV_{pos} resp. PV_{neg} using the actual result as cut-off limit.
- Kappa statistics may deliver similar means for interpretation as regards the correctness of chosen interpretation. Kappa statistics has the advantage of displaying real worth of interpretation (taking into account accidentalness).

The corresponding confidence ranges may be inferred either from the variance estimates by means of the mathematics used or from exercising variation on the input site.

Aspects like sensitivity and validity of the underlying model has no obvious sense for the validation of application as regards individual cases.

The above considerations are limited to static patient situations. When the time and state dependent dynamics of the real world is taken into account the complexity may increase.

Discussion

Decision support systems are currently designed to provide their users with specialized knowledge. They are supposed to be used in situations of great complexity and incomprehensibility or in problem solving situations uncommon to the user. It is, however, a truism to believe that complex problem handling is solved by an unreflecting application of even more complex technology: The legal and professional responsibility resides with the professional. To obtain confidence the legitimacy of every singular application of a Decision Support System has to be proven valid. Therefore, the development of measures and techniques for quality assessment as regards the application of knowledge-based systems on individual cases is a necessity rather than just an academic challenge.

This discipline regards meta-knowledge processing, not in the often used sense of control-structures ("knowledge embedded for control purposes at the inference process", see e.g. the review papers by *Davis & Buchanan, 1977* and *van Harmelen, 1987*), but in the sense of quality assessment[2]: "Assessment of appropriateness in a

---

2   Meta-knowledge is knowledge of knowledge (Aiello et al. 1986), and as knowledge is a conception of causal connections, meta-knowledge is knowledge of the qualities of the conception, e.g. knowledge about the adequacy of the knowledge, when applied or used in any context.

given context", i.e. by establishing a measure for knowledge. From this is seen that application validation is gained by the (users) interpretation of meta-information. Furthermore, the technology for generation and presentation of meta-information may lead to KBSs with a built-in self-constrainment as regards their application.

So the questions are, for the epidemiological validation as well as the case related validation:

- What characteristics of knowledge will explicitly indicate aspects of quality? In other words, what component parts of a KBS may provide the basis for deducing on quality in use?
- Which elements of meta-knowledge are needed in knowledge? In other words, what kind of knowledge (including meta-knowledge) has to be part of a KBS to assure high quality in use?
- How can meta-knowledge be represented unambiguously?
- How is meta-knowledge made measurable and manageable in operation?
- How is it validated?

These issues are sparsely dealt with in the literature, and therefore constitute a research area. The area of chemometrics is one discipline, where the terms are used/evolving (*Deming 1986*) though not explicitly addressed as a part of KBSs.

Acknowledgement

The preparation of this paper has in part been funded from the Commission of European Communities' AIM Programme ("Advanced Informatics in Medicine"), the KAVAS Project (A1021).

References

Aiello, L. et al.: Representation and Use of Meta-Knowledge. Proc. of IEEE, vol. 74, no. 10, 1986, pp. 1304 - 1321.

Brender, J. et al.: Taxonomy for Validation of Knowledge-based Systems. VALID ESPRIT II Project (P2148), February 1989.

Brender, J., McNair, P.: WATCH THE SYSTEM. An Opinion on User Validation of Computer-based Decision Support Systems in Medicine. Accepted for MEDIN-FO 89.

Cannatacci, J.A.: Liability and Responsibility of Medical Expert Systems. Proc. Workshop on Social and Legal Aspects of Medical Informatics, Med Informatics 1989.

Cannatacci, J.A.: Liability and Responsibility of Medical Expert Systems. Complex no.5/88 (TANO A.S., 1988). ISBN 82-518-2523-7.

Commission of the European Communities.: AIM Workplan (Advanced Informatics in Medicine), 24th Oct. 1988.

Davis, R., and Buchanan, B.G.: Meta-Level Knowledge: Overview and Applications. Proc. 5th Intl. Joint Conf. Artif. Intel., IJCAI-77, vol 2, 1977, pp. 920-927.

Deming, S.N.: Chemometrics: An Overview. Clin Chem 32, 1986, pp. 1702-1706.

Feigenbaum, E.A.: Autoknowledge: From File Servers to Knowledge Servers. In: R. Salomon, B. Blum and M. Jørgensen (eds), MEDINFO 86, Proc. 5th Conf. Medical Informatics, 1986, pp. xliii - xlvi.

Gerhardt, W., and Keller, H.: Evaluation of Test Data from Clinical Studies: I. Terminology, Graphic Interpretation, Diagnostic Strategies, and Selection of Sample Groups. II. Critical Review of the Concept of Efficiency, Receiver Operated Characteristics (ROC), and likely Ratios. Scand J Clin Lab Invest 46, 1986, suppl 181.

Lavril, M. et al.: ARTEL: An Expert System in Hypertension for the General Practitioner. In: O. Rienhoff, U. Piccolo and B. Schneider (eds), Expert Systems and Decision Support in Medicine, Proc. 33rd Annual Meeting of the GMDS & EFMI Special Topic Meeting, Peter L. Reichertz Memorial Conference, Lecture Notes in Medical Informatics vol.36 (Springer-Verlag, Berlin, Heidelberg), 1988, pp. 314 - 321.

Michalski, R.S.: How to Learn Imprecise Concepts: A Method for Employing a Two-Tierced Knowledge Representation in Learning. Morgan Kaufmann Publishers, Proc. 4th Intl Workshop on Machine Learning, 1987, pp. 50-58.

Musen, M.A., and Van der Lei, J.: Knowledge Engineering for Clinical Consultation Programs: Modeling the Application Area. Meth Inform Med 28, 1989, pp. 28-35.

O'Keefe, R.m., Balci, O., Smith, E.P.: Validating Expert System Performance. IEEE Expert, winter 1987, pp. 81 - 90.

O'Moore, R.R.: Decision Support Based on Laboratory Data. Meth Inform Med 27, 1988, pp. 187 - 190.

Van Harmelen, F.: A Categorization of Meta-Level Architectures. Department of Artificial Intelligence, University of Edinburgh, DAI Research Paper No. 297, AISB-87 Conf, 1987

Questions from the Discussion:

Andreassen: The problem of detecting whether or not the system is at the borders of its application domain is important. Statistical or probabilistic approaches will provide this information. Such systems say: "I have an answer, but I don't believe in it myself". In my opinion this is not meta-knowledge.

McNair: The problem of detecting whether the system is at the border of its application range (or even beyond this) is extremely important. Without awareness of the system's applicability the user may interpret results as valid although the system is applied beyond its scope. Hence, applicability borders has to be identified and acknowledged for every case before real system application. Preferably this should be a part of the systems functionality itself.

Criteria for application may be explicitly represented as a part of the knowledge base. Implicitly it may be deduced e.g. in probabilistics from a very low likelihood for the case to belong to any possible category. A prerequisite for both approaches is that all categories are well-described in epidemiological demographics.

An applicability statement will conclude on whether the system may at all provide an answer. In your example case, the system states: "I have an answer". Thereby, the system indicates that it is applicable, and the rest of the statement concerns the plausibility of the output statement.

Meta-knowledge is the implicit or explicit knowledge required for the deduction of the referred meta-information.

Blom: A KBS performs a mapping from some set of input data to some output. When embedded knowledge is bad the mapping will be bad. Another failure may be that for some set of inputs, you do not get an output at all. When you don't like that you need more and better knowledge. Hence I see no use for meta-knowledge.

McNair: In order to identify whether knowledge is "bad" or "good" you need some quality measures. These quality measures are "knowledge about knowledge" and therefore constitutes meta-knowledge. When you change a knowledge-base according to the quality indications, you somehow include this meta-knowledge. In the process of operationalization and representation of meta-knowledge as a part of the knowledge-base the concept of meta-knowledge often is limited to explicit control rules. In our opinion, the meta-knowledge concept goes beyond this narrow definition and does not depend on an operational basis, - it is a concept in itself. For instance, the knowledge required for reasoning about application of knowledge we denote as meta-knowledge.

The challenge is that of methodically identifying the component elements of the meta-knowledge concept and of coping with their operationalization and management.

Evaluation of Knowledge Based Systems from the User Perspective[1]

A. Grant[1], C. Parker-Jones[1], R. White[2], D. Cramp[2], A. Barreiro[3], P. Mira[4], A. Artal[5], J. Montero[5]

1 Dept of Chemical Pathology, Leeds University, UK

2 Dept of Med Informatics, Royal Free Hospital, University of London, UK

3 Dept of Electronics, University of Santiago, Spain

4 Dept of Comp Science and Artificial Intelligence, UNED, Madrid, Spain

5 Dept of Medical Oncology, Autonomous University of Madrid, Spain

INTRODUCTION

In the consideration of the development of an evaluation methodology for a knowledge based system, three aspects are given emphasis.

Firstly, user acceptance and utility are regarded as providing the driving force for the objectives of an evaluation programme. The responsibility of the physician is emphasized in this regard.

Secondly, as Medical Informatics is an evolving science, an evaluation methodology for the implementation of information systems in medicine is also in an evolving phase.

Thirdly, "expert" or "knowledge based" systems are regarded as being part of an information system and evaluation is concerned with the integration of a given computerized system into the total information environment, i.e. the real world system in which it is meant to operate. This methodology aims to be applicable to any medical information system, whether it is the development of a simple algorithm or it has been elaborated with the most complex techniques of artificial intelligence. A number of criticisms concerning the evaluation of information systems, not only in medicine, have been recently made (*Riedel & Gordon, 1986, St Johanser & Harbridge, 1986, O'Keefe et al, 1987*). A particular observation based on expert system

---

1   A M Grant is currently with the Department of Clinical Biochemistry Centre hospitalier universitaire de Sherbrooke, Sherbrooke (Quebec) CANADA

conference presentations is the lack of an evaluation component to the experimental design which devalues the presentation of the results (*St Johanser & Harbridge, 1986*). The implication is that evaluation is commonly regarded as secondary to the undertaken technological development, an attitude which is contrary to the objective of successful application in medical practice.

A given research or development programme may have mixed objectives, one domain oriented and one information technology oriented. These objectives must be clearly distinguished to prevent the evaluation standpoint becoming obscured.

A related criticism is that the majority of existing evaluation reports focus on a limited component of the system, usually the validation of the knowledge base, carried out by expert subjective assessment (*Prerau et al, 1985, Weiss et al, 1978, Yu et al, 1984, Gaschnig, 1979, Michel et al, 1986, Miller et al, 1982, Morice et al, 1986, Hickam et al, 1985*). These reports tend to leave implicit how the evaluation exercise might translate into real life practice. It is not enough to have agreement between the expert and the results of the system for the acceptance of its efficiency, and to establish the interest it may have for the user.

As a basis of achieving some understanding behind the difficulties of evaluation of information systems, three key attributes of an evaluation methodology are considered, namely "complex", "dynamic" and "pragmatic".

Under "complex" is presented the view that a clarity of documentation is critical: the structuring of the problem is the first priority of an assessment methodology for without good structuring the statistical assessment, however elegant, is useless.

Under "dynamic", the modular nature of an information system is examined and the need for clearly defined procedures to enable continuing feedback into the design or development process.

Under "pragmatic", the emphasis given is the requirement for a definition of priorities from a user point of view and a recognition of constraints so that the evaluation programme is both valid and achievable. The use of task related measures is endorsed.

This approach to evaluation has been built up in discussion between users and designers in preparation for the clinical evaluation of a prototype work-station which is to assist the physician in following a therapy protocol. This activity is part of the TAO project, "Therapy Advisor for Oncology", a project funded by the European Community as part of the ESPRIT program, "European Strategic Program for Research in Information Technology".

The Complexity of Evaluation

The Analysis of Complexity

The multi-faceted nature of the interaction of an information system with the real world environment in which it is located is well recognized (*Ahituv, 1980*). A major issue to be clearly addressed is how to represent this complexity in a useful way so that both overall and component aspects of a system may be evaluated and be relevant to both designer and user.

Inevitably, a central reliance on model construction is required. An analysis of the general properties of modelling (*Walliser, 1977*) gives a methodology for representation of complexity which acknowledges three basic issues:

- the need for a conceptual representation to enable planning and evaluation according to given objectives;
- the need for a synthetic approach that recognises the properties of dynamic interaction between elements of a system which donate to the total character of the system;
- the need to promote a unifying language across different disciplines.

Three main categories of policy maker interact in the evaluation process of a medical information system, i.e. senior physician, resource manager and system developer/designer. Evaluation methodology and results need to be optimally intelligible between these parties. This means, as should be a practical requisite of model construction (*Walliser, 1977*), an elimination of jargon with a conceptual presentation, often graphical, of the interaction between components and an ability to highlight those aspects that need most attention.

In a first level system analysis pertinent to an information system evaluation, three categories can be distinguished:

- the components of the computerized information system, i.e. database and knowledge-base (including their control elements);
- the boundary between the computerized information system and the clinical unit where it is sited;
- the integration of the clinical unit into its organizational environment, e.g. the hospital.

This categorization is comparable to that which has been earlier suggested in the non-medical domain (*Adelman et al, 1985*); it differs in that medical decision-making is oriented to the profit of the individual patient rather than the organization. This emphasizes the responsibility of the senior physician in the appropriate use of the decision aid.

These categories give a useful separation for evaluation purposes, i.e.:

- – medical decision-making (within the evaluation objective)
  – the decision support performance characteristics of the tool(s) being evaluated;
- the human computer interface;
- the integration into the organizational environment.

It should be noted that the emphasis in (a) is, firstly, on the decision process and, secondly, on the computer tools available to support this process.

From a utility perspective, these categories can be summarized as follows:

- Does it work and is it clinically useful?
- Is it easy to use?
- Does it reduce routine work?

The requirement is to show that the tool fits technically and cost effectively into the total process required for a given set of tasks.

Dynamics of Evaluation

Evaluation of Information Systems has been divided into formative, i.e. during development, and summative, i.e. after development (*Liebowitz, 1986*).

This is a useful distinction but worth exploring: the notion of iterative development required of knowledge based systems (*Freiling et al, 1985*) begs the question, when does formative evaluation become summative? In other words, an information system being installed, particularly if a knowledge based component is included, may have some modules more or less complete and others clearly in a development phase. It is important to note that until now systems being developed for decision support, whether for patient diagnosis or management, have at best only found partial acceptance in practice despite several years of development. Evaluation methodologies so far presented fail to take into account that currently there is an increasingly rapid evolution of information system technology. There is a tendency to focus on summative evaluation, ignoring the chasm currently to be crossed before information systems, become accepted into regular medical practice. A lesson may come from the military domain where it has been noted that despite evaluation being formally part of the methodology of information system introduction, the evaluation often comes too late in the development cycle to provide useful information (*Riedel & Gordon, 1986*).

Iterative development proposed for knowledge based systems recognizes that much knowledge being incorporated into both the overall design and the performance of its reasoning must go through an empirical process of elicitation and refinement. This suggests that an emphasis on summative evaluation, as is naturally the case in other medical assessment areas such as the evaluation of a new pharmaceutical preparation, would be a misguided approach to information system evaluation.

Furthermore, a medical knowledge based system must be constantly maintained so as to be capable of being update as new knowledge is gained. To emphasize this point, a comparison is made here between a drug and an information system.

- A new drug does not change from first laboratory trial to eventual release for general prescription despite several years of assessment. Information system technology can be expected to change enormously over the next years.

- A drug directly affects the patient. An information system is interpreted by the physician it is well recognized that systems should support rather than replace physician decision-making, emphasizing again the key role of the physician in information system evaluation.

- A drug is a single entity. An information system consists of different modules, each of which may be more or less advanced, hence at different stages between formative and summative evaluation.

The danger of using drug development as an analogy for information system evaluation is that it obscures the essentially dynamic nature of information system development.

The Pragmatics of Evaluation

It has been suggested that a limiting factor to the introduction of decision support systems may be the attitude of physicians to the new technology and, in particular, to the possible usurping of the physician's decision-making remit (*Teach & Shortliffe, 1981*).

It is proposed here that it is important to consider the range of issues that contribute to user acceptance and let these be determinants of the objectives of the evaluation methodology.

User Categorization

It is necessary, therefore, to consider the user role in the evaluation process. Several authors (*Wilson, 1988*) have advocated that experts be involved from the start of the design and in subsequent prototype refinement. The complexity of the medical domain is such that medical expertise is required at all stages from design to local implementation of information systems. It is therefore useful in the medical context to define the medical user according to the relationship to system development.

Evaluation Constraints

One possible reason other than complexity and immaturity for the inadequacy of evaluation methodology in the past is that evaluation can be time consuming and resource demanding. Thus, these needs must be accounted for during the planning of the evaluation programme.

It is important to choose a methodology on the one hand satisfactory, on the other hand has a reasonable chance of completion.

The evaluation programme should have these features:

it is realistic to the participant

it is understood by the participant and is not too long

it is appropriately observed

it allows for the participant to qualify and explain the answers to the preset exercise

the information is collated by a person with appropriate expertise which includes developed domain knowledge.

The Development of Task Related Evaluation Criteria

It has been proposed (*Riedel & Gordon, 1986*) that a defect of earlier approaches to information system evaluation is the lack of task-related evaluation criteria. The user carries out a sequence of tasks which use and generate information; these tasks can be analysed into sub-tasks which can form the basis of realistic individual evaluation activities which question how successfully the use of information in the sub-task maps onto the interaction with the information system in relation to this sub-task.

The relation of evaluation to the task is akin to the relation of the knowledge conceptual tools to the task (*Chandrasekaran, 1988*), where the task is categorized according to its knowledge content and inference family and the appropriate tool chosen. Evaluation forms the mirror image of the knowledge computational process. A given task for which computational support is being constructed has two major contingencies namely the class of user who is responsible for the task and also the context of the task.

Task Related Test Material

A patient case can be decomposed into tasks which relate to computer sessions; these form the basis of a library of test material which can be progressively refined (see section on Generation of Task-Related Test Material).

Task Context

Patient Management consists of alternation of diagnosis and therapy over a period of time, the periodicity of physician assessment and possible intervention being related to the severity of illness. After the initial diagnosis at each successive diagnosis, the problem is usually not to make a new diagnosis but to refine within a much smaller set of expected diagnoses which of these is/are the most likely and, also, to determine the extent of the treatment response. Within this set, therefore, the doctor has a conceptual model of the likely response. This personal model, an expert has refined by experience from case exposure as though he had a personal test case library in his memory. At successive diagnosis points on the diagnosis-treatment iteration the doctor's treatment decision depends on the patient state and disease evolution as well as the quality of the available information, thus on the specific context. In particular, if there is a deviation from the expected model of the patient progress then an appropriate response, new investigations and revised therapy plan must be invoked.

The patient case consists of episodes which can be considered hierarchically; each episode consists of the evolution of a particular type of disease or syndrome with its response to treatment and has an associated conceptual model as described above. There is an interrelation between these episodes and hence their associated models. It is evident that the use of evaluation material based on patient cases which contain complete episodes maintains the sensitivity to context and hence the basic issue of "the right information at the right place at the right time".

Categories of User

General Classification

Some distinction can be made between users and beneficiaries in that the system may provide benefits to parties not directly using the system and such benefits need to be measured. The roles of senior and junior physician are considered in some detail.

Users
- Senior Physician
- Junior Physician
- Student
- Nurse
- Secretary
- Patient

Senior Physician
The senior physician is defined for this purpose as someone who has completed the recognized training in a particular medical area and who is practising in this area. This person is responsible for the quality of decision-making on the clinical unit and is conscious that many factors may contribute to the overall patient outcome. A key issue is how to categorize these different factors: it is possible to use the three categories given above for analysis of an information system, also to enable a first level analysis of the factors influencing patient outcome. This should not be surpris-

ing if the ultimate goal of the information system is to optimize patient outcome. Each category is considered in turn.

Medical decision making is the sum of a sequence of decisions which depend on timely supply of correct information, education and previous experience. The senior physician optimally requires a record of sufficient quality of each patient episode to enrich the experience to support future decision-making. Different studies have evaluated how the timely provision of information by a computerized system can improve the performance of medical decision-making (*Wirtschaffer et al, 1981, McDonald et al, 1984*). He is concerned that the factual knowledge and the reasoning of the system is valid and seeks explicit assurance of this in the character of explanation provided.

The human-computer interface designed correctly can present the appropriate pattern of information required for a given medical decision in a particular context (*Politser, 1986*), hence the senior physician is concerned with the optimization of this pattern.

Clinical unit organization requires efficient communication with nursing staff for patient therapy, with administration for resource provision, with other specialties for investigations and specialist diagnosis and treatment and with information sources such as libraries to enable up to date awareness of the medical literature. These different communication requirements have potential impact on information system design.

Junior Physician

The junior physician is defined as someone who has completed the basic medical training and is undergoing training to be an eventual senior physician in an area of medical practice.

For a support to medical decision-making, this person seeks reliability, pertinence, and for it to be educationally useful. The human-computer interface should be fast, the dialogue relevant with low risk of error and there should be access to useful explanation.

From an organizational perspective, much of the work of the junior physician is involved also in organizational aspects of patient care and support for this would be universally welcome.

Beneficiaries

- Patient
- Resource Manager

It should be noted that the two persons responsible for buying the system are the senior physician and the resource manager. Secondly, if the system is not acceptable by any one category of user, then it may fail "a chain depends on its weakest link"!

Methodology

General Evaluation Format

An evaluation phase consists of a number of predefined exercises some of which may take place at the same evaluation session.

The requirements for an individual evaluation exercise are as follows:

- to state clearly the main and sub-objectives of the evaluation exercise;
- to identify the tests and measures to be used;
- to define the time allowed for the complete exercise and schedule the stages within the exercise;
- to identify who is responsible for organizing the evaluation and for collating the data. These persons need to have a clear relation to the "user" and there must be a user ultimately responsible for the exercise;
- to clearly specify the documentation required of the evaluation exercise.

Documentation

Successful documentation is a crucial part of evaluation. Relevant documentation is as follows:

- System specification models (see section on The Analysis of Complexity).

  Practically speaking, there is an aversion of physicians and no doubt other professionals to profuse technical documentation, nevertheless, the components of an information system cannot be discussed and evaluated unless they are clearly specified. The objectives of this approach to documentation are the same as those of developing a conceptual model during the knowledge acquisition process of knowledge based system design (*Breuker & Wielinga, 1989*). An information system should have supporting documentation which consists of annotated models of the different major components. Evaluation results in update of this documentation and is a critical feature of the evaluation process.

- Formats for recording the evaluation exercise. These consist of pre-defined forms to record the different tests which have quantitative and qualitative nature (e.g. time on task measurements, questionnaire response) and to include participant comment per test, time and conditions of exercise and coordinator summary (see section on Consensus Management).

Generation of Task-Related Test Material

The use of task-oriented measures of information system effectiveness as described above gives an opportunity to build a library of test material that compares as closely as possible to the real world situation. Such material also enables parallel studies with real life procedures where data currently being used for a real life problem can simultaneously be put into an evaluation format structured on sets of real life tasks. The evaluation based on task related test material can be oriented to the objectives of different evaluation exercises: the focus needed may be the assessment of the Human Computer Interface rather than the validation of the knowledge content for example.

Test Material Description
Test material can be categorized as follows:
- Its primary task;
- Secondary tasks within the primary task;
- The data content per task or sub-task;
- The judged adequacy (completeness and reliability) of the data content;
- The judged adequacy of representation of the class or subclass of tests required for a given area to be tested;
- The assessment measures that can be applied.

Strong or weak case material is then characterized by:
- class and subclass;
- adequacy of content per task or sub-task;
- applicability and robustness of associated assessment measures.

Test Material is compiled from real patient cases in the domain.

Questionnaires

The quality of the questionnaire relates to the usefulness of the underlying formulated criteria. It may be acceptable to obtain a yes-no response accompanied by the "why?" response. However, it may well be better to attempt a grading of response, e.g. selecting from worst-bad-medium-good-best. The degree of possible refinement depends on the criterion. However, too many scalar choices will only work if the difference between each step on the scale is reasonably clear; often, this will not be the case because of the variation in individual judgement which results in the consensus approach described above. A starting point therefore should usually be a simple scale with 4 or 5 points supported by the "why?" response.

Preparation for an Evaluation Exercise

An evaluation exercise selects the component to be evaluated, the objective, the user category, the task-related test material, the relevant criteria and assessment methods and a planned schedule constructed. Due regard needs to be given to a necessary learning period by the participants.

Phases of Evaluation

The iterative relation of evaluation to development has been discussed in 1.2; the role of the user as regards different phases in 2.9. Four phases are distinguished:
- Initial development, with preliminary evaluation of different component modules.
- Evaluation of the first prototype of the integrated system at designated clinical sites. This should include the use of parallel clinical studies with and without the intended system.
- Wider evaluation at an increased number of sites.
- Formal multi-centre trials.

Combination of data

The notable element of personal judgement behind the response to a questionnaire means that the simple combination of scalar scores (*Liebowitz, 1986*) is unsatisfactory. This must be subject to the consensus management approach.

Work concerning consensus algorithms which generate a combined profile derived from different profiles of individual preference has potential application in this analysis.

Criteria development

At the present time, there are no clearly defined criteria that can be simply taken off the shelf and applied to a given problem. Hence the evaluation process will also be an evaluation of the evaluation methodology itself. It results in an on-going refinement of the most useful criteria, the essential aim being to develop robust criteria and visible assessment techniques set in a methodology. The senior physician and the resource manager should be able to relate to such a methodolgy which also should be satisfactory to system designers and developers.

The evaluation process may, at any stage, lead to results which do not indicate clearly either acceptance or rejection. In this situation, the following must be defined:

Exclusion criteria - these mean the rejection of the information system.

Inclusion criteria - these permit conditional acceptance.

In particular, the system must not cause a reduction in quality of patient care.

Consensus Management

There is a requirement to consider the issues of objectivity and subjectivity. The majority of issues that concern user acceptance cannot simply be quantitated and objectively measured with the application of suitable statistics. These issues require recording of subjective judgement in a structured format where the main focus will be to assess the degree of consensus. The final report of a given evaluation exercise will be the presentation of the consensus view and this must be entrusted to personnel with a high level of medical knowledge who are familiar with the evaluation programme for it needs this combination of knowledge for coordinatory judgemental assessment. The final report will have gone through a process whereby the degree of acceptance of the overall findings has been assessed by appropriate user experts. For each set of qualitative or semi-quantitative tests in the evaluation exercise, it is equally or more important to ask the participant why the given response. The coordinator may glean thus important additional information and insight. Also, it may be better, having carefully delineated the problem to ask sufficient questions from the point of view of criteria development but not too many so as to hinder the participant in responding to the question "why?". For quantitative tests, it is useful for the coordinator to observe the participant during a task to understand the variation in measures obtained.

Thus the management of consensus is an important approach to optimize the information obtained. Consensus management also enables the reduction of bias because:

●the judgemental component of the evaluation is under close surveillance, given appropriate formatting of the evaluation exercise as discussed;

- if different sites are involved, then a consensus is required between the different site coordinators;
- the coordinator must relate the findings to appropriate domain experts before publishing.

The coordinator in addition needs to routinely record following a set of evaluation tests whether unexpected findings have been obtained and also underlying difficulties experienced that could affect the usefulness of the results.

Acknowledgement

This work has been partly funded under the European Community ESPRIT I Programme, P1592, Project TAO, Therapy Advisor for Oncology. Partners are: University of Leeds, Royal Free Hospital, London, England; University of Montpellier, France; University of Santiago, Spain; Medimatica, England; Framentec, France.

References

Adelman L, Rook FW, Lehner PE: User and R & D specialist evaluation of decision support systems. IEEE Trans. Syst., Man, Cybertn, vol SMC 15, 334-342, 1985.

Ahituv N: A systematic approach towards assessing the value of an information system. MIS Quarterly, Dec, 61-75, 1980.

Breuker J, Wielinga B: Models of expertise in knowledge acquisition. In: Topics in Expert System Design, Eds., G Guide, C. Tasso. North Holland Publishing Company, 1989.

Chandrasekaran B: Generic tasks as building blocks for knowledge-based systems: the diagnosis and routine design examples. To appear in: Knowledge Engineering Review, 1988.

Freiling M, Alexander J, Mesick S, Rehfuss S, Schulman S: Starting a knowledge engineering project. A.I. Magazine, fall, 150-164, 1985.

Gaschnig J: Preliminary performance analysis of the prospector consultant system for mineral exploration. In: [vol 1] Proceedings of the Sixth International Joint Conference on Artificial Intelligence, 20-23 August 1979, Tokyo, Japan, p308-310. General Chairman, R Reddy. International Joint Conferences on Artificial Intelligence. c/o IJCAI-79, Computer Science Department, Stanford University, Stanford, California, 94305, USA, 1979.

Hickam DH, Shortliffe EH, Bischoff MB, Scott AC, Jacobs CD: A study of the treatment advice of a computer-based cancer chemotherapy protocol advisor. Annals of Internal Medicine, 101, 928-936, 1985.

Liebowitz J: Useful approach for evaluating expert systems. Expert Systems, 3.2, 86-96, 1986.

McDonald CJ, Hui SL, Smith DM, Tierney WM, Cohen SJ, Weinberger M, McCabe GP: Reminders to physicians from an introspective computer medical record. Annals of Internal Medicine, 100, 130-138, 1984.

Michel C, Botti G, Fieschi M, Joubert M, Casanova P, San Marco JL: Validation of a knowledge base aimed at generalists for diabetes therapeutics: Blind evaluation. In: [vol 1] Avignon 86, The Sixth International Workshop on Expert Systems and their Applications, 28-30 April 1986. Palace of the Popes, Avignon, France, p139-152, p726. Chairman, JC Rault. Agence de l'Informatique, Etablissement Publique National, tour Fiat Cedex 16, 92084, Paris La Defense, France, 1986.

Miller RA, Pople Jr HE, Myers JD: INTERNIST-I An experimental computer-based diagnostic consultant for general internal medicine. New England Journal of Medicine, 307.8, 468-476, 1982.

Morice VP, Degoulet P, Jeunemaitre X, Chatellier G, Devries C, Hemdaqui A, Gascuel O, Boisvieux JF, Menard J: Implementation and assessment of a hypertension expert system. In: [vol 1] Avignon 86, the Sixth International Workshop on Expert Systems and their Applications, 28-30 April 1986. Palace of the Popes, Avignon, France, p561-570, p848. Chairman, JC Rault, Agence de l'Informatique, Etablissement Publique National, tour Fiat Cedex 16, 92084, Paris La Defense, France. (In French), 1986.

O'Keefe RM, Balci O, Smith EP: Validating expert system performance. IEEE Expert, 20.4, 81-89, 1987.

Prerau DS, Gunderson AS, Reinke RE, Goyal SK: The COMPASS expert system: Verification, technology transfer, and expansion. In Proc. of the second conference on artificial intelligence applications, 11-13 Dec 1985, IEEE press, New York, 1985.

Politser PE: How to make laboratory information more informative. Clinical Chemistry, 32.8, 1510-1516, 1986.

Riedel SL, Gordon FP: Utilization-oriented evaluation of decision support systems. IEEE Transactions on Systems, Man, and Cybernetics, SCM 16.6, 980-996, 1986.

St Johanser JT, Harbridge RM: Validating Expert Systems: Problems and Solutions in practice. In KBS 86: Knowledge based systems, 215-229. Online International Ltd, Middlesex, England, 1986.

Teach RL, Shortliffe EH: An analysis of physician attitudes regarding computer-based clinical consultation systems. Computers and Biomedical Research, 14, 542-558, 1981.

Walliser B: Systèmes et Modèles. Editions du Seuil, Paris, 1977.

Weiss S, Kulikowski CA, Safir A: Glaucoma consultation by computer. Computers in Biology and Medicine, 8, 25-40, 1978.

Wilson F: Human factors evaluations in the development and maintenance of interactive computer systems. London HCI Centre, EV/1.1F, 1-31, 1988.

Wirtschaffer DD, Scalise M, Henke C, Gams RA: Do information systems improve the quality of clinical research? Results of a randomized trial in a cooperative multi-institutional cancer group. Computers and Biomedical Research, 14, 78-90, 1981.

Yu VL, Fagan LM, Bennett SW, Clancey WJ, Scott AC, Hannigan JF, Buchanan BG, Cohen SN: An evaluation of MYCIN's advice. In: The [Addison-Wesley Series in Artificial Intelligence] Rule-based expert systems: The MYCIN experiments of the Stanford heuristic programming project, p589-596, p748. Editors B.G. Buchanan and E.H. Shortliffe. Addison-Wesley Publishing Company, Reading, MA, USA, 1984.

Question from the discussion

Andreassen: I agree that an information system is not the same as a pill, but after completion of the system, shouldn't it undergo the same type of evaluation as a pill regarding its impact on patient care?

Grant: In principle, there is a commonality of approach to whatever is evaluated, however, I believe it is very important to emphasize that an information system is dynamically evolving and that the rate of evolution may not be the same for the different components that make up the information system. The relation to patient care is how the physician uses the information system.

Authors Index

List of Participants

Workshop System Engineering in Medicine
16-18 March, 1989
Maastricht, The Netherlands

Dr. S. Andreassen
Aalborg University
Institute of Electronic Systems
Badehusvej 23
DK 9000 Aalborg
DENMARK
Tel: +45-98-1010003 ext 4948
FAX: +45-98-154008

Prof. J. Beneken
University of Technology Eindhoven
Div. of Medical Electrical Engineering
Den Dolech 2
PO Box 513
5600 MB Eindhoven
THE NETHERLANDS
Tel: +31-40-473295
FAX: +31-40-448375
EMAIL: ELEME1@HEITUE5.bitnet

Dr. C. Berzuini
Dipartimento di Informatica e Sistemistica
Universita di Pavia
via Abbiategrasso 209
I-27100 Pavia
ITALY
Tel: +39-382-391350
FAX: +39-382-422881
EMAIL: STEFA@IPVCCN.bitnet

Dr. J.A. Blom
Eindhoven University of Technology
Div. of Medical Electrical Engineering
Den Dolech 2
PO Box 513
NL-5600 MB Eindhoven
THE NETHERLANDS
Tel: +31-40-473287
FAX: +31-40-445187
EMAIL:ELEMHANS@HEITUE5.bitnet

Prof. J. Breuker
University of Amsterdam
Dpt. of Social Science Informatics
Herengracht 196
NL-1016 BS Amsterdam
THE NETHERLANDS
Tel: +31-20-5252149/5253494
FAX: +31-20-5252084
EMAIL: BREUKER@SWIVAX.uucp

Dr. P. F. de Vries Robbé
Academic Hospital Groningen
Oosterhamrikkade 7
NL-9713 KA Groningen
THE NETHERLANDS
Tel: +31-50-612940 / 612579
FAX: +31-50-120974
EMAIL:MIDS@HGRRUG5.bitnet

Dr. A. d'Hollander
Free University of Brussels (U.L.B.)
Dpt. of Anesthesiology C.U.B. ERASME
Route de Lennik, 808
B-1070 Brussels
BELGIUM
Tel: + 32-2-5683919 / 5684363
FAX: + 32-2-5684405

Dr. R. Engelbrecht
GSF-MEDIS Institut
Ingolstädter Landstrasse 1
D-8042 Neuherberg
WEST GERMANY
Tel: + 49-89-3187-5330
FAX: + 49-89-3187-3326
EMAIL: ENGEL@DM0GSF11.bitnet

Dr. J. Fox
Imperial Cancer Research Fund Labora-
tories
PO BOX 123
Lincoln's Inn Fields
London, WC2A 3PX
UNITED KINGDOM
Tel: + 44-71-2420200
FAX: + 44-71-2421510
EMAIL: J_FOX@ICRF.AC.UK

Prof. E. Gelsema
Erasmus University
Dpt. of Medical Informatics
PO Box 1738
NL-3000 DR Rotterdam
THE NETHERLANDS
Tel: + 31-10-4087051
FAX: + 31-10-4362841
EMAIL:GELSEMA@HREUR51.bitnet

Dr. E. Gómez-Aguilera
Universidad Politécnica de Madrid
Dpto. Technología Electronica y Bioinge-
niería
E.T.S.I Telecommunicacion - Ciudad
Universitaria
E-28040 Madrid
SPAIN
Tel: + 34-1-5495700 ext. 298
FAX: + 34-1-2432077
EMAIL:egomez@teb.upm.es

Prof. A. Grant
Dept. of Clinical Biochemistry
Centre hospitalier univeristaire de Sher-
brooke
3001-12th Avenue North
Sherbrooke (Quebec) J1H 5N4
Canada
Tel:
FAX:

Dr T. Groth
Uppsala University
Unit for Biomedical Systems Analysis
PO BOX 2103
S-75002 Uppsala
SWEDEN
Tel: + 46-18-182843
FAX: + 46-18-531202
EMAIL:
      Torgny.Groth@UDAC.UU.SE

Prof. A. Hasman
University of Limburg
Dpt. Medical Informatics and Statistics
PO BOX 616
NL-6200 MD Maastricht
THE NETHERLANDS
Tel: + 31-43-888417 / 888398
FAX: + 31-43-436080
EMAIL:MFMISHAS@HMARL5.bitnet

Dr. S.M. Lavelle
Dpt. of Experimental Medicine
University College
Galway
IRELAND
Tel: +353-91-24411
FAX: +353-91-25700
EMAIL:
        EXMLAVELLE@CS8700.UCG.IE

Dr. P. McNair
Dept. of Clinical Chemistry 339
Hvidovre Hospital
Kettegaard alle 30
DK-2650 Hvidovre
DENMARK
Tel: +45-31-471411 ext 2345
FAX: +45-31-750977

Prof. J. Mira Mira
University of Santiago de Compostela
Faculty of Physics
Dept. of Electronics
Santiago de Compostela
SPAIN
Tel: +34-81-595016
FAX: +34-81-592569
AND:
UNED (Spanish Open University)
Faculty of Sciences
Dept. of Informatics
Seuda del Rey S/R
28040 MADRID
Tel: +34-1-5446000/4492202
FAX: +34-1-5446737

Dr. E. Oliveira
University do Porto
Faculdade de Engenharia
Rua dos Bragas
P-4099 Porto Codex
PORTUGAL
Tel: +351-2-27505
FAX: +351-2-319280

Dr R. O'Moore
Trinity College
Central Laboratories
St. James Hospital
Dublin 8
IRELAND
Tel: +353-1-542088
FAX: +353-1-544494

Prof. Dr. G. Rau
Helmholz- Institut für Biomedizinische
Technik
University of Technology Aachen
Pauwelsstrasse
D-5100 Aachen
WEST GERMANY
Tel: +49-241-807111
FAX: +49-241-8089416

Dr. A. Rossi-Mori
Ist. Tecnologie Biomediche CNR
V. le Marx 15
I-00156 Roma
ITALY
Tel: +39-6-8277101/8273665
FAX: +39-6-822203
EMAIL: MEDEA@IRMKANT.bitnet

Prof. N. Saranummi
Medical Engineering Laboratory
Technical Research Centre of Finland
PO BOX 316
33101 Tampere 10
FINLAND
Tel: +358-31-163300
FAX: +358-31-174102
EMAIL: Saranumm@FINFUN.bitnet

Dr. T. Schecke
RWTH
Helmholz- Institut für Biomedizinische
Technik
Pauwelsstrasse
D-5100 Aachen
WEST GERMANY
Tel: +49-241-807111
FAX: +49-241-8089754

Dr. R. Smeets
University of Limburg
Dpt. Medical Informatics and Statistics
PO BOX 616
NL-6200 MD Maastricht
THE NETHERLANDS
Tel: +31-43-888415 / 888398
FAX: +31-43-436080
EMAIL: MFMISSGR@HMARL5.bitnet

Dr. J.L. Talmon
University of Limburg
Dpt. Medical Informatics and Statistics
PO BOX 616
NL-6200 MD Maastricht
THE NETHERLANDS
Tel: +31-43-888409 / 888398
FAX: +31-43-436080
EMAIL: MFMISTAL@HMARL5.bitnet

Dr. C. E. Thomsen
Aalborg University
Institute of Electronic Systems
Dept of Med. Inform. and Image analysis
Badehusvej 23
DK 9000 Aalborg
DENMARK
Tel: +45-8-138788 ext 278
FAX: +45-8-166150

Dr. G. Tusch
Medical School Hannover
Konstanty-Gutschow-Strasse 8
D-3000 Hannover 61
WEST GERMANY
Tel: +49-511-5322537 /5322540
FAX: +49-511-5323852
EMAIL: TUSCH@DHVMH1.bitnet

Dr. J. van der Lei
Erasmus University
Dpt. of Medical Informatics
PO Box 1738
NL-3000 DR Rotterdam
THE NETHERLANDS
Tel: +31-10-4087048
FAX: +31-10-4088118
EMAIL: VDLEI@HREUR51.bitnet

Prof. O.B. Wigertz
Dept. of Medical Informatics
Linkoping University
S-58183 Linkoping
SWEDEN
Tel: +46-13-227570
FAX: +46-13-104131
EMAIL: OVEW@AMI.LIU.SE

Dr. J. Wyatt
Lecturer in Medical Informatics
National Heart & Lung Institute
Dovehouse street
London SW3 6LY
UNITED KINGDOM
Tel: +44-71-3528121 ext 4351
FAX: +44-71-3763442

Dr. P.E. Zanstra
Academic Hospital Groningen
Oosterhamrikkade 7
NL-9713 KA Groningen
THE NETHERLANDS
Tel: +31-50-612940 / 612579
FAX: +31-50-120974
EMAIL: MIDS@HGRRUG5.bitnet

Lecture Notes in Medical Informatics

Vol. 24: Medical Informatics Europe 1984. Proceedings, 1984. Edited by E H. Roger, J. L. Willems, R. O'Moore and B. Barber. XXVII, 778 pages. 1984.

Vol. 25: Medical Informatics Europe 1985. Edited by F. H. Roger, P. Gronroos, R. TervoPellikka and R. O'Moore. XVII, 823 pages. 1985.

Vol. 26: Methodical Problems in Early Detection Programmes. Proceedings, 1983. Edited by E. Walter and A. Neiß. VIII, 198 pages. 1985.

Vol. 27: E. Mergenthaler, Textbank Systems. VI, 177 pages. 1985.

Vol. 28: Objective Medical Decision Making. Proceedings, 1985. Edited by D. D. Tsiftsis. VII, 229 pages. 1986.

Vol. 29: System Analysis of Ambulatory Care in Selected Countries. Edited by P. L. Reichertz, R. Engelbrecht and U . Piccolo . VI, 197 pages. 1986.

Vol. 30: Present Status of Computer Support in Ambulatory Care. Edited by P.L. Reichertz, R. Engelbrecht and U. Piccolo. VIII, 241 pages. 1987.

Vol. 31: S. J. Duckett, Operations Research for Health Planning and Administration. 111, 165 pages. 1987 .

Vol. 32: G. D. Rennels, A Computational Model of Reasoning from the Clinical Literature. XV, 230 pages. 1987.

Vol. 33: J. Fox, M. Fieschi, R. Engelbrecht (Eds.), AIME 87. European Conference on Artificial Intelligence in Medicine. Proceedings. X, 255 pages. 1987.

Vol. 34: R. Janßen, G. Opelz (Eds.), Acquisition, Analysis and Use of Clinical Transplant Data. Proceedings. IV, 225 pages. 1987.

Vol. 35: R. Hansen, B. G. Solheim, R. R. O'Moore, F. H. Roger (Eds.), Medical Informatics Europe '88. Proceedings. XV, 764 pages. 1988.

Vol. 36: O. Rienhoff, U. Piccolo, B. Schneider (Eds.), Expert Systems and Decision Support in Medicine. Proceedings, 1988. XII, 591 pages. 1988.

Vol. 37: O. Rienhoff, C. F. C. Greinacher (Eds.), A General PACS-RIS Interface. VI, 97 pages. 1988.

Vol. 38: J. Hunter, J. Cookson, J. Wyatt (Eds.), AIME 89. Second European Conference on Artificial Intelligence in Medicine. Proceedings. X, 330 pages. 1989.

Vol. 39: J. J. Salley, J. L. Zimmerman, M.J. Ball (Eds.), Dental Informatics: Strategic Issuesforthe Dental Profession. X, 105 pages. 1990.

Vol. 40: R. O'Moore, S. Bengtsson, J. R. Bryant, J. S. Bryden (Eds.), Medical Informatics Europe '90. Proceedings, 1990. XXV, 820 pages. 1990.

Vol. 41: J. P. Turley, S. K. Newbold (Eds.), Nursing Informatics '91. Pre-Conference Proceedings. VII, 176 pages. 1991.

Vol. 42: E. J. S. Hovenga, K. J. Hannah, K. A. McCormick, J. Ronald (Eds.), Nursing Informatics '91. Proceedings, 1991. XXV, 820 pages. 1991.

Vol. 43: L. Hothorn (Ed.), Statistical Methods in Toxicology. Proceedings, 1991. IV, 159 pages. 1991.

Vol. 44: M. Stefanelli, A. Hasman, M. Fieschi, J. Talmon (Eds.), AIME 91. Proceedings, 1991. VIII, 329 pages. 1991.

Vol. 45: K.-P. Adlassnig, G. Grabner, S. Bengtsson, R. Hansen (Eds.), Medical Informatics Europe 1991. Proceedings, 1991. XXII, 1089 pages. 1991.

Vol. 46: P. B. Marr, R. L. Axford, S. K. Newbold (Eds.), Nursing Informatics '91. Post Conference Proceedings. XV, 200 pages. 1991.

Vol. 47: J. L. Talmon, J. Fox (Eds.), Knowledge Based Systems in Medicine: Methods, Applications and Evaluation. Proceedings, 1989. XI, 330 pages. 1991.